Introduction

During my career as a hypnotherapist and teacher of clinical hypnosis, I have listened to and observed many of the most distinguished experts in the field of hypnosis. Often, I felt that many of the experts focused their efforts on theoretic and analytic teaching and virtually ignored the techniques and underlying principles that enable the practitioner to quickly develop his skill in using hypnosis easily.

Then I heard Dave Elman at work! In August, 1956, shortly after I opened the Hypnotism Training Institute in Los Angeles, one of my students loaned me a tape recording of one of Elman's Classes for physicians. Just a few minutes of listening had an electrifying effect upon me. I knew immediately that Dave Elman had "THE FEVER!"

"The Fever" is a term I use to describe a quality of excitement that ripens into an intense dedication and a lasting devotion to the use of hypnosis as a major treatment modality.

When he was eight years old, Dave saw his father wracked with the pain of terminal cancer. A famous stage hypnotist learned of the situation, and came to visit. In just a few minutes of hypnotic treatment the moaning and groaning was silenced and the pain was relieved. Little Dave was permitted to visit and play with his Dad. Dave Elman never forgot that his father was given relief by a stage hypnotist after the doctors had said there was no way to relieve his suffering.

As a young man, Elman worked briefly as a stage hypnotist, and it was during this period that he developed the rapid induction techniques that made his later teaching demonstrations so extraordinary!

In the ensuing years, Elman became a successful writer, director and producer of network radio programs, and taught these subjects at Columbia University.

He was forty-nine years old when he made the decision to change his profession and become an authority in the teaching of hypnosis. He met with medical specialists, researched the available literature and developed the Dave Elman Course in Clinical Hypnosis.

Although Elman had no advanced degrees and no scientific training, he restricted participation in his training courses to physicians and dentists.

His reputation spread quickly and soon made him the best known and most successful teacher of hypnotism in America.

For the next seventeen years he taught his course to thousands of professionals in every major city in the United States.

This book, originally titled "Findings in Hypnosis," is the summation of the Elman theories and techniques. It was the primary textbook used in his course and has become a classic work in the literature of Hypnotism.

In this major work, Elman strips away the academic and pedantic verbiage and creates a forceful and dynamic presentation of hypnosis as a lightning-fast and amazingly effective tool in a wide range of therapies.

His detailed attention to semantics—voice inflection; and his unique ability to generate mental expectancy form a background for his incredible effectiveness with nearly one hundred per cent of his subjects.

Elman left us only one book and a forty hour set of recordings made in his classes.

The Elman teachings have been a clarifying force and an enriching legacy for me, and I hope that you too may get "the fever" and that your excitement and enthusiasm will help to keep alive the work of

DAVE ELMAN

"MASTER HYPNOTIST"

GIL BOYNE, Director
HYPNOTISM TRAINING INSTITUTE
of
LOS ANGELES, CA.
Dec. 15, 1977

Hypnotherapy

Dave Elman

Westwood Publishing Co.

Glendale, CA

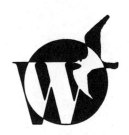

Dedicated to my first lady, Pauline, without whose valuable assistance and persistance, this book would never have been written.

For catalog of HYPNOTISM and MIND
POWER Books, Cassettes and Videocassettes
write to:

WESTWOOD PUBLISHING CO.
700 S. CENTRAL AVE., DEPT. HW
GLENDALE, CA. 91204
818-242-1159

Contents

Introduction
MISCONCEPTIONS, REASONS AND BEGINNINGS

Contents

Contents

MISCONCEPTIONS, REASONS AND BEGINNINGS

DESPITE the efforts of scientific writers and researchers, hypnosis has been wearing a cloak of mysticism for centuries. The very term hypnosis, derived from a Greek root word meaning sleep, is misleading. Hypnosis is related to sleep as night is to day—and is no more like it than night is like day. If you will put aside all preconceived notions and examine hypnosis clinically, you will find that it doesn't look, or "behave," as you thought it would. The way it does behave makes this phenomenon a tremendously valuable medical tool, though misconceptions continually hamper or prevent its use entirely.

The realization of this potential use in healing, and of the damage done by misunderstanding and downright misinformation, prompted me to write this book. I will detail my reasons further in Chapter One, but I wish to emphasize —immediately—the need for hypnotic knowledge and unbiased research if medicine is to take advantage of a great corrective force, the power of the human mind. It is my purpose in this text to impart valuable data to doctors, and also to make an understanding of hypnosis available to the interested laity. This is the only way to remove the mystic cloak. You will therefore find no arcane terminology or esotericisms intruding here.

I have been teaching hypnosis to medical men for years, and have found that many of them seem to think they can become expert hypnotists after a few classroom and practice sessions. Since there is really *no such thing as a hypnotist,* this is obviously impossible. As a practitioner employing this tool, all you can ever do is to show a patient how to go over the hurdle from a normal waking or sleeping state into the peculiar state of mind known as hypnosis. You won't hypnotize him; he will hypnotize himself. This means that those of us using suggestion wield no "power" over any subject. It means that there is nothing I do that you can't learn to do in hypnosis.

A more accurate term than hypnotist is hypnotic opera- tor. As the operator you teach the subject how to achieve the trance state (or other states, which we will go into at the proper time) and then, *if the subject is willing,* you stimulate his imagination—acting, so to speak, as a "dream pilot." It is pleasant to know that you can pilot almost any- one's imagination, stimulating more enjoyable, more intense thoughts than those usually deemed possible.

But, again, do not confuse this piloting ability with power; I stressed the words *if the subject is willing* because consent is imperative. You cannot impart a suggestion un- less the subject is willing to take it. At all times and in all degrees of hypnosis, the subject has complete power of selectivity. He therefore reacts only to suggestions that are reasonable and pleasing to him. You may have seen hypnotic demonstrations in which a subject performed out- landish antics; the fact remains that such a subject *chose* to perform these antics. There have doubtlessly been times in your life when you experienced outlandish dreams. The odd behavior you may have witnessed on the part of a hypnotized person was merely a similar dream induced by the operator, by a dream pilot. And odd or not, it seemed reasonable and pleasing to the subject or he would have rejected the suggestions.

Most modern books on hypnosis stress that the hypno- tized subject is *"in rapport"* with the operator. As a rule, they neglect to add that he is also *in rapport* with himself— for he can give himself autosuggestions—and with the whole world. Therefore, the subject may easily take rea- sonable and pleasing suggestions from persons other than the operator, unless the operator has first implanted a nega- tive reaction to such suggestions. Also bear in mind the fact that just because the subject is amenable to suggestions, he is not going to let anyone "control" him. I repeat that in every stage of hypnosis, the subject is in control and can select the suggestions he will accept. If the crisis of an unwanted suggestion arises, the subject will either arouse himself from the trance state or continue in it but simply refuse to act on the suggestion.

Under hypnosis, a person has control of more than his selectivity, or will power; he is in control of all his faculties except one. He can hear, see, feel, smell, taste, speak. Though he may sometimes look unconscious, he is completely aware and can therefore cooperate. The single exception to this control is what I call the critical faculty. If you give him a suggestion which pleases him and which seems emotionally and morally reasonable to him, he will accept it despite the fact that under ordinary circumstances he might consider it an impossible suggestion. For example, you can suggest anesthesia, erasing pain without a chemical agent. Or you can induce total recall, even back to as early an age as say, three years, and even when the subject ordinarily has a poor memory. In regressing a patient during hypnoanalysis, you lead the mental process still a step further, inducing abreaction; this is the reliving of a past experience rather than mere recall. The suspension of the critical faculty does not contradict the statement that the patient is in complete control of himself and has full selectivity; he accepts such a suggestion because it is pleasing, it is good for him. But his critical faculty—the disbelief that such fantastic feats are possible—is bypassed in hypnosis.

To state it another way, in hypnosis the body and mind are equally suggestible, operating as a harmonious unit. Hypnosis has an effect on the unconscious as well as the conscious mind, and on the autonomic nervous system, too. When you pilot a person into the suggestible state and provide him with pleasing dreams, his sensations upon "awaking" will be physical as well as mental. Having had a pleasant experience, he will feel refreshed and invigorated.

These general truths notwithstanding, every individual reacts differently under suggestion. To use hypnosis successfully, you must be able to respond to a variety of reactions, and your knowledge of the phenomenon should therefore be profound. If a doctor is to help a patient, he should not let himself be taken by surprise.

No one can learn hypnosis thoroughly by merely observing it. You must experience it yourself to know how different it is from the descriptions generally found in books. You will find hypnosis a pleasant state, and as you learn more about it, you will not only wish to experience it for yourself but you will also be able to hypnotize yourself. There is no such thing as not being hypnotizable.

Since selectivity prevails in the hypnotic state, and the law of self-preservation will not let a subject accept a harmful suggestion, no one has ever been injured by hypnosis. Numerous hypotheses have been formulated to the effect that a subject might be induced to hurt himself, knowingly or unknowingly, or might be "fooled" into committing a crime. Yet there is no case on record of any such happening. We have conducted thousands of tests, and in all cases, one of two things happens when an improper suggestion is given: The subject either rejects the suggestion or completely terminates the trance state. I repeat this fact because it is so important to the acceptance of hypnosis as a valuable and safe medical tool.

The three requisites for hypnosis are (1) the consent of the subject; (2) communication between the operator and subject, and (3) freedom from fear, or reluctance on the subject's part to trust the operator. Since these are the only requisites, it is obvious that those authors are wrong who say that any particular technique—fixation, for instance —is the only reliable way to induce trance. Actually, there is no limit to the number of techniques that can be used to trigger the desired response; you might say that there is no way in which you cannot hypnotize a person once you know how to utilize suggestion.

It can be seen from the foregoing (all of which will be treated in detail at the proper points in this work) that there is a great deal of misinformation in what has been written about hypnosis. In view of this, I feel that I must answer here questions the reader may have as to my qualifications for writing about the subject and the basis for my interest in it.

The first question is, fortunately, easy to answer. I have been teaching hypnosis to medical men (physicians, dentists and podiatrists) for more than a dozen years. I do not hold a medical degree, and therefore do not administer treatments to patients, although at the physician's request and with the physician in attendance, I have hypnotized thousands of patients and assisted doctors with such hypnotic instrumentations as hypnoanalysis and deep anesthesia. I have delivered lectures to members of hospital staffs and have also lectured to many thousands of doctors in private practice. I aided in the demonstration of a delivery without chemical anesthesia for a medical film. And I count among my successful students many eminent doctors, including the heads of several state medical societies. I recount these facts not as a bid for credit or recognition of any kind, but so that readers will be able to study this book without the hindrance of wondering whether the author (as in so many books on the subject) is in reality an authority.

The second question—the original basis for my interest in the subject—cannot be answered in a single paragraph. I have had an intense involvement with the subject since early childhood, and it probably stemmed from an incident that took place when I was about six years old. My father, who was a student of hypnosis, had by that time already told me a good deal about it. Then one day he took me to visit a family living a few blocks from us (in Fargo, North Dakota). A young girl in this family had a pronounced stutter, but when my father hypnotized her, the stutter vanished. Then, when the trance was terminated, her speech difficulty immediately returned. My interest in hypnosis was awakened, although it was not until much later that I learned how stutters can be permanently corrected by means of suggestion.

An even more important incident occurred in 1908, when I was eight years old and my father was forty-two. He had become acquainted with one of the great hypnotists of the era, a master performer who had a reputation for performing astounding feats. This man learned that my father was dying of cancer and was suffering intense pain. He came to our house, went into the sickroom and in a few minutes alleviated this pain. I had not been allowed to go into the room until then, but after the hypnotist came out, I was permitted to enter. Just before this, I had been sitting near the door and had heard my father groaning. Now I went in and he played with me. It was the last time he ever played with me, but so far as I know he was absolutely pain-free for some time after the hypnotist's visit.

A few weeks later he was dead. I have never forgotten that for a while before his death he was given relief that had not been deemed possible by his doctors. Of course, I didn't understand at the time how many other medical uses hypnosis has, but my interest in the subject became—and remained —profound.

Soon afterward, I attended a performance given by the same hypnotist, and he allowed me to assist him. He told the subjects on stage that I would shake hands with them, and that as I did so each one would go into a deep state of hypnosis. I shook their hands—and it worked. Afterward, I tried to produce the same effect, without success of course, on my mother, my brothers and sisters, my schoolmates. At first, I couldn't understand my failure, but I began reading every book on the subject that I could find in the library. The only point on which all these books seemed to agree was that fixation could be used reliably to hypnotize: you must have the subject stare at a light or a brilliant object, the authors instructed, for a period lasting anywhere from three minutes to two hours, in order to produce a trance.

Since neither my father nor the hypnotist had used a light, this dogmatic statement puzzled me. I tried staring at a light myself, but only made one important discovery: looking at a light for an hour can be rather boring.

All the light achieved was to tire my eyes. Perhaps, I thought, this was necessary for fast, deep hypnosis. So I asked my own eye doctor about it. He explained that the human eye sees in leaps and darts. If you prevent the eyes from following the natural habit of leaping and darting, the muscles quickly tire. As a demonstration, he placed his hand just above my eyes and very close to my forehead; then he brought his hand down slowly, instructing me to keep watching it as he did so. By the time his hand was under my chin, I realized that my eyes felt very sleepy. Now I knew how to tire a person's eyes quickly—without using fixation. This, I believe, was the birth of rapid conditioning in hypnosis. By adopting this doctor's demonstration as part of my technique, I could do in a few seconds what the fixation-light did in two or three hours. You will find that this hand-lowering technique consistently speeds hypnotic induction.

I began to have many successes in my attempts to hypnotize friends—adults as well as children. I didn't give up experimenting until, during my early teens, the father of a girl whom I had dated told me not to see her again. He had heard that a hypnotic subject could be seduced by the opera-

tor! This bit of misinformation could, I calculated make me
the least popular boy in Fargo, so I laid hypnosis aside and
did not return to it for many years.

* However, I had already learned some valuable facts that
were not generally known. Hypnosis could be used to alleviate intractible pain. It could be produced almost instantaneously. The greatest obstacle in obtaining the state was
any fear on the part of the subject—even a fear at a level
below conscious awareness. Even today, many textbooks
assert that a certain percentage of people will be found
unhypnotizable, when the truth is that the removal of fear
permits any person to be hypnotized. The other discoveries
described above were likewise not to be found in the writings
of the experts.

When I returned to the subject as an adult, I tried to
go on learning by maintaining the same open-minded attitude
of experimentation—accepting no theories or dogmas without
the strongest supporting clinical evidence. Such an attitude
is, I believe, essential for anyone who wishes to participate
in the improvement of the medical arts. Perhaps I am
merely rewording the old saw that experience is the best
teacher. At any rate I insist that my students learn by
watching and doing, rather than by only listening to lectures
or reading unsubstantiated theories.

I have attempted to incorporate the same principle into
the writing of this book. In discussing any given technique,
finding, theory or application of hypnosis, there is at least
one excerpt—usually more—from a tape-recorded hypnotic
session involving the operator, the patient and attending
doctors. Confidences and identities have of course been withheld where ethics so dictated, but the editing has been slight.
While extraneous material that necessarily intruded on tapes
now and then (entrances or exits of doctors in an audience,
coughs, statements of addresses and names, interruptions,
etc.) have been pared away, the participants are permitted
to speak as they spoke. If a person used a colloquialism or
a bit of bad grammar, it has only been changed on those
occasions calling for a clarification of meaning. After all, a
person's personality, emotions and responses are expressed
in the words he actually uses, not in a technician's or gram-
marian's alterations.

Bracketed descriptions of non-verbal actions or communications (such as [Patient nods . . . or refuses to answer . . . or begins to smile . . . or coughs . . . or opens his eyes] and the like) are included, in the manner of stage directions. This is done, first, for the sake of clarity, and second—and more important—because the observation of reactions is vital to the successful medical application of hypnosis. Having made the introductory remarks that I think are important to a proper study of the subject, it is time to begin finding out about hypnosis. I have only one note to add before launching the study proper; my heartfelt thanks to the thousands of doctors who have been my students. Just as I have been their teacher, they have taught me. .

Chapter 1

MY FIRST IMPORTANT FINDINGS

I TEACH hypnosis to men in all branches of medicine. Naturally, I use many teaching aids, including recordings, copious outlines and notes, but I have never relied on any textbook. The idea of writing a book of my own on the subject has been suggested to me by physicians, dentists and podiatrists. Now, finally, I am acting upon the suggestion. Why? An explanation can be found in two communications I recently received, while recuperating from a serious illness.

The first one was a telegram which came all the way from California. It was from someone I do not know and who has never studied with me. It reads: "Are you going to teach in Los Angeles soon? I am a psychiatrist. What do you suggest? Sincerely."

The second was a letter from a doctor in another field. He lives in Detroit and is a former student of mine. He studied with me about seven years ago. He wrote, in part: "I'm certain that none of the doctors in Detroit who have been your students were aware that you were ill, for your name is often mentioned with fondness by all your former students and had but one known, I'm certain that all of us would have heard about it . . . All of us hope that when you are fully recovered Detroit will be on your itinerary. We'll be looking forward to seeing you . . . I've bought everything you have recorded in order that my boys will have access to as much of your work as possible in the years to come . . . I know what an insight you gave me into the human mind and I am only sorry that it is not assured that they are going to have the same advantage, Dave. If your course leaves this earth with you it will be a great tragedy. I am most sincere."

Naturally, these two communications, together with many others of a similar nature, have deeply affected me. These friends, both known and unknown, deserve consideration. So do all the medical practitioners who work so hard

1

to alleviate suffering. So do their patients. If my knowledge can help in any way, this book will have served a fine cause.

First, I wish to make clear certain limitations in my discussion of medical topics: I am not a doctor. There are no degrees after my name. Being a layman, I make no claim to *medical* knowledge. However, several hundred psychiatrists have been my students. Circumstances have enabled me to work with literally thousands of physicians, dentists and podiatrists. I began teaching doctors the professional use of hypnosis many years ago, and I made it plain to every doctor who attended my classes that I have no medical knowledge; all I could teach them was professional hypnosis, and once they knew what could be done with hypnosis, they would have to attach their own knowledge to what I taught them in order to come up with something valuable. This is still the case today. What I offer here is not an exploration into medicine but a history of my findings in hypnosis. My work with medical men has enabled me to do important research.

Not long after I began teaching, doctors began asking me to help them with patients who had no organic pathology and yet were quite ill. There was no medical explanation for their illness. Let me give you an example that led to a very important discovery.

It was in 1950 that a psychiatrist in one of my classes told me about a woman patient who was suffering severe pain of an unexplained nature. Every medical test had been made, and the tests showed the patient was in good health. Yet the pain was intense, and the psychiatrist was at a loss to help. Would hypnosis reveal the cause of her condition?

I asked the psychiatrist to bring this woman to my home and I would see what could be done. I questioned her at great length and learned that she had not known such a pain prior to an operation for a gall bladder condition. The pain had begun almost immediately after the operation, and yet she had recovered from the operation quite easily.

I succeeded in getting the patient into the state of hypnosis known as somnambulism, and learned that her statements were true. There had been no comparable pain prior to the operation. My probing only confirmed what the psychiatrist had already told me.

The psychiatrist asked if I would be willing to work

again with the same patient at his office. I agreed to do so.
When I arrived, he was busy with another case and asked if
I would get started with the patient while waiting for him.
He left the room, and the patient readily accepted the state
of somnambulism.

We covered much of the same ground, and then it
occurred to me that if the pain had only begun after the
operation, its cause must be in the operation itself. But the
patient had been deeply anesthetized during the surgery.
How could I learn what had happened in the operating room?
I decided to get the woman into a much deeper phase of
hypnosis. I call this phase hypno-sleep. Recent research
has confirmed the fact that it is a deeper state of hypnosis
than has ever been deemed possible. It was in this deep
state of hypnosis that I had the patient relive her experiences
as she was being taken to the operating room.

Further questioning revealed that she could relive the
entire operation, telling me exactly what had occurred in the
operating room while she was unconscious and had apparently lost her sense of hearing. She could tell me exactly
what the anesthetist, the surgeon and his assistants said,
even after the chemical anesthesia had taken full effect. One
of the things she had heard which seemed to affect her violently in the abreaction (the reliving of the experience) was
what the surgeon had said after making the incision and
exposing the gall bladder to view. He had remarked, "Take
a look at that gall bladder! She'll never be the same after
this."

I asked the patient what that statement meant to her
and she answered, "I think it meant that I would never be
a well woman after the operation." I explained to her that
the doctor really meant this as an encouraging statement,
but had unfortunately used the wrong words, that the pain
which she was suffering would subside—and before the visit
was over the pain had completely vanished. She was now
pain-free for the first time since her operation. Subsequent
reports from the psychiatrist were to the effect that the
patient was getting along beautifully.

It had never occurred to me that a patient could relive
what had occurred during complete anesthesia. Like everyone else I thought that such a patient could neither hear nor
remember what was going on around him at that time. Now,

inadvertently, I had stumbled upon an amazing fact. Here was a patient who could not only hear under chemical anesthesia, but who could afterward relive the things going on around her during the operation. I decided to see if it was possible to do this with other patients. Perhaps many unexplained "illnesses" could have been caused by indiscreet remarks made by a surgeon, anesthetist or nurse during surgery. I induced other patients to relive their operations under hypnosis and give me the details. To my surprise, person after person was able to give me information which he apparently did not have at a conscious level, and upon checking with the doctors, I found this information to be absolutely accurate.

I then passed this discovery on to my students, all of whom were doctors, with the suggestion that when treating a patient for illness of unknown origin after surgery, they look to the operating room for the cause. After I obtained sufficient reports from doctors who were able to duplicate what I had done, I began to stress in the classroom that doctors and their assistants should be careful of what they say even though the patient is unconscious and apparently unable to hear them.

It also occurred to me that if the patient could be influenced by unfortunate remarks in the operating room, he could be similarly influenced by good suggestions given to him when he was in deep anesthesia. This made possible the following important finding: The patient can be given suggestions to maintain anesthesia even after the *chemical* effects of anesthesia are gone, thus making recovery much easier. This was my first important finding in the use of hypnosis; it has been substantiated by many surgeons and psychiatrists.

Interestingly enough, a few years ago I learned that a doctor on the West Coast was beginning experiments along the same lines and had made similar discoveries. This doctor was not a student of mine and we didn't meet until two years ago. He has sent me several very interesting papers which have been published in medical journals, again confirming that a patient can hear while under chemical anesthesia.

In this connection, I recall an incident that was tape-recorded in the classroom. It happened in San Antonio, Texas. I was giving this information to my students when one of the doctors in the class vehemently disagreed with me, but conceded that if what I said was possible, it was an important contribution to medical knowledge. He remarked that a few years previously he had undergone major surgery, and didn't have the slightest recollection of what went on after the anesthetic was given to him. I asked him if he would like to relive that operation and learn exactly what happened. He said he would like to try it, but didn't believe anything would come of it.

I put him into the state which I call hypno-sleep and had him relive the operation in detail. During the abreaction, he exclaimed, "So that's why they are making such a long incision." After rousing him from the state, we spent the balance of the session discussing this doctor's operation, the things he didn't know about it before the hypnosis and the things he now knew and understood. He was most enthusiastic. He sent the tape-recording he had made to the West Coast doctor who was doing research in this area, and has since sent the tape-recording to me. A transcript of that hypoanalysis will be found in a later chapter of this book, when we discuss the phase of hypnosis known as hypnosleep.

It will probably be many years before doctors all over the world accept the fact that patients under complete general anesthesia retain their sense of hearing and that the mind is functioning even if it is at an awareness below the level of consciousness. Yet papers have been written by doctors of excellent repute substantiating these facts—which have been proven in over two hundred cases. When mental activity under anesthesia is accepted, it may well lead to further valuable findings.

Since the mind functions at a level below conscious awareness when the patient is unconscious, it is reasonable to pose this question: "Is there any possibility that a person who is made unconscious by an accident or any other means still retains his sense of hearing, and that the victim's mind is still working even though the consciousness is below the level of awareness?" I believe further research is indicated though I make no claims at this writing that such is the case.

Before describing a second important finding I made through hypnosis, it is worth mentioning that classroom incidents have been accurately recorded while they were taking place. For several years my wife, who is an expert at shorthand, transcribed every word said in class. Later, we began tape-recording class sessions. In this way I could review each session privately, learning what doctors needed to know about hypnosis in order to use it effectively. The technique also enabled me to spot any mistakes I might have made in my teaching and correct them during the next class.

Let us go now to that second important finding made shortly after I began teaching doctors the professional use of hypnosis. One night, an industrial physician attending the classes announced with great enthusiasm that in twenty-four hours, with the use of hypnosis, he had relieved two male patients of impotence. The other doctors in class were inclined to scoff at his pronouncement. Still, he insisted that he had already helped both men. Here is what he said: "There had been a slight accident at the plant and I was binding the lesions of one of the victims. As he was leaving the office, he said to me, 'I wish you could fix up my real problem as well as you fixed up these minor things.' I asked him what his real problem was and he answered, 'Impotence, and I've had it for several years.' I asked him how it had started and he told me it began after his first vacation away from his wife. He'd gone down to Florida and while there he'd had relations with a strange woman and had contracted gonorrhea. He went to a doctor and was quickly cured, but he had such a feeling of guilt that he didn't have the heart to go back home to New Jersey. It was ten weeks after the doctor told him he was cured before he could get up enough nerve to go back home. When he did he was unable to resume family relations. He'd had a very unhappy marriage ever since.

"I hypnotized the man and told him he had punished himself long enough. I stressed that by punishing himself he was also punishing his wife and destroying a happy marriage; that from now on, he would cease punishing himself and would find himself quite able to resume family relations that very night. Then I brought him out of the somnambulism, and gave him a little more encouragement and sent him away.

"Next morning he came into my office, bringing another man from the plant with him. He said, 'Doctor, it worked so well for me, maybe you can help my friend. He's got the same trouble, and he's had it quite a while.'

"I asked the second man to tell me about his troubles and he told me, 'I got married a few years ago. I was forty-five years old and I was marrying a girl of twenty-one. On our wedding night, the fellows began to kid me. They said I could never make good with a girl of twenty-one—that I was an old buck and couldn't possibly be a real husband for a young girl who was less than half my age. I must have believed them because we've been married for over four years and we still haven't been able to consummate our marriage.'

"I put this second patient into somnambulism and went over his story again, and then I told him that he would be as potent as anybody for the rest of his life, and that he would be able to consummate his marriage immediately. I roused him from the state, talked to him a bit further on the subject, and he was able to report to me that the condition was completely corrected and the marriage had been consummated."

The doctor told the story well. So well, in fact, that the other doctors changed their attitude and asked me what I knew about using hypnosis to correct impotence. I told them that I knew very little about it but that if it had been successful in those two cases, it might be successful in many instances. I advised them to try it and see. They tried it only on cases where all pathology had been ruled out. Pretty soon the doctors began to report successes. They noted that while many cases of impotence are caused by the use of certain medications, by pathology or surgery, about ninety percent of all impotence has an emotional basis. In those cases where emotional disturbance was to blame, they were successful many times.

Occasionally, however, the phone would ring and a doctor would say to me something like, "It worked in two cases, but it has not worked at all on the third man I tried it on. What did I do wrong?" I told these doctors that I hadn't the slightest idea what they'd done wrong, and I didn't know why it had worked for some and not for others. Then they began asking me whether I would come to their offices and see if I could find out why they had occasionally failed. These calls would come in sometimes three or four a day. When I went to the doctors' offices and watched them work, the reasons for failure quickly became apparent. They were succeeding in almost every case where the patient knew the cause of the impotence at conscious level—as in the instances already given. They were unsuccessful when the patient was unable to tell the doctor the cause. By means of hypno-analysis, we then determined the causes of the impotence, and once discovered, the patient's trouble could be readily relieved. The results were spectacular. Soon, I was work-ing with more impotence cases than I could handle, for every time a doctor was unsuccessful I would be called in to do hypnoanalysis.

I think it was less than a year later that one of the doctors in class asked, "Hypnotic techniques seem to work so well in problems of impotence, why wouldn't they work equally well with frigidity when there is no pathology pres-ent? Frigidity is, of course, the female counterpart of the male problem."

They gave the idea a trial, and the calls began to come in from enthusiastic doctors saying that they had been able to correct frigidity by means of hypnotic techniques. When these reports were made in class, there would always be one or two doctors who would say, "Well, maybe you were suc-cessful, but I wasn't. I tried it and it didn't work. What did I do wrong?" It was easy to see that the same situation existed in frigidity as existed in impotence: Whenever the patient knew the cause of the frigidity at conscious level, it was quite easy to relieve; but when the patient was unable to state the cause, the doctors would fail. Again, hypno-analysis was the answer. A long series of hypnoanalysis was begun on women and the results were gratifying. We would uncover the cause of the frigidity, give the patient insight regarding the problem, then bring her out of the state and discuss it thoroughly. One after another, these women were able to report that they were no longer troubled with frigidity.

I can safely say that in the first four or five years of teaching I never failed to correct an impotence case. The results were not quite so consistent, however, with cases of frigidity, and I firmly believe that the reason for my inability to achieve as spectacular results was the natural reserve of the female. A man will reveal all his sexual problems hon-estly to another man. But a very modest woman, whether she realizes it or not, often holds back information which the doctor vitally needs in order to help her. When a woman doctor is working with frigidity cases, she finds that a woman will tell all of her problems and thus make recovery from frigidity easier to relieve. This has been borne out by many reports I have had from female doctors. There is one doctor in particular who told me quite seriously, "I used to think I was a general practitioner. Now I find that my time is taken up day and night with frigidity problems and that what you have taught me has enabled me to hit a very high percentage of success."

Doctors might well be guided by these findings—namely, that after pathology has been ruled out there are only two types of impotence and only two types of frigidity. Type A is where the cause of the impotence or frigidity is known at conscious level, and type B is where the cause of the impotence or frigidity is not known at conscious level but is retained in the mind by an awareness below the level of consciousness.

* * *

It is my belief that these discoveries, and others on which I shall report, can be well utilized by the doctors who read this book. The public enthusiasm for writings about medicine shows that such findings are also interesting to the layman. I shall therefore describe and document them fully.

Among the calls for help that I have received from my students (physicians and dentists), one was particularly interesting: This was the situation as revealed to me over the telephone by an obstetrician: "I have a patient in the hospital who has been in a catatonic state for about seventy-two hours. The woman is pregnant. She is sitting up in bed and none of us seem to be able to get through to her. Several psychiatrists have been called in and after consultation they decided the only medical treatment that would help her is shock therapy. The Mother Superior at the hospital is violently opposed to shock therapy in this case because she is under the impression that if the woman is given a number of shock treatments, she will probably miscarry. So she will not permit shock therapy in this case. Is there anything you can do to help this patient?"

Naturally, I reminded the obstetrician that I was not a doctor, and was not supposed to work in a hospital. He said, "Dave, this is an emergency and the psychiatrists have asked me to call you. You are being given permission to work with this patient at the hospital under the direction of the psychiatrists and myself. We will be there with you."

I didn't know whether I could help the patient, but I was certainly willing to try since it was going to be done under medical supervision. I was shown the patient's hospital chart; I didn't understand it at all, but the obstetrician explained to me just what the data on the chart revealed. He also introduced me to several of the psychiatrists. Then the obstetrician and a couple of the psychiatrists took me into the room where the patient was sitting upright in bed. She was staring straight ahead at the wall, not moving a muscle, and she didn't even turn her head when I approached her bed.

I stood silent for a moment, not knowing what to do. Then I said to her, "You must have had a lot of trouble to put you into such a terrible state." So far as I can remember, that was all I said to her but I did say it in a very sympathetic voice. She slowly turned her head toward me and said, "I have." Then she began to cry. I asked her, "Won't you tell me what the trouble is? Maybe I can help you." She said, "I don't think anybody can help me" and she just went on crying. I said, "If you will just follow my instructions, maybe it will be easier for you to talk and tell me just what is bothering you. Would you be willing to follow my instructions?" In the midst of her tears, she said, "I'll do anything if you can help me."

I put her into hypnosis and then got this amazing story from her. It seemed that she was the mother of a three or four-year-old child. Her husband was a veteran of the Second World War who worked nights, coming home at about 2:00 A.M. When he was in the army, he had been given a very short leave before being sent overseas. He was only able to be home with his wife for one night. It was on this night that she became pregnant with her first child. Her husband was overseas when the baby was born. Then the war ended and he came home. He began to tease is wife, saying "Are you sure I am the father?" He may have said this teasingly, but the wife was never certain whether he was really joking or meant what he said.

They lived happily for several years, during which time whenever he had a few drinks he would bring up the subject again. Then she became pregnant a second time, and after several months had passed, went to see the obstetrician to confirm her pregnancy. When the obstetrician told her she was really pregnant she was very happy. She went home, intending to give her husband the good news. Expecting her husband home from work about 2:00 A.M., she waited up for him, but he didn't come home until five o'clock in the morning. He had had a few drinks and was quite high. Before she could tell him about the pregnancy, she asked him what had kept him so late, and he said to her, "I went to see the doctor today and he gave me some terrible news. The doctor said that I am not only impotent but I am completely sterile."

Now the poor woman was in a terrible dilemma. What was he going to say about the second baby? That was when she became so emotionally disturbed that she landed in the hospital in a catatonic state.

In deep hypnosis, I got her thoughts. They went something like this: "If he was impotent and sterile, how in the world did I get pregnant? He is the only man I have ever been with. What is my husband going to say when he finds out I'm pregnant?"

The obstetrician and I did our best to placate her, and we told her we would speak to her husband. When we brought her out of the hypnosis she was no longer catatonic, but she was still a very disturbed woman. The doctor got in touch with her husband, and that night my wife and I and the obstetrician met the husband in the doctor's home. The doctor questioned him about his impotence and sterility, wanting to know what doctor had given him this diagnosis and when. The husband laughed and said, "I'm not impotent or sterile. No doctor told me that. I got drunk and stayed out too late and I thought this would be a funny alibi, so I made it up on the way home." The doctor and I were appalled. Then the doctor laced into the husband. He told him this sort of thing was not funny, and of the damage that had been done. By now, the husband was upset and kept protesting that he had only been teasing in the same manner as he had teased all these years about his first baby, knowing full well the baby was his.

Then the doctor said, "I'm going to take you over to the hospital and you're going to tell your wife the true story, and I'm going to be there to hear you tell it." Result: The woman got well and later delivered a fine, healthy baby.

This incident illustrated another important finding, as important as it is simple: There are times when a kind word will break through to a patient when all other forms of therapy have failed.

Chapter 2

WHY I STARTED TEACHING HYPNOSIS

IN WRITING this book, it is my aim to do more than entertain. It is my desire to teach, to make known certain findings. I am confident that the doctors among you, after reading about my observations, will test their validity through clinical research, and will thereby prove the truth of my theories. If I succeed in having you regard this book as informative, as a text worthy of study, I will have fulfilled my purpose.

I have often found that teaching—that is, the imparting of insights that enable a student to assimilate, store and use knowledge—is best accomplished by a narrative of the teacher's experiences. It may be well, therefore, to complete your introduction to my discoveries by recounting a few more of my early experiences.

I have never told the full story of how I happened to go back to the practice of hypnosis after abondoning it during my youth for what were then socially strategic reasons. Although I gave up hypnosis at the age of fourteen, I went on studying the subject. I used to lie awake at night analyzing what I had done with hypnosis. I wondered why I had been able to make certain things happen that apparently no one had thought of doing before. I kept wondering what made these things successful.

It was at about this time that I became stage struck. I am an extrovert by nature, and I like the feeling of standing before an audience, doing something to amaze people. If I couldn't do it with hypnosis, I was certainly going to do it somehow—and so I became a performer. Being a music lover, I began writing songs that never became popular. When one of these songs was finally accepted by W. C. Handy, I came to New York thinking that I would become a famous song writer under his tutelage. I began working for him as a song plugger, plugging not only his songs, but my own.

Eventually I took a job in radio as a writer, performer

and producer for CBS and was soon succeeding in a very substantial way. I didn't have to depend on hypnosis for a
living, and I didn't mention my knowledge to anyone. In
1937, I conceived the idea for a radio show called Dave
Elman's Hobby Lobby. The success of the show was instantaneous. In 1941 I was changing sponsors. The Colgate-
Palmolive-Peet Company bought the show, and we were
making preparations for the first performance. The director
of the show said to me, "We have to make this first show
sensational. What is the most sensational hobby that we
could put on the air?" I told him I had just received a letter
from a printer in Philadelphia who claimed his hobby was
hypnotism and who offered to go on the air and hypnotize
people who were sitting in another room. "If he can do it,"
the director commented, "He'll make a sensational spot for
the opening show."

The man arrived from Philadelphia, and I put him
through some grueling tests. This man knew the subject
of hypnosis very well, but he didn't realize he was going
through a test by a man who also knew the subject. He
met the test beautifully, and I was considerably impressed
by him. The only thing that worried me was that he said
it would take him at least three to six minutes to accomplish the feat, and I felt that if he took more than three
minutes, there would be an awfully dull spot on the show.
I gave him an audition which proved that he could perform
the feat in three minutes. This increased my respect for him
considerably. We put him on the air and the nationwide
acceptance was fantastic. The performance was given the
Variety award for being the most dramatic radio show
of 1941.

My wife at that time worked as my secretary, and, of
course, observed my work with the hypnotist. She said to
me, "You showed that hypnotist what to do, didn't you?
I think you know much more about the subject than you
pretend to." Suddenly, my knowledge had become a help
rather than a hindrance.

From that time on, I would occasionally do hypnotic
demonstrations, either for charity or at very nominal fees.
One day I put on a show for a well-known fraternal organiza-
tion in Passaic, New Jersey. The demonstration was highly
successful. Many doctors were there that night and some of

them asked if they could talk with me. The gist of the conversation was to the effect that these men had studied hypnosis and were trying to use it in their medical and dental practices, but were very unsuccessful with it. They volunteered the information that some of my subjects were patients on whom they had attempted, and failed, to gain the state of hypnosis. They asked, "What do you know about hypnosis that we don't know?" I answered, "Apparently we have studied the subject from different angles. If you had studied it as I have, you would be just as successful as I am."

One of the doctors asked if I would be willing to teach them. Never having done any teaching, I was reluctant; I hadn't the slightest idea what they would have to know Some doctors can be very persistent, and I soon found that whenever I made a public appearance in New Jersey, one or more of them would be at the meeting. They would seek me out and ask, "When are you going to start teaching us hypnosis?"

I was between sponsors and I had a lot of time on my hands. I wondered if I could write a course on the subject that would enable doctors to use hypnosis on a professional basis as I used it.

One of these doctors, an oral surgeon who has since passed away, said to me one day, "Mr. Elman, a group of dentists in Newark, New Jersey, is studying hypnosis. Would you like to go over and see just what's being taught to these men?" I accompanied him to the meeting—and was completely astounded at the misinformation which was being given to these sincere men. The teacher was a very fine gentleman and a sincere teacher. He just didn't know the subject he was trying to teach. Now as then, misinformation is broadcast as gospel in many hypnosis lectures. I decided that if this was the way physicians and dentists were being taught the subject, something had to be done about it. I went home and prepared a course in hypnosis for the medical and dental professions which I have been teaching ever since. For the sake of medical progress, let's put this teaching to use.

*   *   *

When I make the statement that everybody has been placed on the threshold of hypnosis thousands of times and that everybody has hypnotized himself again and again without knowing it, the reaction is usually one of consternation. I can understand the disbelief that many people will have regarding the above statement, but let us analyze a few simple manifestations of hypnosis.

Take the person who is superstitious. That person may firmly believe that Friday the thirteenth is unlucky. He is so firmly convinced that Friday the thirteenth is an unlucky day that he will postpone business arrangements or pleasure engagements to prevent their turning out disastrously. Common sense tells us that Friday the thirteenth is just like any other day. There is no reason for a belief that this date is different from others. The person who believes Friday the thirteenth is an unlucky day has hypnotized himself, for he has bypassed the critical faculty of his mind—that is, his sense of judgment—and has implanted, unknowingly perhaps, a process of selective thinking. The person who carries a rabbit's foot, believing it to be an emblem of good luck, is in the same category. He, too, has bypassed his sense of judgment and has implanted selective thinking.

Other simple manifestations of hypnosis, made on the assumption that hypnosis is merely a state of mind, include *every* bypass of the critical faculty and the implanting of selective thinking. The examples are almost countless. In several states, an attempt is being made to ban the practice of hypnosis by other than the medical professions. Such laws would be an attempt to control the thinking of the people. Even if they are put into effect, they can't be enforced, because you can't outlaw what goes on in the minds of people. For example, a person who has been in an accident, and is feeling pain, gives himself a suggestion that there will be no pain. This is most definitely hypnosis. Can any law prevent this? No one has hypnotized the accident victim, but he has hypnotized himself. Who can stop him?

There is also a silly notion that the use of hypnosis should be restricted to psychiatrists. Who is going to prevent the physician or the dentist from giving patients suggestions for their welfare? He can do this in excellent fashion without the *obvious* use of hypnosis, but nevertheless he is using hypnosis, and who can possibly stop him?

When you attempt to outlaw hypnosis, you are attempting to outlaw such effective therapy as the sterile hypo.

Doctors praise the use of sterile hypos in glowing terms. This applies even to doctors who have no knowledge of hypnosis and insist they don't use hypnosis. Yet a sterile hypo contains no actual medication; it is the very suggestion of its use that helps the patient—i.e., hypnosis. How in the world can you possibly outlaw placebos? Yet, if you outlaw hypnosis, you certainly must include placebos.

Are you one of those people who think they have never been hypnotized? Perhaps you wouldn't "allow" yourself to be hypnotized. If so, you are laboring under completely false illusions. There isn't a person alive of normal intelligence and over the age of two who has not been hypnotized, and if you are in your later years, you have been hypnotized many times. If you doubt this, you don't know what hypnosis is.

Did you ever close your eyes and begin to dream? Perhaps you visualized some pleasant incident in which you had participated some time ago. For example, you might have closed your eyes and visualized a pleasant vacation spot. You knew very well that you were not actually at the vacation spot in your recollection, but the scene was quite vivid in your mind's eye. If you have done that you have not only put yourself on the threshold of hypnosis, bypassing your critical faculty—but if you have actually said to yourself, "It's just as if I were there right now," and placed yourself there mentally, you were hypnotized. You not only bypassed your critical faculty but implanted selective thinking. Everyone in the world has probably done this time and time again. Sometimes dreams are so startling that you wake yourself. You don't realize it, but this, too, was hypnosis. You knew the dream was not real, yet it seemed very real to you. If, while you were asleep and dreaming, someone said, "Now you won't feel anything," you would accept the suggestion and find yourself completely anesthetized. If you are willing to test this statement, you will be amazed to find that the experiment is quite successful. Many doctors who are adept in the use of hypnosis have used this simplified technique and have reported success with it. Make sure, however, that when tests are made the patient is fast asleep and that the words of the doctor don't rouse him from his slumber.

When a person rejects hypnosis, it simply means he has refused to bypass his critical faculty and thereby make the implanting of selective thinking impossible. It doesn't mean he can't be hypnotized or won't be hypnotized, but simply that he refused to follow instructions. If he does follow properly given instructions, hypnosis is possible for him just as it is for everyone.

It will sometimes be found that the induction of hypnosis attached to sleep is faster and easier than induction when the subject is awake. This is because the subject is "pre-relaxed" when you begin. The techniques—and possibilities—of *hypnosis attached to sleep* will be detailed in the chapter of that title. But it is important, meanwhile, that you bear in mind the facts outlined above as they will have a bearing on your further study.

Chapter 3

HOW TO STUDY HYPNOSIS

I START my teaching with a lecture on "How to Study Hypnosis." Here is what I tell each doctor: If you decide to take up this subject, you are giving of your time and effort to learn how to use a tool that can be of inestimable value to you in your practice. You can learn to use it properly if you follow instructions. First and foremost, do your homework. Doing it will not take precious time away from your busy office and hospital hours. Instead it will give you *extra* time to increase your practice and your leisure hours, because you will be able to do more with each patient in less time. Therefore, as you begin practicing, limit your induction period to one minute for each patient. When you take longer than a minute to introduce the subject of relaxation and gain the hypnotic state, you are wasting time. It is my firm conviction that if hypnosis is to have a respectable place in medicine and dentistry, it must be available to the doctor almost instantly. If he can't use hypnosis on a more or less instantaneous basis, it has no practical value in the average doctor's office. It is a rare doctor who can afford to spend from three minutes to two hours on the doubtful assumption that he might be able to succeed in obtaining hypnosis if he keeps trying long enough. So, at the beginning, use one minute for each patient and one minute only. Don't take any more time than that—and you shouldn't even need the full minute to gain the state.

On the other hand, don't expect to have perfect results from the start. If you have excellent results in your first few tries, you are nonetheless bound to meet with failure later on. The best student has a combination of successes and failures while learning. It is my firm belief that in this subject you learn more from your failures than you do from your successes. If your first ten attempts are all successes, and then you fail, it may be a blow to your ego. After such an experience, a doctor often finds it difficult to continue improving his technique. But if you fail the first two or three times and then succeed, and then perhaps fail another time, then suc-

ceed twice and then have another failure, and then succeed
three or four or five times—then you get to the point where
you don't fail at all. You have become a good student. The
man who fails a few times among those first ten is going to
progress well because he's going to find out what he did that
was wrong. If instructions are followed, he will become
adept in a short time.

Failure to obtain the hypnotic state during the first few
attempts is often caused by a lack of confidence. The
remedy: Try again. As your studies continue and you are
taught new methods, try *every* new method you are taught.
Don't form the bad habit of using one technique only. There
are many from which to choose. As you go along, select
those techniques that seem most natural to you and that
obtain the state most rapidly and deeply for you.

Occasionally, a doctor will say at the second or even the
third session, "No, Mr. Elman, I haven't started practicing
yet. I'm waiting to learn more about the subject." This is
the phoniest excuse for laziness or timidity in the world, and
your teacher knows it. You can only learn more about the
subject by starting at the beginning. You can't start in the
middle and go both ways. It's impossible.

Each time you endeavor to induce the state in someone,
you are adding to your knowledge. While timid students
are waiting to learn more, their colleagues are going ahead
rapidly, learning more and more about the subject by putting
into practice what they've learned at each class, together
with what they've learned at each previous practice session
in their own offices and at the hospital. Every patient with
whom you work presents a new experience—a chance to observe individual reaction, a chance to correct the faults you
were able to notice in previous inductions. And the man
who learns by a combination of instruction and experience—
in other words, by practicing—achieves a far greater success
than the man who tries to learn by theory alone.

Some years ago, one of my physician students was, to
put it charitably, a hesitant practicer. Despite my warnings
about this pitfall, he kept postponing any attempt to put my
teachings into operation. Finally, during the ninth class
session, he said, "Mr. Elman, I have an important announcement to make. This week I hypnotized two people." By that
time, every man in the room had probably hypnotized a

couple of hundred people. And this man still had to make the mistakes that they would make no more.

There are certain things you should not do, at least at the start. After three or four weeks have gone by, you can forget these don'ts: Don't try to hypnotize your wife, or members of your family, or friends you see socially; these people know you are studying hypnosis, and will put up an instinctive objection to becoming your guinea pigs. Don't try to hypnotize people who "defy" you to put them into the state; hypnosis is a *consent* state and, obviously, the person who defies does not consent. Don't try to prove the value of hypnosis to a skeptic; at this early stage, you will be arguing from a position of weakness. Later on, when you know enough about hypnosis, you can argue from a position of strength.

It is also very important that you don't treat the subject of hypnosis as a joke or a parlor game. Hypnosis is a scientific study when it's properly conducted, and if you respect hypnosis as you should, you will not use it for parlor tricks. It has a great value in medicine. You must intend to use it that way if you—and your patients—are to get the maximum benefit from it.

This, I think, is very important, too: Don't get ahead of yourself. In this book, I am going to explain the proper techniques to use, just as I do in actual classes. Don't skip lessons and attempt more advanced techniques. Don't attempt *any* procedures until you have thoroughly digested it, and preferably not just from a text but with a capable teacher. Practice what you've been taught in each lesson. Go no further, and you will learn more from each lesson. Every phase of the subject is covered in proper order for you to absorb it. If you try to get ahead of yourself, you're bound to run into things that puzzle and mystify you. As these things are covered and explained, the puzzlement leaves, you understand the subject more fully and you're ready for those reactions that require a deeper knowledge of human reaction to the power of suggestion.

Once I asked my students for their reports at the second session and everybody gave me a report except one man. "I didn't write down my homework," he said, "but I have a wonderful report to make. This week I succeeded in using hypnosis exclusively to deliver a woman and it worked beau-

tifully. Perfectly. I had one hundred percent success
with it."

I guess he expected an ovation, but instead he heard
these words: "Doctor, I'm awfully sorry you did that. With
your present inadequate knowledge, if you had perfect success, it was a complete accident. You don't know *why* you
succeeded, and when you try it again, you'll fail because you
don't have sufficient knowledge to carry a woman through
delivery at this point. Then you'll try it a third time and fail,
and by the time you've tried it about four times and failed,
you'll decide that hypnosis can't be relied upon, and you won't
make a good student at all. On the other hand, if you go
along with the course, when I tell you that you are well
enough equipped now to do a delivery, *then* you'll be able to
help, to some extent at least, every woman who comes into
the delivery room."

Hypnosis can be used on every patient who comes into
your office, if for no other reason than to relax the patient.
There is no one who cannot benefit from relaxation, and until
you have learned to go further into the subject, your patient
should be taught the immediate benefits of relaxation and the
relief of anxiety.

When you begin practicing, endeavor to obtain a state
of relaxation on at least ten of your patients using the relaxation approach and the handshake technique. While doing so,
look for the signs of hypnosis. Hypnosis gives off five signs.
These signs are subtle, minute. If you don't know what to
look for, the signs could all be there without your detecting
one of them. When you know hypnosis, however, you can
spot all five signs at a glance. Here are the five signs of
hypnosis, all of which you must carefully observe: (1) body
warmth; (2) fluttering of the eyelids; (3) increased lacrimation; (4) the whites of the eyes getting red or pinkish;
(5) the eyeballs going up into the head. We will go into
further detail regarding these signs in a later chapter. For
the time being, it is merely important for you to bear them in
mind and memorize them so that they will be quickly recognized when they occur.

A bad habit pattern can keep you from becoming adept
and can keep you from becoming a good student. Begin
practicing the methodical restraint I advised a moment ago
by not jumping ahead.

Chapter 4

INTERESTING FACTS ABOUT HYPNOSIS

IN VIEW of the countless volumes that have been written about the history of hypnosis, it would be pointless for me to attempt a capsule history in this book. A few historic highlights that have had an effect on the teaching—and learning—of hypnosis do, however, have a place here.

A couple of hundred years ago, a Viennese physician named F. A. Mesmer watched a street magician perform an act with lodestones, or magnets. The magician declared that he could make a spectator do his bidding by touching him with one of these magnets. And he proceeded to put on a demonstration that proved he really could do it. The secret was the power of suggestion, of course. Mesmer believed the magnets actually had a power of their own, however, and out of this belief he developed his theory of magnetism. Good health, he claimed, depended on the direction of magnetic flow, which could easily be reversed.

At one time three thousand patients a day begged to see him, and in order to accommodate them all he had to change his technique. His first technique was to place a tub in the middle of a large room from which protruded a number of so-called "magnetic rods." People sat around the tub holding on to these magnetic rods and believed that the magnetic flow in their bodies would be corrected, thus accomplishing a cure. It was the power of suggestion at work. It was impossible to accommodate three thousand patients a day around these tubs and so he went out into the yard, touched a tree with his so-called magnetic rod and declared the tree to be magnetized. Now, all people had to do was to touch the magnetized tree and they would be miraculously cured of their ills. It was the power of suggestion, again at work. When Benjamin Franklin was in France, he watched a demonstration and pronounced this verdict: "If these people get well at all, they seem to get well by their own imaginings." (Evidently, Franklin understood something of hysterical symptoms and mob psychology.)

Thereafter, mesmerism suffered a decided drop in popularity. But patients in an obvious hypnotic (or "mesmeric") state had been observed, and many doctors studied mesmerism in secret. One of these was an English physician named James Braid. By accident, a patient of Braid's entered the first stage of mesmerism while staring at a fixed light as he waited for an eye examination to begin. Because of the contempt in which mesmerism was then held (the date was 1840), Braid coined a new term—hypnotism—derived from the Greek word for sleep. And he published a paper about obtaining hypnotism through fixation. This paper was published in 165 different languages and dialects.

The next important incident involved J. M. Charcot, an early psychiatrist whose teachings influenced Freud. After watching hypnotic demonstrations performed by a very poor operator, on three psychotic patients, Charcot—brilliant though he usually was—came to the conclusion that hypnosis was only successful with psychotic or pre-psychotic patients. To prove this theory, he put on demonstrations for physicians, using psychotics. These demonstrations became so popular that crowds of laymen began attending them . . . and at least one stage performer believed the same thing could be done with sane people and proved it by adapting the technique for his own use.

Braid's fixation method and its derivatives—monotony, rhythm, imitation and levitation—are still being used. The result was great success for stage performers and frequent failure for doctors. The performer had a chance to practice on thousands of people, with the advantage of stage lighting to help him apply fixation. The doctor had one patient at a time, time-consuming techniques and a suspicion that the whole business might prove to be nonsense.

These historic incidents have led to two deplorable conditions in the teaching of hypnosis today. First, even fairly modern texts have insisted that the only reliable technique is fixation. Second, they have insisted that fixation requires anywhere from three minutes to two hours for induction, and that stage performers who succeed faster than that are faking. As you will see, neither of these beliefs is true.

Chapter 5

THE HANDSHAKE TECHNIQUE

L ET US start with the handshake technique. When I was a comparative beginner in hypnosis, my technique was to walk up to the subject and say: "I'm going to shake your hand three times. The first time your eyes will get tired . . . let them. The second time, they'll want to close . . . let them. The third time they will lock and you won't be able to open them . . . *Want* that to happen, and watch it happen . . . Now, one . . . two . . . now close your eyes . . . now three . . . and they're locked and you'll find they just won't work, no matter how hard you try. The harder you try, the less they'll work. Test them, and you'll find they won't work at all . . . That's right. Now, that's perfect eye-closure."

I used to think that was hypnosis. Later, I realized it was merely the opening wedge into hypnosis, and this is an important finding, as you will see.

As soon as I learned how to tire a person's eyes very quickly, my technique improved to the place where I was getting approximately nine out of ten successes instead of five out of ten. I would shake hands with a person as I placed my other hand in front of his forehead, with the little finger of my left hand next to his face. Then I would say, "Keep your eyes on my hand as I bring it down under your chin," and I would then bring my hand down along the profile of his face until it was under his chin. "Now, close your eyes and relax the muscles around your eyes, relax them to the point where they will not work. When you're sure they won't work, test them." And by this simple device, I would get excellent eye-closure.

Those of you who have taken other courses in hypnosis have been told that once you have obtained eye-closure you have obtained hypnosis, and can go on from there. The fact of the matter is that just because you have eye-closure you do not necessarily have hypnosis. That is why so many novices are unsuccessful. They don't realize that it takes more than eye-closure to establish hypnosis. Most textbooks, because they are based on incorrect assumptions about such establishment, go astray here.

If you were to read a hundred books on hypnosis, trying to find a definition of the subject, you would be completely confused because you would find that every author—doctors included—has a definition that disagrees with all the others. This is a situation very much like that of the three blind men who were asked to describe an elephant. Like the blind men, each author describes only what he has touched, and describes it from a different viewpoint. None has seen the elephant hypnosis as it actually is, yet each one of them is sure that he is right. Most of them will agree that hypnosis is a state of high suggestibility, but then they begin to disagree, going off in every direction. Most of them start with the words, "Hypnosis is a condition in which . . ." and since hypnosis is not a "condition," the rest of their findings are bound to be inaccurate.

One of the first things I discovered was that hypnosis is a state of mind. Now, what is the difference between a condition and a state of mind? In the first place, you are not in a hypnotic condition as you read these words. If I wanted to put you into a so-called hypnotic condition, I would have to change your present condition. Not many people are willing to have their condition changed. A question of semantics perhaps, but an important one since the *state* of mind, unlike its condition, frequently and easily changes. The state of mind of hypnosis can be obtained instantaneously, for a state of mind is merely a mood, and I maintain that hypnosis is merely a mood. Your condition probably hasn't changed today, but how many moods have you had since you got up this morning?

I would like to give you an axiomatic definition which will stand up to careful clinical examination: "Hypnosis is a state of mind in which the critical faculty of the human is bypassed, and selective thinking established." The critical faculty of your mind is that part which passes judgment. It distinguishes between the concepts of hot and cold, sweet and sour, large and small, dark and light. If we can bypass this critical faculty in such a way that you no longer distinguish between hot and cold, sweet and sour, we can substitute selective thinking for conventional judgment making.

Practically all textbooks declare that you must first obtain eye-closure if you wish to obtain hypnosis, and that eye-closure can usually be obtained by the methods called fixation, monotony, rhythm, imitation or levitation. I'll show you a simple way to bypass your critical faculty, and obtain eye-closure, without these methods. Close your eyes and pretend you can't open them. Keep on pretending, and while you are pretending, try to open your eyes. You'll find that it is impossible, if you are concentrating hard on the pretense. Now you know very well that you can open your eyes any time you change your mind and stop pretending. All the time you were pretending that you could not open your eyes, your sense of judgment was completely suspended concerning that particular action. You have obtained the same eye-closure that you would if you had used the techniques of fixation, monotony, rhythm, imitation or levitation. This can be done instantaneously.

But does it mean that you are hypnotized? Indeed, it does not. It is merely the entering wedge, and hypnosis is not obtained until selective thinking is firmly established.

Selective thinking is whatever you believe *wholeheartedly*. For example, if you are led to believe that you will feel no pain, and you believe it completely, you will have no pain. Let the slghtest doubt come in and the selective thinking vanishes; the critical faculty is no longer bypassed. You will feel pain at normal level. Selective thinking vanishes not only when doubt enters the picture but when fear does. When a woman delivers a baby under hypnotic suggestion as the anesthesia agent, she feels no pain. However, should the doctor, nurse or any attendant make an unfortunate remark—for example, that "The pains should be really strong now"—she will then feel pain strongly, and lose the value of the hypnotic anesthesia. The introduction of fear causes a defensive reaction that brings the critical faculty back into focus.

Now let us return to the eye-closing pretense. If I were to say, "Close your eyes and pretend you can't open them," and you followed instructions, your critical faculty would be bypassed, but I must go further to accomplish hypnosis. I must also firmly establish selective thinking. Therefore, I would say to you, "So long as you keep pretending that you can't open your eyes, you will feel nothing. Nothing will bother you, no matter what the doctor does." If I say this convincingly enough and you believe it completely, I have established selective thinking while your critical faculty was inoperative, and the result is complete anesthesia. An understanding of this simple process enables me to stand quite often before a large audience of doctors and make this statement· "I want some doctor to come up to this chair, and I want that doctor to be the biggest skeptic in the room. I won't hypnotize him. I'll let him hypnotize himself, and I'll prove to him by so doing, the value of hypnosis."

This usually brings forth a skeptic—someone who believes that hypnosis is of no value and has no place in medicine or dentistry. He sits down in the chair and I then ask him, "What is your favorite game or sport?" He answers. Then I say to him, "Now, all I want you to do is to close your eyes and visualize yourself actively engaged in this sport."

We will say for example, that the sport is swimming. Then I say to him, "Can you see yourself swimming?" When he says, "Yes" I tell him that so long as he continues to see himself swimming nothing that is done will bother him." At this point, I call upon another doctor in the audience—preferably a dentist—to take a sharp sterile dental probe and make a severe test on the doctor who thinks that hypnosis is of no value in medicine or dentistry. The man in the chair learns to his amazement that he has complete anesthesia. Most of those who undergo this test will stand up in astonishment and say, "No real test was made on me. I didn't feel anything." Every doctor in the room knows that he has undergone a severe test. Both participating doctors are members of the community, and this demonstration cannot be "rigged" in any way.

Why does it work? Because when the man visualizes himself swimming, he is not really swimming, he is merely bypassing his critical faculty; and when I add the words, "So long as you keep on swimming, you won't feel anything," I establish selective thinking. The two steps were made so adroitly that he didn't realize he was subjected to selective thinking.

The realization that both steps can be made instantly and effectively is perhaps the key to why my students have shown consistently rapid advancement and have been so outstandingly successful in the use of hypnosis. It has always

been my contention that if hypnosis is going to be of value
in the several branches of medicine, it must be available to
the doctor on an instantaneous basis. Fixation, monotony,
rhythm, imitation and levitation have been proved unreliable
since the year 1840. No ruling by any group of medical men
is going to make them suddenly become reliable. The doctor
wants hypnosis here and now, and if it isn't available here
and now, he quickly discards any attempt to use it. That is
why I stress the importance of rapid induction. When doctors
discard the unreliable techniques and learn hypnosis on a
scientific level, it will achieve its proper medical status. It
will be taught as a required course in medical schools
throughout the world. And it will be taught as carefully and
thoroughly as any other item in the curriculum.

Many doctors wonder why I am so vehemently opposed
to "three-day courses" in hypnosis. I have studied the subject for many years, and even today, I can learn new things
about it. There is much more research to be done, and it is
my earnest hope that what I have to say will stimulate further research. If a man who has studied hypnosis more than
half a century is not in a position to say that he knows it
all, how can a man who has studied it only three days expect
to know enough about the subject to use it as a medical tool,
to be employed in the treatment of his patients?

Having now mentioned both some facts and fallacies regarding the handshake, eye-closure, fixation—and the study
of hypnosis in general, I want to explain a basic technique for
improvement in fast induction. This technique is simply the
properly applied handshake, coupled with recognition of the
five signs of hypnosis. At the same time, we will give some
thought to the importance (and ease) of autosuggestion.

There are several good reasons why the handshake technique is particularly valuable to the doctor beginning the
study of scientific hypnosis. The first reason is that it enables the operator to observe at close range the person on
whom he is working. Observation is a most important phase
in the study. Another reason is that the handshake is a
gesture of friendship. It creates an immediate rapport which
is essential. You already know that bringing the left hand
down over the profile of the patient's face is a technique for
tiring the eyes quickly, and therefore you are still using the
fixation technique.

The right hand contains the first sign of hypnosis. Hypnosis give off five signs, and in that handclasp you find the very first one, body warmth. The advanced student, and usually even the inexperienced operator can immediately tell from the handclasp whether or not the patient is receptive to suggestion. A cold hand says that the person is cold to the subject; a hot, wet hand says that the patient is liable to resist. A warm hand tells you that you should be successful immediately.

An orthopedic surgeon by the name of Eugene H. Reading told me several years ago that he was able to discover something even more valuable in the use of the handshake technique. He claims that his study of hypnosis has enabled him to learn that the radial pulse often becomes imperceptible as the patient goes into hypnosis. It is very easy to test the radial pulse when using the handshake technique. This finding by Doctor Reading is very important, and I don't believe you will find it mentioned in any textbook. Despite my intense study of hypnosis and the reading of innumerable books, I can find no trace of anyone having mentioned it before. You are at liberty to test for this sign and learn for yourself whether or not Doctor Reading's conclusions constitute valuable progress in the research still necessary in the subject of hypnosis.

Let us now discuss the other signs of hypnosis which can be observed when you use the handshake technique. In addition to the body warmth, you should see the fluttering of the eyelids, increased lacrimation, the whites of the eyes getting red, and in many people, the eyeballs going up into the head. The astute student who fails to see at least some of these signs will not venture further with the patient at that sitting.

There is another group of signs frequently mentioned in the textbooks erroneously. They only occur when fear is engendered in the patient by the realization that hypnosis is being used, and then only if the patient is afraid of hypnosis. Notice how these signs comprise a fear syndrome. They are: faster pulse, faster heartbeat and increased respiration. These signs can be observed in a person who is afraid of anything, and therefore they are *not* hypnotic signs.

True hypnotic signs cannot be aped, imitated or pretended. For example, you cannot imitate or pretend body warmth; it has to be there. You cannot imitate fluttering eyelids. Try it for yourself and notice how after a second or two the eyelids no longer flutter. In hypnosis, the fluttering eyelids occur almost constantly as the induction proceeds. There are very few people who can, at will, cause their eyes to tear, nor can you at will cause the whites of your eyes to redden. Try to make your eyeballs turn up into your head. You will find it difficult to do—but in hypnosis those eyes in many cases turn upward into the head.

Before we discuss other techniques, I think it is important for the person who wants to study hypnosis properly to know the subject of autosuggestion. Most authorities agree that all hypnosis is autohypnosis and autohypnosis is autosuggestion, so that when I teach you autosuggestion, I am in reality teaching you how to hypnotize yourself. If you can get these effects on other people, certainly you ought to be able to get them on yourself. For example, if I must have painful dental work or medical work done, I don't let the doctor use anesthesia. I tell him, "Doctor, I can anesthetize myself. In fact, I can get better anesthesia than you can give me." And immediately I will proceed to give myself a suggestion and I will have complete anesthesia. I have had six gingival cavities prepared and filled under autosuggestion. Dentists will agree that deep gingival cavities are usually pretty troublesome, and I didn't even feel the work being done. I have had a growth removed from my face that the doctor thought might be malignant, and he wanted to have a biopsy taken. He told me, "I'll have to go very, very deep on this, so you'd better have anesthesia for it." I said, "No doctor, I can give myself better anesthesia than you could possibly give me." After it was all over, the doctor said, "I don't know how it is possible for you not to have felt more than you felt. Don't you have feelings?" I have also had a rectal abscess opened, and those of you who are in medicine know that the rectal area is one of the most difficult areas of the human body to anesthetize. The proctologist said to me afterwards, "Mr. Elman, how did you do that? I've never seen such good anesthesia in my life." And all I did was to give myself a suggestion. When I say that I want you to be able to do the same thing, I'm not indulging in wishful thinking or exaggeration. There are people all over the world who can use autosuggestion as well as I can, and many are even better at it.

Anything that's valuable is certainly worth practicing, and the only way you're going to be able to learn autohypnosis on a permanent basis is to practice it. Anesthesia isn't the only thing you can use autosuggestion for. Many of you in medicine and dentistry work awfully hard. To face those last few patients at the end of the day, when you wish you didn't have to see any more people, when you'd like to have the pep you had in the morning—give yourself a suggestion, and you're as peppy as you were in the morning; the last few people are as easy to treat as the first. But after the last patient leaves the office or after you leave the hospital and your work is done and nature says that you don't need the suggestion any more—the critical faculty takes over, and you do feel the difference. Then you realize how valuable the autosuggestion has been.

Another way that you can use it is for getting rid of headaches or other aches and pains. Women who are troubled with dysmenorrhea, get rid of the dysmenorrhea. Suggestion will do it. You'll be able to alleviate aches and pains —even organic aches and pains. You'll never *mask* a symptom, but you'll be able to *alleviate* it. You can get rid of a toothache. You'll know the toothache is there, but it won't hurt so much. You'll still know you should go to the dentist, but the pain will be lessened. To know that anesthesia is available at your command gives you a wonderful feeling of achievement.

To obtain the state of mind in which autosuggestion is possible, you must do to yourself exactly what you would do to the patient. You must first bypass your own critical faculty and you must then establish selective thinking. This, of course, is a rather simple way to explain autohypnosis, but it will stand up to any scientific investigation.

How are you to bypass your own critical faculty? The way I do it is to close my eyes and pretend I can't open them. I then test to make certain that I have complete eye-closure. Until I have obtained eye-closure, however, I won't go any further. Once the eye-closure is firmly established, I then give myself the suggestion which comprises selective thinking. This might be a suggestion for anesthesia, to relieve a feeling of weariness, to be able to concentrate on my work, to relieve aches and pains of any type or sort, etc.

I usually help myself establish autosuggestion by a cue word. I choose the word "green" because green, in my mind, is God's color. It connotes the pleasantest visions in the minds of the most people.

Here are your instructions: Say the word green and close your eyes. Test for eye-closure. When you are sure you have eye-closure, use the symbol word "green" again, knowing that the instant you say it your suggestion will take full and complete effect. Then test to make sure that the suggestion has taken full effect. To release the eye muscles, say the word "green" once again, and your eyes will open.

It takes about four seconds to anesthetize yourself. But you must practice. Autosuggestion is a priceless possession. In one of my early classes a doctor told me this story. He said, "I am a polio victim. I contracted the disease when I was about fourteen years of age. I'm in dentistry, and I have to stand on my legs all day. Every once in a while my knee has a habit of going out of position. It isn't very strong. About twice a year, it just goes out of position, and when it does, I have to cancel all appointments for two or three days while I'm waiting for my leg to be able to support my body once again. The other night I was sound asleep and I woke up with a start. Apparently I had moved in some way and I had thrown the leg out of position and the pain was absolutely unbearable. I said to myself, 'If what Dave Elman has taught me about autosuggestion is right, I ought to be able to control that knee with autosuggestion. Green, green, green' . . . and I give you my word, that knee went right back into position. I don't know what caused it, but I woke up my wife because I was so excited by the realization that I was able to use autosuggestion that way. And Mr. Elman, I didn't have to cancel my appointments the next day and everything has been going beautifully. Autosuggestion is wonderful."

I would like to tell you about the most startling demonstration of autosuggestion that I ever saw. I had been teaching in Washington, D. C., and one night a doctor brought his three-year-old daughter to class. It seems the little girl had been troubled with a rash that appeared every time she was emotionally disturbed.

The father very proudly told me that he had taught his little girl autosuggestion in order to control the itching which occurred whenever the rash was present. He said to me, "Would you like to see my daughter demonstrate her knowledge of autosuggestion?" I didn't believe it was possible for a youngster of that age to have enough intelligence to use autosuggestion properly. Perhaps my disbelief showed in my voice, for he said to the child, "Show Mr. Elman how you play that game when you get a rash and want to stop the itching." The little child said, "First I have to have the itch and feel as if I want to scratch." Her father said, "All right, make believe you have the itch and want to scratch. Then what do you do?" She said, "Well, now I make believe I have the itch and I want to scratch, so I close my eyes like this." She closed her eyes and continued, "But I must make sure that I can't open them, so I play the game of make-believe and now while I'm making believe that I can't open them, I try to open them, like this." And she made a visible effort to open her eyes, without success. She went on, "Now I know I can't open my eyes, so I say to myself, "I won't itch any more and so I won't want to scratch. Then I wait a little bit and I open my eyes when I stop playing the game, like this"—and she opened her eyes—"and now I don't itch and I don't want to scratch."

When the class had assembled, I told the doctors about this amazing little child. One of them said, "Mr. Elman, I find that hard to believe. I have been practicing autosuggestion all week without success, and I certainly want to master it." I asked the father of the child if he would let his daughter demonstrate before the group of doctors and he agreed. Then he said to his daughter, "Honey, all these people here are doctors just like Daddy, and they want to learn to play the game you play when you have the rash. Would you be a good girl and stand up here in front of the room and show them how you do it, and as you do it, tell them how." She said, "All right, Daddy," and repeated her perfect demonstration. I asked her father if she always remembered to do this when the rash appeared, and he told me that occasionally when the rash appeared she would forget and start scratching, whereupon he or her mother would remind her to play the game. Then she would immediately go through the autosuggestion routine, and there would be no more scratching and the rash would disappear.

I decided to see if I could learn the cause of the rash, and so I did hypoanalysis on this little girl. She accepted hypnosis readily. The story she revealed showed how much a little child loved her father. She described how a couple of years before when her father was going away somewhere, her mother was crying. (I learned from the father that at the time he was an army doctor and was leaving home to report for duty.) All she could understand was that Daddy was going away and Mother was unhappy about it—more unhappy than the child had ever known her mother to be. It affected her so that she found herself crying, and eventually cried herself to sleep. When she awoke, the rash was there and she itched all over. The itch was so severe that she had to scratch and the mechanical irritation made the situation worse. The child went on to say that her mother put something on the affected area, and there were times when the itching was not so bad, but there were other times when it seemed to get worse. Further questioning brought out the fact that when Daddy came home on leave the itching was not apparent but after he left it came back. This happened several times.

I felt I had found the cause, and now I tried to explain to the child what had brought about the itching. I explained to her that each time Daddy went away, it made her sad and upset her, and when she was upset the rash appeared. She refused to accept this explanation. She said, "My Daddy never made me sad. He loves me and he wouldn't do that to me."

No matter how I tried to explain she always got back to the fact that she didn't believe Daddy could possibly be the cause of any rash or anything else that would cause her discomfort. The love of that child for her father was beautiful to see but I was saddened by the fact that I was unable to give the child an insight that would end her discomfort permanently.

Let me repeat again that this demonstration of autosuggestion by a three-year-old child was the best demonstration of autosuggestion I have ever seen; if a three-year-old child can learn autosuggestion, it is not beyond the capabilities of any adult.

Chapter 6

PRELIMINARY INSTRUCTIONS

IF YOU tried the experiment involving the eye-closure pretense on yourself, you must have noticed a conflict in your mind. One part of your brain seemed to be saying, "You can't open your eyes." Another seemed to be saying, "Nonsense."

Doubt—skepticism—is a natural human reaction, and often a valuable one. The same can be said of fear. However, doubt and fear can defeat you if you don't know how to avoid or overcome these reactions.

Much depends on your approach to the patient. First, in introducing your patient to hypnosis, don't use the *word* hypnosis. Give the patient the benefit of the state without ever using the word. Why should you generate the fear associated with the word in the minds of the uninformed? Those who object that this isn't cricket ought to ask themselves whether they tell their patients what's in every prescription.

Now let me show you a good approach to, say, a dental patient. The dentist might say this: "You know every time you come to the office, I notice how tense you get, and when you sit tensely you have to feel discomfort more because that's the nature of tension. If I could teach you how to relax, your visits to this office could be made very easy and I'm sure you know that. How would you like to *enjoy* a dental visit for a change instead of being all tense about it? All right, I'm going to show you how to relax. Take a long, deep breath. That's it. Now let me have your hand. Now watch this left hand come down over the profile of your face. Now close your eyes. Relax those eye muscles to the point where they won't work, and when you're sure they won't work, test them to make sure they won't work. That's right. Stay like that and let that feeling of relaxation that you have in your eye muscles go right down to the toes. I'm going to lift your hand and drop it and if it's really as relaxed as

it should be, it'll just plump down like a wet dishrag. Look
at that relaxation. Now, I'm going ahead with our dental
treatment, and nothing I do in this office will bother or disturb you from this moment on. You'll know I'm working
there, but if you'll just hold on to this relaxation, you won't
feel a thing. You won't mind a thing that I do. You'll
know that I'm working there but that's about all."

And with that, the dentist can go ahead with his work.

It's taken him about thirty seconds to perform the entire
induction. Try it for yourself. You will get such fast results
that you will be able to do about two or three times as much
work as you ordinarily would be able to do, because the
patient isn't raring back and fighting you. Suppose you have
some difficult work to do. You can give him chemical anesthesia now if you haven't enough faith in yourself to be able
to do this without it. But give him some novocain or zyl-
caine or whatever you use after relaxing him and you'll find
that he doesn't object to it at all; you'll find that you have
a much more tractible patient. The wonderful thing for the
dentist to know is that even if the patient opens his eyes
(and he has to open them to use the cuspidor) you can say,
"Now, I want you to open your eyes—rinse your mouth—
get rid of that debris, and then when you lean back you'll
relax more than ever." Instead of *losing* the state when this
happens, you actually can intensify it.

The following is an excerpt from a tape-recording of a
first class session. Immediately preceding the opening words,
I had bypassed the critical faculty of a doctor-student and
had established selective thinking—i.e., I had hypnotized
him. And I had led him to expect that I would test the
hypnotic anesthesia I had produced by having a dentist probe
his mouth. Here is the conversation:

DOCTOR: Did you do anything to my mouth?

ELMAN: No, I didn't, but I'll show you something.
          Close your eyes again. Close them just like
          you had them. Relax just like you were. Let's
          have some dentist—well, here, [speaking to a
          dentist] you didn't make that test yet, come on
          . . . [again addressing doctor] Close your eyes,
          please . . . [to dentist] You go ahead and make
          a test, and you'll find now that he won't feel

anything.   He'll know that you're working
there, but that's all . . . What did you feel?

DOCTOR: Oh, just something—nothing bad.

ELMAN: Now, gentlemen, did you see what he did?   He
let it [a sharp dental probe] hang there.   He
let it hang from your gingival area.   Isn't that
correct?   Isn't that where you had it?

DENTIST: Sure.

ELMAN: And the gingival area is a pretty sensitive area
of the mouth, doctor, and you would have just
hit the ceiling under ordinary circumstances.
I want to show you that you're like anybody
else.   Everybody is amenable to suggestion if
you'll realize it when you work with them
. . . You're in dermatology.   Doctor, just start
[working] as though there was a patient in
your office coming in for some painful derma-
tological treatment and you want to make this
treatment easy for him.

DOCTOR: Let's say I'm going to take a mole off his lower lip.

ELMAN: All right.

DOCTOR: You want me to go ahead?

ELMAN: Yes, yes.   Use the same approach that I did,
and don't worry if I stop you, because you're
the first man up and the first man up always
gets the brunt of the criticism, you know that.
But you seemed to do all right yourself, so now
you know what has to be done to the next man.

DOCTOR: Do you want me to take this off your lip?   Have
you ever had one of these removed before?

2nd DOCTOR: [acting as patient]:   No.

DOCTOR: Well, do you think they hurt?

2nd DOCTOR: Yes.

DOCTOR: Well, I think if you'll relax we can do this
without hurting you.

ELMAN: Now doctor, may I just make a little suggestion here. Never use the word hurt while you're using hypnosis. Hurt—pain—knife—needle —sharp—incision—stitches—any word that implants a picture of pain—leave that out. In other words, "I think we can do this without you feeling it at all." Something like that— "without it bothering you a bit"—but don't implant a picture of pain because you make them very suggestible as you work with hypnosis, and your word has painted a picture. So watch your wording at the very start.

DOCTOR: If you relax, we can do this in a very pleasant manner. That's better. Now, try to just let yourself go. As I bring my hand down over your eyes, let your eyes close—right on down —now close them. That's fine. Keep them closed. Make sure that they're closed and see that you can't open them. That's right. Be sure they won't open. Now then, let that feeling pass all over your body. Just let it go down to the tips of your toes. Now doesn't that feel good?

ELMAN: No, no, you don't make a test yet, doctor. Give a suggestion before you do: "Just stay completely relaxed—we're going to make a little test here and you won't feel it or you won't notice it"—and he won't because right now you know where his threshold is. Look, that threshold has practically vanished so you know he's not going to feel it as he normally would. Now what sort of test do you want to make?

DOCTOR: I want to use a pair of pliers or a pair of forceps.

ELMAN: Now, you see that would paint a picture— you see what I mean? And even in clowning when you're doing this you *don't* clown because you see what you do if you paint a picture in his mind that he's going to feel this.

Then your test will not be valid. So, when you ask for an instrument, just say, "Give me that gadget," or something, you know what I mean. Now, stroke the area that you're going to make the test on and you'll find that he won't even feel it.

DOCTOR: I'm just going to make a little test here. Stay relaxed.

ELMAN: Now, I want you to see this and I want you to notice how little he notices this. See. Now, you know that ordinarily, doctor, that would make a person react, but how much did he feel it?

DOCTOR: Very little. There's still an indentation.

ELMAN: Yes, well, you gave him pretty good pressure. [to doctor serving as patient] You know, he used an allis clamp on you and he had it right down there to the third notch. Now, [to doctor who applied clamp] let me tell you, doctor, the friendliness was good. I wouldn't ask questions—I would make it a statement—"notice how good that feels." But I wouldn't say, "Doesn't that feel good?" because some patients will feel required to answer you, and snap out of the state. So let them stay relaxed. Luckily, he worked with you and he didn't feel like he should come out of the state, so he stayed in it. That was excellent for a first time through. The reason you have to bring them out with health suggestions is that this is an autosuggestible state. And should he suggest to himself that having the state made him concentrate like the devil and so he's got an earache, a toe ache or a bellyache or something as a result, an autosuggestion has been implanted. You eliminate all chance of a negative autosuggestion by saying, "When you open your eyes you're going to feel wonderful."

Chapter 7

TWO-FINGER EYE-CLOSURE METHOD

SEMANTICS OF HYPNOSIS

THE two-finger eye-closure method is the fastest technique ever devised for obtaining hypnosis. It is a development of the Doctor H. Bernheim and Doctor Liebault technique used seventy years ago. They used it in its ten-minute format, but the method is equally effective when made to work instantaneously. Because results are obtained so quickly, it might be thought that the technique produces only light hypnosis. On the contrary, there are reports by hundreds of doctors in medicine, psychiatry and dentistry who have done extended work using this technique. A better method has been devised for working with adults, as you will see, but there is no better technique for children.

I am going to show you the technique as applied to youngsters first. In this excerpt from a class recording, a woman is serving as a "child patient" for the purpose of demonstration. A dentist is practicing the induction:

DENTIST: Jean, I guess you play a lot with your dolls when you're home. And you probably pretend a lot with them, isn't that right? Well, we have a little game of pretend too. And if you can learn to play this little game of pretend, nothing that happens in the dentist's office will bother or disturb. You just won't feel anything that we're doing if you learn to play this little game. Would you like to learn it?

PATIENT: Yes.

DENTIST: All right, open your eyes wide. I'm going to show you this little game. I'm going to pull your eyes shut with my forefinger and my thumb, like this. [Gently places thumb and finger on eyelids and draws them down.] Now you pretend with your whole heart and soul

41

that you can't open your eyes. That's all you have to do. Just pretend that. Now, I will take my hand away [removes hand] and you pretend so hard that when you try to open your eyes they just won't work. Now try to make them work while you're pretending. Try hard. They just won't work, see. Now just because you're pretending like that, anything we do in this office won't bother or disturb you at all. In your mind you can be home playing with your dolls and you won't feel anything I have to do.

ELMAN: And now, doctor [addressing second dentist], you're in dentistry. Will you come up here please and make a test inside her mouth, and you'll find that it doesn't bother her at all. I want you to see the absolute anesthesia that you get with this technique . . . Don't be afraid to make a good substantial test. She won't feel it . . . Did you make a good test, doctor?

DOCTOR: Yes.

ELMAN: She has better anesthesia than any anesthesia that's ever given in a dental office because she has such a perfect state of hypnosis . . . Now [addressing patient] when I have you open your eyes, your mouth is going to feel better than it's felt all day and all week and you're going to feel so good. Open your eyes and see how good you feel. How do you feel?

PATIENT: Fine.

ELMAN: What did you feel while the doctor was working in your mouth?

PATIENT: Nothing. Let me ask you something. Why do I remember what you said?

ELMAN: Because you aren't unconscious in hypnosis. It's not sleep, you know. I must have contact with you, otherwise you couldn't follow instructions.

*   *   *

In the above instance, hypnosis was obtained immediately. The patient was a grown woman, acting the part of a child in a dentist's office. She had a vivid enough imagination so that she was able to see herself as a child—and could be approached at a child's level for the purpose of demonstration. The "let's-pretend" or "let's-play-a-game" approach works very well with young children. With older ones, or with adults, it is generally wise to use a more sophisticated type of indirection to bypass the critical faculty. It can be seen in another class excerpt:

ELMAN: [Addressing patient]: Every time you come to this office, I notice how tense you get, and if I could teach you how to relax, you wouldn't mind anything we have to do. Suppose I teach you how to relax. Would you like that?

PATIENT: Yes.

ELMAN: Take a good long deep breath. Now open your eyes wide. I'm going to pull your eyelids shut with my forefinger and my thumb. Now I want you to relax the muscles that are underneath my fingers. Now I will take my hand away. Relax your eye muscles to the point where they just won't work. Then, when you're sure those eye muscles won't work, test them and make sure they won't work. Test them hard. That's right. Now let that feeling of relaxation go right down to your toes, and when I lift your hand and drop it, that hand will be so relaxed it will just plop down into your lap. And just let it plop. That's it . . . Now [addressing class], in order not to have her feel discomfort, it is necessary that you do give the proper suggestions. This is where you put in your selective thinking . . . [to patient again] Any work that I do from this point on in your mouth or any other part of your body, you just won't mind. Just stay relaxed like that. Make sure at all times that your eye muscles won't work and you have relaxation all through your body and you won't feel a thing . . . [to class] Now, gentlemen,

I'm going to show you the degree of anesthesia
that she has already as a result of that suggestion . . . [to patient] I'm going to stroke
your arm in the area where I'm going to work
and you just won't feel anything. You'll know
I'm working there, but nothing will bother,
nothing will disturb. I'm ready to do my
work now and you have complete anesthesia
in your right arm . . . [to class] Watch me
make this test . . . That was an allis clamp to
the third notch . . . [to patient] Now, when
I have you open your eyes notice how good
you feel. Open your eyes. How do you feel?

PATIENT: Fine.

ELMAN: What did you feel?

PATIENT: Well, I felt you do something. But I didn't
feel any pain.

*   *   *

This approach was used in East Chicago at St. Cathar-
ine's Hospital to set a compound fracture on a twelve-year-old
boy. The doctor had intended to reduce this fracture with
the aid of chemical anesthesia. The only anesthetist on duty,
however, was working on another emergency case upstairs.
Finally, the doctor couldn't stand the suffering of this boy
any more, and he used the method described above to produce anesthesia. He then proceeded to reduce the compound
fracture. In the midst of the work, the anesthetist came
downstairs, prepared to give chemical anesthesia. He was
amazed to find his services were unnecessary, and soon afterward became my student. This approach is recommended
for the emergency victim because it is so fast; you generally
get hypnosis within five seconds.

It should be noted that you suggest muscle relaxation
only with an adult, not with a child. The child bypasses his
critical faculty so quickly that usually when you use this
technique with a child, you need only to say, "Pretend you
can't open your eyes," and he pretends and relaxes automatically. It's just as though he went into a sound sleep. But
he doesn't really sleep. This technique is often used for
induction for surgical purposes.

It is, of course, important to obtain deep hypnosis. You can deepen the child's state by having him pretend to smell beautiful roses or you can say, "What's your favorite game when you're home?" or "What do you like to watch on television?" You can actually have the child watch a television show or play a game mentally while you're doing painful dental or medical work on him. Suppose you suggest to the child that he go on a trip to the moon in a space ship. When you're through working with him and you want to bring the child back to earth, say, "All right, you can come back from that space trip now. Come back to earth now. And when you do I want you to open your eyes and notice how good you feel. Open your eyes. How do you feel?" (Be sure to notice the redness of the eyes, the increased lacrimation and the eyelids fluttering.)

Sometimes the patient must open his eyes during an examination, perhaps to roll up his sleeve for an injection of some sort. While his eyes are still shut and he's pretending he can't open them, you say something on this order: "Anything that we do in this office from now on will not bother or disturb you at all. In a couple of seconds I'm going to have you open your eyes and get your arm ready so that I can work with it, and then we'll play this game again and you'll see that you won't feel anything that I have to do. Now, you open your eyes and get your arm ready."

To demonstrate the usefulness of this technique let me reproduce an excerpt from a letter which I have recently received from an anesthesiologist in Florida. The patient's name has been fictionalized in order to preserve ethical privacy; "Re: Patient Tommy Haines, age six. The patient was admitted to the hospital during the evening of July 27th with a broken left humerus. I sat beside the child in the operating room, never having seen him before. He was a very frightened little boy. However, he was not hysterical nor was he frantic. I talked with him and began playing pretend games. The child responded readily to the games and was shortly watching his favorite program on television. I told him that while he was watching television his mother would bring him a bowl of pretty flowers and he would be able to smell them. At this time I began blowing cyclopropane gas in his face. Frankly, this stuff stinks, though the child nodded in agreement that it smelled good. During this induction period rapid recovery suggestions were given. The child was shortly asleep and a two hour operation was completed. Everything went fine and the surgery was completed very late in the evening. I saw the child the next afternoon and he was getting along so well, and was so completely happy, that his doctor decided to let him go home. This was one to two days earlier than usual. Tommy told his parents how much he enjoyed playing games with me and made the statement, 'I played a game with Doctor Nickell and I won because I fell asleep before he did.' "

Some doctors have the impression that following the very rapid technique of two-finger eye-closure described above, the hypnosis is light. In most instances it is actually deep. To demonstrate this, I frequently hypnotize a doctor by the two-finger method, and show the class proof as follows:

ELMAN: [to hypnotized doctor]: When I lift your hand and drop it, I want the telephone number of your office to disappear from your mind, and you'll find that it will drop out as I drop the hand. Now when you try to think of your telephone number, it just goes further and further away and you just can't find it at all. Now when you try to find it, it just isn't there. Try to find it and you'll see that's just exactly what happens. You can't find it at all. Gone completely. Let it be gone completely. Gone, isn't it?

DOCTOR: Yes.

ELMAN: Now there you have somnambulism Suggested amnesia is the test for it. So you see it isn't as light hypnosis as you thought. It's much deeper . . . [to patient] I'll lift your hand again and drop it and your telephone number will come right back and then you'll open your eyes and you'll feel wonderful. How do you feel?

DOCTOR: Fine.

ELMAN: Isn't that a nice feeling? Where'd the number go?

DOCTOR: I don't know. It just disappeared temporarily, that's all.

*   *   *

If you give your suggestions properly, you get anesthesia in somnambulism. Too many doctors are anxious to get to work before they have implanted the selective thinking. That is the reason for their many failures. They don't realize that without the implanting of selective thinking they don't have anything but deep relaxation to work with: they don't have hypnosis. Make it a rule to implant selective thinking, and at the termination of the hypnosis to leave the suggestion of a feeling of well-being.

The above description of suggested amnesia brings us to the matter of certain tests for hypnosis. Even though doctors see the five signs of hypnosis, discussed previously, they are still not always satisfied that they have a hypnotized patient. New students will sometimes ask me to prove a state of hypnosis by making the subject's arm rigid, just as they've seen it done on the stage. Regardless of the misinformation given in three-day hypnosis courses, stage hypnotists use the rigid arm technique as a deepening device, not as a test. Let me show you the way it is used in medicine today:

ELMAN: [to hypnotized patient] Close your eyes; just pretend you can't open them. I'm going to take your arm and I want you to extend it and make it rigid as I count to three. Make that so rigid you can't bend it. One—make it rigid —two, like steel—three, now you can't bend it no matter how hard you try. When you try, it just won't work at all. Test it. You'll find you can't bend it at all. Now you've got the rigid arm.

At this point, doctors tend to assume the patient is ready for therapy. He's not ready for therapy; he's merely got a rigid arm. It doesn't mean he'll take another suggestion. You want to get depth. That's what the stage operator used the rigid arm for. So the complete technique was used like this, and it looked dramatic on the stage:

ELMAN: [to patient]: Now when I have you relax the arm, you'll go much deeper . . . Now you can

PATIENT: relax. Relax and you'll go much deeper. Can
              you feel that depth? Can you feel yourself
              going deeper? You can answer. Can you
              feel it?

PATIENT: Yes.

                        *   *   *

That's the way the stage operator used it to get depth.
It is not a good technique to use in a doctor's office. It is not
a good test. It does not take a medical education to know
the semantics of good patient relationship and having stiff
arms in the office is certainly no way to handle a patient.
If you want to get depth and to find out if the patient is
hypnotized at the same time, do it the scientific way. You
already know that the patient's eyelids should flutter, that
the whites of the eyes should get red and that there should
be increased lacrimation. Demonstrating on a patient again,
I now say this:

ELMAN: [to patient]: Now, when I tell you to, I want
              you to open your eyes and let me look at them
              for a couple of seconds. When I tell you to,
              open your eyes, keep them open till I tell you
              to close them and then you'll go much deeper,
              and let yourself go much deeper. Now open
              your eyes.

When you follow this procedure, you will see the signs
—the increased lacrimation, the whites of the eyes getting
pink. And you say to the patient: "Now close your eyes
again and notice how much deeper you go, and let yourself
go deeper. Can you feel that? Now, open and close your
eyes again and you'll go about ten times deeper. That's right,
let yourself go. Feel that?"

When you do this, it will be obvious that the patient is
immediately becoming more deeply hypnotized. It is a device to get greater depth, and you can use it again and again
and again, getting greater depth as you do.

A physician often has to have the patient go from room
to room for various examinations—might want to have him
take x-rays in one room, putting him into some outlandish
position for the x-rays, and then might want to go into some
other room for something else. The doctor wants him relaxed

in the second room and the third room and so on. It is
therefore invaluable to know that the patient can open his
eyes and, instead of losing hypnosis, will become more deeply
hypnotized.

Remember at all times that you are working with a person who hears and understands everything you are saying.
You are talking to a person who is perfectly conscious when
he's in deep hypnosis. Therefore, don't make the mistake
of the old-time practitioners and talk down to your patient.
Talk across to him. He isn't beneath your dignity. He's
a human being with whom you are in rapport. Therefore,
do not violate his sense of dignity by being condescending
or patronizing. Talk to him just as if he were not in the
suggestible state; it will increase the rapport and he will be
far more willing to take your suggestions. I have had doctors in my classes say, *"You can't open your eyes. You can't.
You can't."* The usual reaction of the patient is to prove how
fast he can open his eyes. You don't talk to a patient like
that, any more than you use such words as hurt and pain.
Stay away from all words or phrases that paint an unpleasant picture: cut, needle, knife, incision, stitches, rip out the
stitches, sharp, etc. Usually, the patient knows when he's
going to get an injection, stitches or an incision. Why remind him of the unpleasantness he must go through? It is
a good idea to keep the patient apprised of what you are
about, but you can do this with words such as procedure,
treatment, etc. Also bear in mind that iatrogenic illnesses
are caused by surgeons, anesthetists, assistants and nurses
using the wrong words in the operating room. Remember
that the patient never loses his sense of hearing. Therefore,
never say anything disturbing in the operating room.

Here is another example of the importance of words:
Which would you rather have—medicine or medication?
Medication, I'm sure. Then why ever write out a prescription for medicine? You'll be surprised how much more effective your prescriptions will be when you say to the patient,
"I'm going to write out a prescription for some medication.
I want you to take it and have it filled and you're going to
feel so much better as a result of it." That word medication,
changed from the simple word medicine, will do your patient
a vast amount of good. If you doubt it, try it.

At all times be reasonable in your suggestions, as you

are in your words. Don't say anything that sounds prepos-
terous to the patient. Don't be extravagant in your claims
of what you are going to do. We're stating here elementary
principles in the giving of suggestion. Throughout my
teaching, in this text as well as in the classroom, reference
is made to the proper method of giving more complicated
suggestions. And as you learn more about semantics, you
will learn how often and how much you can help your patients with your words.

Chapter 8

HYPNOSIS AS AN ADJUNCT TO CHEMICAL ANESTHESIA

THE most learned man in the history of medical hypnosis was Doctor Henry Munro, who lived and practiced in Omaha, Nebraska, at the turn of the century. In 1900 there was practically no preoperative medication. There was very little to alleviate surgical shock. Even today the average person faces surgery with apprehension, but in 1900, the situation was much worse. One in four hundred people died on the operating room table as a result of the *anesthesia*— not the surgery.

The fears of patients were much greater than they are today. One man knew something about those fears and tried to alleviate them. Doctor Murno had a good method for alleviating fears. He would get his patients into the hypnotic state, discuss their fears with them, and tell them that when they went into the operating room knowing they were going to recover, they would have a quick recovery and would feel a lot better. He was the first to give preoperative talks in hypnosis.

One man came in for surgery who was filled with apprehension. The surgery had to be done, so Doctor Munro hypnotized him, removed his fears and said, "Well, you'll never be in better condition for the surgery than right now, so let's go ahead." Ether was the anesthesia agent then most commonly used. With about ten percent of the usual amount of ether, Doctor Munro was amazed to find that he had perfect surgical anesthesia, and he went ahead and performed the surgery. He thought this was luck and would probably not happen again. But a month later, a woman came in for surgery. She was very nervous. Doctor Munro hynotized her and, with about twenty-five percent of the usual amount of ether, again he was able to get perfect surgical anesthesia —banishing the excitement stage of ether entirely. One of his observations was that such patients recovered easily and quickly; the postoperative recovery was almost miraculous. He drew the conclusion that he might be able to get the same

51

excellent results with every patient through hypnosis. He had about a hundred surgical cases in succession in which he was able to do surgery with from ten to twenty-five percent of the usual amount of chemical anesthesia. He had made a great discovery, but other doctors ridiculed him.

He arranged a group of lecture dates, one of which took him to Rochester, Minnesota. Before the lecture that night, he had dinner with two of the doctors who were working at St. Mary's Hospital—the Mayo brothers. It was before the days of their clinic.

Doctor Munro was telling the Mayo brothers about his discovery. The Mayo brothers decided his discovery was worth testing. If the patient didn't get the necessary anesthesia, all they had to do would be to use more ether. If it worked they'd have a valuable medical aid.

When they got back to St. Mary's Hospital, the Mayo brothers started Case Number One of Seventeen Thousand deep abdominal surgical procedures, without a single death or injury directly traceable to the anesthetic. The eyes of the world focused on the Mayo brothers, and success was theirs. This was the only place in the world where a patient didn't have to take a chance on dying from anesthesia. Anyone who needed surgery could be confident of living through the operation.

Alice Magaw, the anesthetist of the Mayo brothers, was very proud of her work. She wrote an article for the Obstetrical Journal of May, 1906. That Journal was not widely circulated. Many doctors did not get it in 1906, and the story remained obscure. I know about it because Doctor Munro occasionally visited my father (we lived in Fargo, North Dakota, which is not far from Rochester) and I heard the two men discussing it. But, strangely, the Mayo brothers never said that they used hypnosis.

Here is a technique similar to that which Doctor Munro showed the Mayo brothers; you will see it is very simple to use. You're in the operating room. Say to the patient, "We're going to start the anesthesia in just a minute, and to make this procedure very easy for you, I want you to do just as I tell you. Open your eyes wide. I'm going to pull them shut, like this. Now pretend you can't open your eyes. That's all you have to do. Pretend you can't open your eyes. We're going to start the anesthesia, and in a little while you'll wake up in your room upstairs. The operation will be over and you'll be on the road to recovery. Just keep on pretending you can't open your eyes and we'll go ahead and start the anesthesia." That is all that is necessary. This is a by-pass of the critical faculty and it implants selective thinking. Try it, and you will be amazed at what you are able to do with it.

The fourth edition of Doctor Henry Munro's book "Suggestive Therapeutics" contains a careful documentation of every fact I have told you. I make this documentation available to all my students, but some doctors are still hesitant to use the Mayo technique.

A doctor who was president of the Anesthetists of New Jersey was one of my students. At the third class session, he arrived early and told me this story: "All this week I have used the technique you described and have been working with from twenty-five to thirty-five percent of the usual amount of pentothal that I would normally use in surgery. I will not turn a patient over to a surgeon if that patient does not have complete surgical anesthesia. Henry Munro was absolutely right. You get perfect surgical anesthesia with twenty-five to thirty-five percent of what is usually used. This is just as important today as it was in 1900. Today we have only an occasional death, but we also have an occasional injury of some kind, traceable to anesthesia. If I can stay seventy-five percent away from the saturation point, I never have to worry about an injury from anesthesia. As an anesthetist, I can tell you this is very important."

As more and more doctor-students began using the technique which had been ignored all these years, anesthetists would get up in class and tell of their experience with the Mayo technique. Surgeons and anesthetists tell me they have never varied this technique—that they use it for every surgical procedure.

I could give you case history after case history of surgeons and anesthetists who have used this technique. I have been told by quite a few doctors in OB-Gyn that it works beautifully, when you're first learning hypnosis, and still using chemical anesthesia, to carry a patient through a complete delivery without her feeling a solitary thing.

What about the man in dentistry or the doctor giving local anesthesia? He says to himself, "This applies to gen-

eral anesthesia but doesn't apply to local." Yes, it does.
Take your ampule of xylocaine, and instead of giving the
patient the full ampule, cut it down and give ninety percent.
You'll get just as good a result as you did with one-hundred
percent. With your next patient, cut it down to eighty percent, then seventy, sixty, fifty, forty percent—and you'll find
that because of the selective thinking you've implanted you'll
soon get to the point where you will be working with a drop or
less of xylocaine or novocain or whatever it is you are using,
and get just as good an anesthesia as with an entire ampule.

I feel very proud of the fact that I, as a layman, brought
the attention of physicians to Doctor Munro's great discovery.
Doctors have too long ignored his findings. Here is the documentation that can be found in the fourth edition of Doctor
Henry Munro's wonderful book, "Suggestive Therapeutics."

"Let us now look into the facts bearing evidence of the
value of the employment of suggestion as an adjunct in the
administration of anesthetics and the safety of the method
to the patient.

"Alice Magaw, Dr. W. J. Mayo's anesthetist at Rochester,
Minnesota, who has, with possibly one exception, anesthetized more patients than any other person in the world, has
an unbroken record of approximately seventeen thousand
surgical anesthesias without a single death directly from
the anesthetic.

"No other surgical clinic in the world has been so constantly witnessed by surgeons during the last several years,
and no other clinic presents a greater number of difficult
cases to be operated upon, or those that are more unfit for
favorable results from the administration of anesthetics.

"At St. Mary's Hospital, in the personalities of Alice
Magaw and Miss Henderson, the anesthetists of W. J. and
C. H. Mayo, at Rochester, Minnesota, we see the results from
the outcome of surgical work done with a minimum amount
of the drug employed for anesthesia and the free and intelligent use of suggestion as an adjunct to its administration.

"It was with no small degree of pleasure that, upon a
visit to Rochester during the month of November, 1907, I
found these women actually putting into practice one particular phase of psychotherapy that I had so strongly urged
upon surgeons during the eight years previous.

"Both Alice Magaw and Miss Henderson were highly

appreciative of that particular part of my lecture to the Physicians' Club of Rochester wherein I urged the importance of the employment of suggestion as an adjunct in the administration of anesthetics, and cited their everyday work as an illustration of complete surgical anesthesia with the use of but little ether, and the employment of suggestion to meet the requirements of the individual patient as an adjunct. Moreover, these women were free to say that they knew from everyday experience that what I had to say in reference to the use of suggestion as an adjunct in the administration of anesthetics was true.

"In the Journal of Surgery, Gynecology and Obstetrics of December, 1906, Alice Magaw says: 'Suggestion is a great aid in producing a comfortable narcosis. The anesthetist must be able to inspire confidence in the patient, and a great deal depends on the manner of approach . . . The secondary or subconscious self is particularly susceptible to suggestive influence; therefore, during the administration, the anesthetist should make those suggestions that will be most pleasing to this particular subject. Patients should be prepared for each stage of the anesthesia with an explanation of how the anesthetic is expected to affect him—"talk him to sleep" with the addition of as little ether as possible.'

"By the employment of suggestion scientifically and earnestly, very little ether is required to produce surgical anesthesia, and even less chloroform, to keep the patient surgically anesthetized.

"I do not exaggerate in the least when I assert that it is quite the common occurrence for an anesthetist who does not understand the use of suggestion to use from ten to twenty times the amount of ether in anesthetizing a patient than is used by Alice Magaw and Miss Henderson, who make use of suggestion in every possible way in a given operation.

"Nor is the anesthesia where such enormous quantities of ether are employed one iota more satisfactory from the surgeon's point of view than is secured by the Mayos. On the contrary, there is no period of excitement, no struggling of the patient that demands restraint, comparatively little stertorous breathing, no feeling of the pulse, and no hypodermics administered in the course of the operation, and, more yet, an unbroken record of approximately seventeen thousand cases without a single death from the anesthetic.

"But the significance of the employment of suggestion
as an adjunct to the administration of anesthetics goes far
beyond the danger to the patient directly and immediately
during the course of the operation. The surgeon who does
not have his patient's reserved energies so weakened and
exhausted, and the patient's brain and nerve centers presid-
ing over all physiological processes so seriously and permanently injured, as is the case with the Mayos, on account of
the employment of suggestion to obviate the necessity of such
enormous quantities of the anesthetic, simply has more recu-
perative power left in the cells of the organism upon which
the hope for a favorable outcome from a major operation is
based, and surgical operations upon patients with the minimum amount of poison from the anesthetic to combat are
unquestionably attended with better results than where
larger quantities of the drug are used.

"Inherent within the protoplasmic mechanism of the human organism is an untapped reservoir of available energy,
which is either utilized by the judicious employment of suggestion for the welfare of the patient, or it is exhausted,
perverted, or wasted by the indiscreet use of the anesthetic."

You will find that this technique works with every type
of chemical anesthesia. In a class at Forest Hills, Long
Island, one of the doctors read an open letter to me from
Doctor Fein, head of the Queens County General Hospital.
The letter invited me to speak to a special staff meeting. The
doctor who read the letter explained the reason for the invita-
tion: "I have my Boards in anesthesia, and I specialize in
nitrous oxide particularly. When you told us about this technique, I wondered how well it would work with nitrous
oxide. Let me tell you why that's important. You showed
us a technique whereby we could cut down the amount of
nitrous oxide, and with the first fifty cases I tried it on, I have
never had to go above thirty-five percent nitrous oxide and
sixty-five percent oxygen, and I can start my patient at that
point and decrease from there. When I took the statistics
on the fifty cases to Doctor Fein, he said, 'That's the finest
set of statistics on nitrous oxide that I've ever seen.' I told
him where I'd learned the technique, and he wants you to
talk to the staff."

I talked to the staff, and afterwards gave the same talk
before the Queens County Medical Society.

Chapter 9

COUNTLESS METHODS OF INDUCTION

THE ways of inducing hypnosis are almost countless. And while some methods take longer than others, they can all be used to produce the deep state known as somnambulism.

A student of Mesmer's, one Marquis de Puseygur, discovered the state of somnambulism by accident. Like Mesmer, he used a supposedly magnetic tree. One day, he found that a young boy had tied himself to this tree. As the Marquis watched, the boy slowly closed his eyes and apparently fell asleep.

The Marquis, extremely frightened, ordered the boy to untie his knots, and to his great surprise, the lad, without opening his eyes, did as he was bid. Continuing his experiment, the Marquis ordered the boy to walk forward and the boy walked forward. He ordered the boy to stop and he stopped. After a few more orders of this kind which the boy followed—even the order to open his eyes and wake up —Puseygur proclaimed his discovery to be somnambulism because he saw this boy walking and executing orders while apparently asleep.

That is how the use of the word somnambulism originated in connection with hypnosis. The term has been used ever since to denote a specific hypnotic state. It is interesting to note that the boy went into true somnambulism by himself, without instructions from anyone, proving how easy the hypnotic procedure really is.

The methods of achieving the trance state are limited only by your own imagination. There is no way in which you cannot hypnotize a patient, provided you know the art of suggestion. The old-time practitioners used the fixation method. That is, they had the subject stare at either a light or a brilliant object and sought to tire the muscles around the eyes, thus achieving eye-closure. Since eye-closure is the first goal at which you must aim, all you need is a device that will cause it. *Any* device will cause it, provided you know the art of suggestion and provided the person expects

to be hypnotized. Substitute the word 'relaxed' for 'hypnotized' and every patient who needs the therapeutic values
of hypnosis can be relaxed instantly. This applies even to
patients who have never been previously conditioned. The
devices employed to achieve the trance state are used as
catalysts. Therefore we call this the catalyst method of
achieving trance. Here is an excerpt from a teaching session
which will enable you to understand what I mean:

ELMAN: I want someone who hasn't been here before.
              All right, sit right there. You don't have to
              move from your chair. I'm going to take three
              puffs on this cigarette. With the first puff your
              eyes are going to get tired, the second puff
              you're going to want to close your eyes, but
              wait until the third puff, at which time close
              them. They will lock and you won't be able
              to open them. Want that to happen—expect
              it to happen—and watch it happen . . . Here's
              the first puff—notice how tired your eyes are
              getting and let them get tired. Now they'll
              get so tired you'll want to close them but don't
              let them close yet. Now when I take the third
              puff they'll close and lock—let them. Now
              close them. You'll find they're locked . . . The
              harder you test them the less they'll work.
              Test them and you'll find you can't make them
              work. They just won't work at all. That's
              right. Now when I snap my fingers you'll be
              able to open them very readily. All right,
              you can open them . . . Now there is eye-
              closure achieved by puffing on a cigarette.
              Let's try it another way . . . Some one else who
              hasn't been up here, please . . . All right, want
              this to happen, expect it to happen and watch
              it happen. I'm going to take a drink of water
              —just one swallow—and when I do, your eyes
              will close, they will lock and you won't be able
              to open them. Want this to happen and watch
              it happen. Close your eyes and you'll find now
              they're locked. They won't work at all. Test
              them and you'll find that you can't make them

work. The harder you try, the less they'll work . . . When I snap my fingers they'll open very readily. Now you can open them. Now you find eye-closure achieved by taking a puff on a cigarette, eye-closure achieved by taking a drink from a glass of water. I'm showing you this on unconditioned people. If they want eye-closure they can get it.

Let's have another person who hasn't been here before . . . I'm going to tap my head—that's all I'll do—and when I tap my head your eyes will close and lock and you won't be able to open them. Want it to happen and watch it happen . . . Now close your eyes—you'll find they're locked already and when you test them they won't work at all. Test them and you'll see they won't. There we have perfect eye-closure again . . . All right, you can open your eyes now.

It must be perfectly apparent to you that if I can do that with a cigarette, with a glass of water, with a pat on the head, I can also do it by whistling a tune, singing a song, doing a jig, turning my back, walking out of the room, or any other way. Why? What happened? He wanted eye-closure so he followed instructions. Anyone can do the very same thing.

Someone will always say, "If you can hypnotize by any means within your imagination, hypnotize by doing nothing at all because nothing is something in this instance and becomes a method by which to hypnotize. Can you do it?" Of course you can do it. But you must know the theory behind it. I must get over to the person the fact that I want the eye-closure to occur . . . We'll just prove it with everyone in the room. I won't do anything, and every one of you get eye-closure . . . Just try it . . . Did you notice the number who got eye-closure? I see so many of you testing so I know you got it. The only ones who didn't get it are those who didn't try it.

It isn't necessary to tap your head . . . to mop your brow . . . to light a cigarette. It isn't necessary to do any of these things. You don't have to bring your hand down in front of the person's eyes. You don't have to use the two-finger eye-closure method. You can do nothing but convey the idea of eye-closure and still get as good an eye-closure as you can possibly get. Now we're armed with information which we didn't have before, and armed with this information that you can get eye-closure by merely conveying the idea, we should be able to get a better state of hypnosis than any we have worked with up to this point, and we can. Let me show you how that technique is arrived at.

I used to allow my students one minute to get the light state, two additional minutes to get the deep state. That has ended. Students of mine now must get the deep state of hypnosis within one minute . . . We will practice the three-minute routine tonight, but as you get more adept with hypnosis, I want you to be able to cut it down to one minute from the time that you begin working with your patient . . . You will be working with deep hypnosis—not the relaxation stage, not the pre-hypnotic stage —with deep hypnosis . . . and I want you to work to that end and practice to that end. Only by making hypnosis possible in its deeper stages within a matter of minutes are we going to be successful in making hypnosis an import-ant part of medicine . . . So, while we are going to practice the three-minute routine tonight, I am going to show you as we go along how to get it within one minute, and I want every doctor in class to be able to do it within one minute. Let's have someone come up here who hasn't been here before and I'll go on from there . . .

[to patient]: Will you just take a good long deep breath and close your eyes. Now relax the muscles around your eyes to the point where those eye muscles won't work and when you're sure they won't work, test them and make sure they won't work . . . No, you're making sure they *will* work. Relax them to the point where they will not work and when you're sure they won't work, test them. Test them hard. Get complete relaxation in those muscles around the eyes . . . Now let that feeling of relaxation go right down to your toes . . . In just a moment we're going to do this again and when we do it the second time you're going to be able to relax ten times as much as you're relaxed already. Now open your eyes. Close your eyes. Completely relax—let yourself be covered with a blanket of relaxation. Now the third time we do it you'll be able to double the relaxation which you have. Open your eyes—now relax. I'm going to lift your hand and drop it and if you've followed orders up to this point that hand will be just as limp as a dishrag and will just plop into your lap . . . No, let me lift it—don't you lift it—let it be heavy—that's good—but let's open and close the eyes again and double that relaxation and send it right down to your toes. Let that hand be heavy as lead . . . You'll feel it when you've got the real relaxation . . . Now you've got it. Youl could feel that, couldn't you?

PATIENT:　Yes.

ELMAN:　That's complete physical relaxation, but I want to show you how you can get mental relaxation as well as physical, so I'm going to ask you to start counting—when I tell you to —from a hundred backwards. Each time you say a number, double your relaxation, and by the time you get down to ninety-eight you'll be so relaxed there won't be any more numbers . . . Start with the idea of making that happen and watch it happen. Count out loud, please.

PATIENT:　One hundred.

ELMAN: Double your relaxation and watch the numbers start disappearing.

PATIENT: Ninety-nine.

ELMAN: Watch the numbers start disappearing.

PATIENT: Ninety-eight

ELMAN: Now they'll be gone . . . Make it happen. You've got to do it, I can't do it. Make them disappear, dispel them, make them vanish. Are they all gone?

PATIENT: Yes.

ELMAN: This is the state of somnambulism, attested to by the fact that he was able to dispel those numbers . . . I'm going to let the patient tell you just how he feels . . . Stay as relaxed as you are, and tell the folks exactly what the feeling is from inside the state . . . How do you feel?

PATIENT: Warm.

ELMAN: The first sign of hypnosis—warm . . . What else? Is it a pleasant feeling?

PATIENT: It's not unpleasant—detached.

ELMAN: In other words, in this state the patient feels like all is well with the world and anything within reason seems possible, and therefore the patient accepts your suggestions almost without criticism. If it's a pleasant suggestion for the good of the patient, he will accept your suggestion unquestioningly. If he has doubts about it being good for himself, he'll reject it . . . Do you think anybody could persuade you to do anything against your ethics or your code of morals at this point?

PATIENT: No.

ELMAN: It is nonsense that if you get a person hypnotized you can get him to do something he wouldn't ordinarily do. The person in hypnosis—and the patient will verify what I am saying—has greater awareness than the person not in hypnosis.

PATIENT: That's right.

ELMAN: Now, I want you to see that when you give a suggestion which is reasonable and pleasing, the suggestion is taken instantly. For medical purposes now, I am going to numb his hand. Watch how fast that hand becomes numb so long as he remains in the state . . . I'm going to stroke your hand and I want you to notice how quickly it becomes numb. Now that area will be completely numb and you'll have no feeling in it whatsoever . . . How's the hand?

PATIENT: It feels numb.

ELMAN: You see how fast the selective thinking occurs once you get the state. If it is necessary for his hand to get more numb, there are ways to make it so numb that you can get an anesthesia equivalent to any chemical anesthesia which you could possibly use . . . Now we're all through and when I have him open his eyes the anesthesia will be gone. Notice how good your hands feel and notice how good you feel . . . All right, open your eyes . . . How do you feel?

PATIENT: Good.

ELMAN: Notice the signs. He had a much deeper state of hypnosis than any that you have worked with so far. Occasionally, every one of you who has done your practicing the way you're supposed to has stumbled into the state without realizing it because the longer patients are in the state, the deeper they go. Some of you have had somnambulism right in your own offices already. But now the idea is to have it at will . . .

*   *   *

You should get somnambulism every time you try for it unless there's an out-and-out rejection by the patient. In each case, the critical faculty is bypassed, and selective thinking established after the somnambulism is achieved . . . following the same procedure, however, you sometimes get a response that is quite different—as in the case of another patient with whom I am now working—

PATIENT: I can still think of the next number.

ELMAN: If you can, make that number disappear.

PATIENT: Each time I've tried to say a number, I reach for the next one at the same time.

ELMAN: That's all right. What's your first name?

PATIENT: Ken.

ELMAN: Kent or Ken?

PATIENT: K-E-N.

ELMAN: K-E-N. I've written that on your finger just like it was on a blackboard, and in your mind's eye you can see it as clear as on a blackboard. Isn't that right?

PATIENT: Yes.

ELMAN: Now I'm going to do something I think you'll like. I'm going to erase it from your finger and from the blackboard and from your mind all at the same time. I rub it off your finger and it is completely gone . . . Now try to tell me what I took off your hand.

PATIENT: Can't find it. It's gone. Can't remember it.

ELMAN: That's a test for resistance . . . He passed the test beautifully. I knew there was no resistance. He was finding it difficult to make the numbers disappear because the next one came in, but done this way he was just able to make that name disappear from his finger so easily. Now, [to patient] will you describe the feeling from inside the state?

PATIENT: My name.

ELMAN: You brought it back?

PATIENT: It never left.

ELMAN: Then why didn't you tell me what it was that
           I took off your hand?

PATIENT: Too darn tired.

ELMAN: This is the artificial state of somnambulism
           because he has what is known as aphasia—an
           unwillingness—an inability—a desire not to
           speak. He said, "Too darn tired." That indi-
           cates aphasia. When you get aphasia, you get
           a state of hypnosis that is not nearly as effec-
           tive as true somnambulism. And if you want
           to do difficult operative procedures on him at
           this point you will not be able to do so. I call
           this state artificial somnambulism. He's got
           to make those numbers or that name disappear
           before we have the true state because aphasia
           is one thing, amnesia is another. And I want
           to make sure that the amnesia is there. So [to
           patient] make those numbers completely dis-
           appear . . . Banish them . . . Are they gone?

PATIENT: No.

ELMAN: Make them disappear. I'm going to lift your
           hand and drop it, and when I do, the rest of
           those numbers will drop out. Want them to
           drop out and watch them go . . . Gone?

PATIENT: Yes.

ELMAN: Now they're gone . . . Why do I check so care-
           fully? Because I expect students to check
           carefully. I would have had failure with al-
           most anything I tried with him so long as he
           held on to those numbers and had an unwill-
           ingness, an inability to speak. The instant he
           makes those numbers disappear, he can feel
           that difference . . . I regard the state of true
           somnambulism as a very desirable state. I
           wouldn't do painful procedures on a patient
           who didn't have true somnambulism because

all he would get would be analgesia. It is a positive scientific fact that when you get artificial somnambulism you can't get anesthesia with it. When you're first working with hypnosis you encounter artificial somnambulism quite frequently. You must learn how to dispel it. You have to cause artificial somnambulism to turn into true somnambulism before you get the results you want. Even after you are adept with hypnotic techniques you will occasionally encounter artificial somnambulism. Learn to recognize it for what it is and don't try to do difficult work with it. The lifting and dropping of the hand is a good technique for changing artificial to true somnambulism.

Chapter 10

WAKING HYPNOSIS AND WAKING
SUGGESTION

BEFORE we discuss further the deepening techniques in hypnosis, I think it is necessary that you know a phase of hypnosis which is seldom mentioned in the textbooks, and then inadequately described. To do this properly we'll begin with a story about my eldest son.

When Jackie was five years old he developed the habit of waking up after about two hours of sleep. He usually awoke from his sleep screaming. When my wife went to comfort him he said, "I had such a bad dream it frightened me." She would talk to him for a little while and then suggest that he go back to sleep. He refused to go back to sleep for fear he would have the same bad dream. After much coaxing, he would try to fall asleep, but without success for quite a long while.

One night on arriving home I found him awake and crying bitterly. He told me about the bad dreams. I told him, "You don't have to be frightened by bad dreams. There's an awfully good cure for them that my Daddy used for me. My Daddy bought me some dream medicine, and after I took it I didn't have bad dreams any more. It's quite a while since he gave me that dream medicine and I don't know whether they make it any more, but I'll be glad to call up the drug store to find out if they have any." He said, "Oh, Daddy, will you please do that. If they haven't got it maybe they can order some."

I left the bedroom and went into another room where the telephone was. I pretended to phone the drug store. Then I hung up the receiver and went into my son's room and said, "The druggist told me he'd have it delivered right away and all we have to do is wait a few minutes and it will be here."

I excused myself and went into the other room and told my wife to go out into the hall and ring our doorbell, but to do it very quietly so that all Jackie would hear would be the doorbell and not the sound of her going out into the hall. Then I returned to my son. Pretty soon the doorbell rang and I said, "That must be the dream medicine. I'll get it for you."

I made a pretext of answering the doorbell, opening the door quite noisily and thanking the imaginary delivery boy for being so prompt with it. I called out to my son, "The dream medicine is here. I'll bring it to you as soon as I unwrap the package." Then I went into the bathroom and filled an empty medicine bottle with clear water. I stuck a label on the bottle and printed on it "Dream Medicine." Then I took an ordinary glass and filled it with water. I brought the medicine bottle and the glass of water into my son's room and said to him, "This is kind of bitter so you'd better be ready to take this water after I give you a teaspoonful of the medicine." I poured a teaspoonful and gave it to my son, quickly following it with a glass of water. Then I kissed him goodnight and told him he would be asleep in a minute—and he was. He didn't have bad dreams after that, for every night he would ask for his dream medicine before going to bed and then he would sleep all through the night.

He got to the point where he said to me rather proudly that he believed he could take the dream medicine without a chaser. I said to him, "That's wonderful. Let's try it just once to see if you can." And so he took a teaspoonful of clear water from the medicine bottle and said, "I did it, Daddy, and I didn't mind it a bit."

We used dream medicine for all three of our children and here is an interesting fact. I discussed the dream medicine recently with my second son, Bob, who is thirty-three years old. I asked him if he remembered the dream medicine, and he did. Then I asked him if he knew this was a form of hypnosis. He said, "Dad, I've known it was hypnosis for many years, but let me tell you something that I think will amuse you. Ever since you gave me that dream medicine, I've been in the habit of taking a sip of water just before I go to bed and then I sleep soundly all through the night. After I was married, my wife got into the habit of taking a small sip of water before going to bed. That dream medicine must have been powerful because I've been using it successfully as long as I can remember."

The story of the dream medicine illustrates a phenomenon known as waking hypnosis.

Because of the never-ending confusion in the literature of hypnosis about two distinct phenomena—waking suggestion and waking hypnosis—I'm going to attempt to clarify these two completely different states. Waking hypnosis can be one of your most valuable allies in medicine or dentistry. In fact, it is my firm belief that no one can know hypnosis without knowing waking hypnosis.

The true use of waking hypnosis should be this: When you find resistance to the trance state, use waking hypnosis. Where you are trying to save time, use waking hypnosis. You'll get your short-range results just as well. But where time is not of the essence, you will find that in the long run the trance state will serve you better for many purposes than the waking state.

Here's a definition of waking suggestion: *A waking suggestion is a suggestion given in the normal state of consciousness which does not precipitate a waking state of hypnosis.* For example: Someone in the room yawns. Somebody sees him yawn, and he yawns, too. Another person sees him yawn, and the third person yawns, and pretty soon you have a room full of yawning people. That is waking suggestion. Every one of us has seen this occur. There is no bypass of the critical faculty involved.

Another form of waking suggestion is this: I might say to you, "Doctor, won't you be seated," or, "Come in, Mrs. Jones." Either of those statements is a waking suggestion. There is no waking hypnosis involved because there is no bypass of the critical faculty.

Now let me show you the difference between waking suggestion and waking hypnosis: *When hypnotic effects are achieved without the use of the trance state, such hypnotic effects are called waking hypnosis. In every case, it involves a bypass of the critical faculty and the implanting of selective thinking.*

Let me show you an example of waking hypnosis at work. Here is a classroom demonstration, performed with a doctor previously unknown to the teacher.

ELMAN: Doctor, do you like to go to the dentist?

DOCTOR: No, I don't.

ELMAN: Watch this. I'm going to stroke your jaw
              three times. You will lose all feeling in the
              side of the jaw that I stroke . . . One, two, three
              . . . And now will some man in dentistry come
              up here, please . . . You're going to find a most
              amazing thing has taken place . . . Take any of
              those instruments at all—go inside on the right
              side of his jaw, and he won't be able to find
              any feeling there whatsoever . . . I think the
              man here is going to be amazed because I un-
              derstand he's an anesthetist himself . . . He's
              got perfect anesthesia—right?

DOCTOR: What did he do?

ELMAN: He gouged you hard enough so that ordinarily
              you would have hit the ceiling, doctor. That's
              what he went in with . . . Thank you, that's
              all I need you for now.

DOCTOR: How long will this last?

ELMAN: It will last as long as you would need to be in
              the dental chair. It would last for two hours,
              three hours, four hours. As long as he had to
              work on you. And I can assure you it's just as
              good anesthesia as you would get with xylo-
              caine or anything else . . .

(Doctor in audience says he was at the dentist today and now
has anesthesia on one side of his face. He would like to have
anesthesia on the other side.)

ELMAN: All right, doctor. Please come up here. If
              you have anesthesia on one side, I'm going to
              prove to you that hypnotic anesthesia can be
              even better than chemical anesthesia. Watch
              this—I want to make a test on both sides. I'm
              going to stroke his jaw three times and he will
              lose all feeling on this side of the face. One,
              two, and now, that jaw will be completely
              numb when I say—three . . . All right, [to an-
              other doctor in audience] doctor, come up
              please . . . I want you to work on either side
              because he has chemical anesthesia on one side,

hypnotic anesthesia on the other. See if you can find any difference. See which you like best for your anesthesia. [Doctor makes test.] There's more anesthesia from the hypnotic anesthesia than from the chemical anesthesia . . . Doctor, will you tell them that, please.

DOCTOR: That's true.

ELMAN: Those of us who know waking hypnosis and how to use it know the power of it—for that anesthesia which he gets is better than a chemical anesthesia. Let me show you waking hypnosis from another standpoint.

ELMAN: [Now addresses doctor in audience, tells him to stand up in front of his seat.] Will you give us your name and address, please. [Doctor gives his name and address and Elman repeats it.] All right, I'm going to snap my fingers and you'll find that you can't think of your name or address. [Snaps fingers.] Try to say it now and you'll find it's gone. Try hard. [Doctor is unable to say his name and address.] All right, now you can say it. [Doctor now says his name and address.] Now, why did it work? I said to him, "Want this to happen," and he rather liked the idea of it happening. He said to himself, "I wonder if that could happen to me?" Isn't that right, sir?

DOCTOR: That's right.

*   *   *

Every effect obtainable with the trance state is obtainable in many people with waking hypnosis. In the above demonstration, I got anesthesia, stronger anesthesia than you can get chemically. I also got temporary amnesia in another person. In the trance state, somnambulism is necessary to attain amnesia. I attained amnesia with the gentleman in the above demonstration, and therefore I had somnambulism in the waking state. He was hypnotized.

In the study of waking hypnosis and waking suggestion, all posthypnotic phenomena are excluded because waking hypnosis is not posthypnotic. It may be achieved on patients who have never known the trance state. Again and again, waking hypnosis is used as a lever to enter the deep trance state. Therefore, a knowledge of waking suggestion and waking hypnosis will make you a better operator.

Now let me show you waking hypnosis in group thinking. A whole group of people can be hypnotized in the following experiment. In the presence of a number of people, crack and break open a perfectly fresh egg. Make a wry face and exclaim, "Phew, that egg smells rotten. I wouldn't eat that for a million dollars. Oh boy, is that terrible. Smell that, will you somebody?" Now pass that egg around for the people to smell. Person after person will say, "That egg smells terrible." And some will say, "Why, it even looks bad." These people have been hallucinated into believing that the fresh egg is bad. To all intents and purposes, they have been completely hypnotized. Many will contend that these people have not been hypnotized, for they were not in the trance state at all. Well, let us examine the facts. You have learned that hypnosis is a state of mind in which the critical faculty is bypassed, thus making selective thinking possible. You have been asked to practice obtaining the state on yourself and others in order to increase your ability to urge a suggestion so strongly on your patients that you bypass the critical faculty—that is, the ability to judge selected matters accurately, and replace the patients' judgment in these selected matters with your own. When you achieve that state of mind, you have hypnosis. And now you're learning that you do not need the trance state to achieve actual hypnosis and hypnotic effects.

Consider the case of the egg again. When you made the exclamation, "Phew, that egg smells rotten. I wouldn't eat it for a million dollars," you made a positive statement of apparent fact, which your hearers accepted at face value. Respect for your judgment caused them to believe what you said even before they smelled the egg. Having minimized their ability to judge the egg fairly, you asked them to judge it, and they did so—not with their critical faculties, but with yours. You accomplished hypnosis. You hallucinated two of their senses—that of sight and that of smell. You accomplished hypnosis as effectively as a trance can render it. If subsequently the hallucination were not exposed, your hearers would remain convinced to the end of their days that the egg was in an advanced state of putrefaction.

Another experiment can be performed easily on a single individual. Suppose you were to see a smart-looking nurse in a trim uniform, and were to say to her, "Miss So-and-so, do you mind turning around once? There's something about that uniform that puzzles me." The nurse would follow your instructions. Then suppose you were to gaze at her critically for a moment, and say, "Hmm, turn around the other way, won't you, please. I was wondering what was wrong. Thank you so much. Good day." At this point you could walk away without saying anything more, and you would have precipitated hypnosis. Despite assurances from other nurses that her uniform was quite in order, the nurse whom you appeared to criticize would be certain that her dress was too long, too short, too small, too big, or that it bulged or didn't bulge in the wrong or right places. And the longer she wore it, the more she would question her own judgment as to the uniform's fitness. When her ability to judge the uniform was sufficiently minimized, she would substitute what she believed to be your considered judgment for her own. Without the aid of the trance state, you would have bypassed her critical faculty, and implanted a hypnotic suggestion so firmly that she would only be satisfied when she changed uniforms.

Let's leave waking hypnosis for a little bit now and go back to waking suggestion. Every man in dentistry will tell you that he has seen patients come into his office suffering the pangs of toothache. As the patient walks in, the pain subsides. He fears the dentist more than he fears the toothache. Soon, he decides the tooth doesn't ache at all. The thought of the dentist drives the pain away.

Here's another example: An accident patient is rushed to the hospital. He seems to be in bad shape. He's a mixture of shock and panic. In the emergency room, he hears the reassuring words, "Not serious. He'll make it. He'll do all right," and that instant he begins to respond. Those magic words "not serious" have probably saved thousands of lives. And those of you who have worked in the emergency rooms of hospitals have seen this happen and wondered why it happened. Waking suggestion did the trick. This phenomenon is not waking hypnosis, but waking suggestion. Conversely,

the doctor says to the patient, "This is going to hurt a bit."
The patient tenses up and what should have been a minor
procedure becomes an almost major one—pain induced by
suggestion.   Every student in medical or dental school is
informed by his professors, "Never take the patients by surprise; keep them apprised of what you are doing at every
step." The doctor's way of warning them in an easy way
is to say, "This is going to be a bit uncomfortable, this is
going to hurt a bit, but I'll try to go easy on you," and he
thinks he's going easy on the patient, when as a matter of
fact, he is making it about ten times tougher. Instead of
saying, "This is going to hurt a bit," say, "Well, now I have
some work to do on your arm; I don't think you'll mind this,"
and immediately the minor procedure is made so easy for the
patient that he really doesn't feel it.   This is waking suggestion—bordering, perhaps, on waking hypnosis, and used
constructively.

Lack of sympathy in psychosomatic ailments is frequently found to be a great cause of patient distress. The
fact that his doctor has said, "Well, we can't find a thing the
matter with you. It must be in your mind," causes patient
after patient to feel that he is headed for insanity. Psychiatrists have confirmed this many times in discussing their
problems with me. They have said: "Doctors send patients
to us that way. That's the way they introduce the patient to
the psychiatrist. And it means we must work about six
months longer with the patient because of the improper introduction to psychiatry that the doctor has made."

Sympathetic treatment of psychosomatic aches and pains
gives the patient the necessary attitude to aid in his recovery.
There isn't one man in psychiatry who will not agree with
that statement.

Let's go back to waking hypnosis and show examples in
medicine and dentistry. There are few doctors who have not
found it advisable at times to administer or order administered the very common sterile hypo. It is useful in a variety
of cases. It's a waking hypnotic technique. There are so
many other things that medicine could have taken from hypnosis, but didn't take, which would also have been vastly
beneficial. For example, there wasn't a doctor in the nine-
teenth century, I guess, who didn't know this stunt that I'm
going to show you now. This is probably the most useful

adjunct to the physician or dentist working with a "gagger."
I'd like to show you a valuable technique for stopping a person from gagging. This demonstration took place in a class,
and the "patient" was a doctor who tended to gag during
oral examinations:

ELMAN: Doctor, come up here and examine this gentleman's throat any way you want to, and try
               to make him gag after I show him what to
               do . . . [to patient] Hold that pencil tightly
               with both hands, and you'll find you can't gag
               so long as you hold that pencil tightly. Watch
               this . . . [to examining doctor] make any examination you want to. You won't be able to
               make him gag so long as he holds the pencil
               . . . You use that technique doctor, and I promise that you can have dental work done—
               you can have medical work done. Just hold
               on to the pencil—that's all—hold on to the
               pencil with both hands. And you'll have the
               nicest result.

                    *   *   *

The "patient" in this demonstration finally gagged when
the uvula was touched; that's the trigger mechanism of nature to make you gag. So nature's trigger mechanism was
not suggested away. But I did suggest away the trigger mechanism that in the past made this man's uvula react long
before the doctor got to it. Ninety-seven patients out of a
hundred who gag, will be benefitted by this technique.

Who is the person who won't be benefitted by this technique? The person who gags because of a traumatic incident
in his past. Recently, one of my students, a psychiatrist, said
to me, "Mr. Elman, my wife has a rare illness. It's effect is a
lack of saliva. For twenty-five years she hasn't had any
saliva, and because of it she got pyorrhea—lost all her teeth
—she gets cracks in her lips that are so severe they require
medical attention." I said to him, "Doctor, she must have
secreted *some* saliva over the years or she couldn't have
digested her food. She couldn't have lived without saliva for
twenty-five years." He replied, "Well, she secretes very, very
little of it."

I pointed out to him that what she did secrete must be pretty good as she was otherwise in good health. Then I mentioned to him the possibility that her difficulty might have an emotional basis. "Oh no," he said. "After all, she's the wife of a psychiatrist. She has had psychiatric nurse's training. So I'm positive it isn't on an emotional basis. But I would like you to help her if you could. She can't wear her dentures. Because she doesn't secrete enough saliva, the dentures burn her mouth and after she wears them for perhaps a day, she has to go three or four days without them." He asked, if despite his doubts, I would try to help her. Ten minutes of hypoanalysis revealed this:

Twenty-five years ago she had an arrested case of TB. Her throat had been affected, but now she had to have her tonsils out. The doctors in charge preferred to have a specialist perform the surgery. They called in a specialist from a distant area. However, she got the strange notion that the specialist's hands were dirty. She was under local anesthetic and awake, and insisted that he rewash his hands. Perhaps this hallucination of uncleanliness was triggered by fear of the operation. At any rate, she then got the notion that if his hands were dirty, his medical instruments must also be dirty. She made him resterilize them, but the operation was to her a horrible one, to say the least, and afterward she was slow in making a recovery. Now every time anything foreign comes into her mouth, there is no saliva. Have you ever noticed that when you're afraid your mouth gets very dry? One of the common symptoms of great fear with many people is lack of saliva. I am of the opinion that she is abreacting to the tonsilectomy of twenty-five years ago and that she has never had anything but an emotional problem, an almost constant panic whenever anything comes near her mouth. Foreign objects such as dentures would, at a level below conscious awareness, remind her of medical instruments coming at her throat. I'm positive we'll achieve gratifying results in this case and she'll be able to wear dentures without discomfort. There was a definite traumatic incident there, and her husband said to me afterwards, "I never, never would have suspected that this situation could arise from an emotional problem."

When you find a person who has had a traumatic incident such as this, the patient, even though he holds the

pencil, will not get relief from the gagging. Fortunately, this
is rare, and, the pencil catalyst will work beautifully in about
ninety-seven cases out of a hundred. It's strictly a hypnotic.

Many cases of impotence have been relieved by doctors
who prescribed sugar pills, with the assurance to the patient
that "this will make you as potent as a young bull." It is
interesting to note that physicians and dentists make use of
waking hypnosis almost every day, but are completely unaware of it. One of the intents of this course is to bring to
the students' attention the scientific utilization of such
techniques.

Now, if there is such a thing as waking hypnosis, if it
was possible for me to produce anesthesia in an anesthetist
and amnesia in another doctor, there must have been a rational key to the process. The thoughts that went through
the anesthetist's mind ran something like this: "I've seen
Mr. Elman succeed, and he would be a fool to attempt anything that was likely to fail before an audience of doctors.
Wouldn't he be an idiot to say I was anesthetized if I wasn't
anesthetized? He must know what he's talking about. I
must be anesthetized."

Therefore, he locked his mind around the idea that he
was anesthetized, and so he was. It happened as simply as
that. Why did another man get complete amnesia for a few
seconds? Simply because he liked the idea of it's happening.
He said to himself: "Wouldn't it be interesting if that really
happened." He had amnesia because his mind said, "I'd
enjoy that. I'd like to see what the effect is like." The minute he thought that, his critical faculty was bypassed, substitute judgment was used, and he had amnesia. Following the
demonstration described above, the doctor who experienced
amnesia confirmed this hypothesis.

There is a specific and reliable way to attain waking
hypnosis, (there must be, for I don't miss very often with
it and my doctors don't miss very often either). This is the
key to the process: *The mind of the subject must lock itself
around a given idea.*

The crying child is certain that if mother kisses her the
pain will disappear. The nurse is certain that the judgment
of the doctor concerning her uniform is infallible; the people
present at the egg experiment are certain that the first person
who passed judgment on the egg was correct; the anesthetist

was certain that I would be the biggest fool in the world if he
wasn't anesthetized so he was sure in his own mind that he
was anesthetized.   His mind had locked around the idea and
therefore he had anesthesia.

To cause the human mind to lock around a given idea,
suggestions in the waking state must be given with complete
confidence, with absolute assurance.   They must leave no
room for doubt.   If doubt creeps in, the suggestion usually
becomes ineffective.   Therefore, give the suggestions in a
manner which implies that what you have said is as certain
of happening as the dawn.   Leave no room for doubt.   Every
one of the people in the experiments described locked his
mind around a given idea that had the appearance of a cer-
tainty.   *First, the mind of the subject must lock itself around
a given idea.*

*Second, the suggestion must be one which the patient
wants.*

Any patient suffering intense pain wants relief.   He's
apt to quickly take suggestions for the alleviation of his distress.   Any patient facing the prospect of pain—the dental
patient is an excellent example—is ready for waking hypnosis.   The emotionally disturbed patient is usually ready to
listen to the practitioner who shows sympathy and understanding.   All these people will take suggestions because
they *want* suggestions.   Now, how do you convey these
suggestions?

*Let the patient hear those words which he is anxious
to hear.*

At this point I am going to describe a remarkable experiment which I perform before doctors, and which would not
be as likely to succeed before laymen.   Here is the experiment, as recorded in class:

"Every one of you knows that this [holding up pitcher]
is merely ice water and nothing else.   And every one of you
knows that these are cotton swabs [holding them up].   And
every one of you knows that ice water does not anesthetize,
and that cotton swabs do not anesthetize.   And I'll even tell
you that the words I'm going to use are fakes.   All the words
I'm going to use are phony words.   But these are surgical
instruments, gentlemen, that have *sharp* ends, and they are
just as sharp as any needles that you have ever seen, and
they hurt like the devil.   So you see, even my semantics are

bad—yet, using incorrect semantics, using ice water for my anesthesia agent, using cotton swabs, using words that are fakes, every one of you is going to be anesthetized by what I'm going to do now. Now listen to the words I use and I think you will love this, because this is a true application of waking hypnosis, and you'll see why it works . . . [addresses physician]: Doctor, you know that some of the drug houses have come up with something really new and interesting. You know what they do? They put the anesthesia right into the alcohol now—and when I swab you with this, you'll become completely anesthetized, and now when I go to work on that area, you'll know that I'm working there, but nothing will bother, nothing will disturb. Watch, doctor, [applying surgical clamp]. What did you feel then? Anything in the way of discomfort?"

DOCTOR: Nothing.

ELMAN: I would like you to do that to the next doctor. You'll find that it will work on him just like it worked on you . . . Most people can't even tolerate that for a second. And if you can get to the place where you can hold it on there and swing it around, and it doesn't bother, and you know you could leave it there a minute and it wouldn't bother, you're getting to the place where you're getting pretty good anesthesia . . . [addressing doctor who has risen to ask why same experiment might fail before laymen]. Since the day you began practice, how often you have wished—when you swabbed a patient preparatory to giving him an injection or preparatory to working with something that you knew was going to be uncomfortable— how you have wished that you could anesthetize at the same time you swabbed. And when I came up with the words, "They put the anesthesia right into the alcohol," I was really echoing what you have been thinking below the level of conscious awareness since the day you got into practice. These words are particularly welcome to the doctor's ears. He says to himself, "All I've got to do is say that I get anesthesia. Let's try it." And because he gets the anesthesia, he is amazed, but he forgets that he is receptive to the suggestion. If I do this same thing before a group of laymen, I'll tell you what will happen every time (and I've quit doing it before them for this reason). About the second person I do it to will say, "Oh, that's a lot of nonsense. It can't possibly work." And after that, everybody begins to feel it. But you'll never hear that reaction in a group of doctors, because the doctor says, "Oh, brother, how I'd like to make this work."

*   *   *

While many of my doctor-students have used waking hypnosis beautifully, perhaps one of the greatest exponents of its use is a student of mine in the Midwest. He said to me a few weeks after we had the class session described above, "I wonder how many of your students can say that they have actually done deep abdominal surgery with waking hypnosis. I used the exact technique you taught us and I got such perfect anesthesia that I was able to go ahead and do surgery on a cardiac case where I couldn't have used much anesthesia anyhow, but in this way, I avoided the use of *any* anesthesia."

Here was the technique he used on the deep abdominal surgical case he described to me. He asked the patient, "Have you ever been anesthetized before?" When the patient said he had, the doctor continued. "Well, I'm glad to hear it because we have a capsule here which follows the exact nerve pattern of the previous anesthesia. All I have to do is have you swallow this and you'll be completely anesthetized in every area where you were anesthetized before. In about thirty seconds you'll have complete anesthesia wherever you had it before." He had the patient swallow the capsule. Seconds later, he was able to take towel clips and attach them to any part of his body without the patient feeling them. He went ahead and did the surgery. "When I could see that he didn't feel the towel clips," he told me, "I knew he wouldn't feel the incision either, so I just went to work. I had tested with towel clips in tender portions of his anatomy. If he had felt it, I wouldn't have gone ahead with the surgery. Since he didn't feel the towel clips, I went ahead and did the surgery." Subsequently, this doctor reported similar success on four more cases handled this way.

With minor variations, you put waking hypnosis to use in medical or dental practice in the same way. Here's a class scene in which I worked with a woman who had ordinarily dreaded dental work:

ELMAN: Doctor, swab the inside of her mouth. Give her the same story about how they put the anesthesia—the very same thing that you did before—and you'll get perfect anesthesia in her mouth. [Doctor proceeds: test is made.] Satisfied, doctor? Sure. Well, that's how you can use waking hypnosis in dentistry . . . [addressing patient] And madam, may I ask, did you feel anything at all?

PATIENT: No. Nothing.

DOCTOR: Can you drill with that?

ELMAN: You can drill and everything else with that. And you'll have just as good anesthesia as you ever had with chemical anesthesia . . . Now, remember, you must *lock the mind of the patient around the idea.* Don't think you can simply say, "Well, now, you're going to be completely anesthetized," and start doing the work. Because if the patient's mind isn't locked around the idea, you will be unsuccessful. You must lock the mind of the patient around a given idea, and the idea must be one to which the patient is receptive. Every patient wants anesthesia, so they're particularly receptive to the idea.

* * *

Now how would you use it in other branches of medicine? One of my former students, who is adept in the use of waking hypnosis, came back to class one night and before a group of other doctors, told this story:

A manufacturer of a nationally known product for the alleviation of pain had an accident. He got his hand caught in a lawn mower and the laceration required quite a few stitches. It was a very painful accident. The doctor told the manufacturer he had just received a wonderful preparation from Vienna that would anesthetize his entire hand, so that he wouldn't even feel the sutures being made. He then proceeded to cleanse and swab the area with a placebo and asked the manufacturer to tell him when the hand was completely numb. In a few seconds, the manufacturer said, "My hand is completely without feeling now, doctor." Then the doctor proceeded to do the suturing, and when he was finished he said, "That anesthesia will stay with you until your hand begins to heal. You won't have any discomfort."

The patient was amazed. "I didn't feel a thing," he said. "The pain is gone completely and I wouldn't even know that I had a damaged hand unless I looked at it. What's the name of that product you're using? I'd like to analyze it and put it out for use in this country. Give me a small sample of it to take to the lab for chemical analysis."

The doctor did a little fast thinking and answered, "I can't give you any. I just used it all up on you."

Chapter 11

APPLICATIONS OF WAKING HYPNOSIS

A SPECIALIST in radiology once told me that he was hesitant to use waking hypnosis in preparing patients for barium enemas. Though he considered the barium enema to be radiology's most unpleasant procedure, he felt that the approach I suggested amounted to deceiving the patients.

He usually told them, "I have to put you through a procedure that isn't very comfortable, but I'll make it as easy for you as I can."

I contended that he was telling patients a lie, since the procedure doesn't have to be uncomfortable. If I were the radiologist, I said, I would approach patients in this manner: "You're fortunate that you're here today. The doctor who referred you tells me that you've been having a lot of distress lately. I need some x-rays, and in order to get them, I'm going to coat the lining of your stomach with the most soothing medication ever devised."

The radiologist refused to tell patients anything so "absurd" until one day he had to work on a man who was already in terrible discomfort. Out of desperation, he tried my approach. The patient was relieved, and, in fact, actually enjoyed the barium enema. The radiologist now uses this approach consistently. The only problem he has encountered is that some patients so thoroughly enjoy the "soothing medication" that they retain the barium and refuse to let it go. He solves this by telling them it will feel as beneficial leaving as it did entering.

Another doctor learned a variation of this technique for doing internal examinations on tense women patients. A gynecologist taught him to tell such a patient that a new preparation had just arrived from Vienna—an anesthetic especially designed for such examinations. He would then swab her externally with a bit of medical jelly (squeezed out beforehand and left in a jar or on a spatula). After waiting a couple of minutes for the placebo to "take effect," the examination could proceed without further trouble.

A urologist recommends a similar approach for such procedures as cystoscopy. The doctor touches the tip of the canal with a lubricant. Then he puts the lubricant on his instruments. But he tells the patient this lubricant is an anesthetic, and that nothing will be felt during or after the procedure.

A proctologist said, "I never thought there was such a thing as painless proctology until I began using waking hypnosis."

All of the above instances are examples of applications for waking hypnosis. Recently, one doctor told me that the only problem he encounters with the technique, now that he's learned its proper applications, involves nurses rather than patients. In biopsies and the like, it frightens the nurses a little when the doctor doesn't pick up the novocain —just starts cutting. My answer to this is that nurses and assistants should be taught what to expect in cases where hypnosis is used, and how to act properly in the presence of hypnotized patients.

One application of waking hypnosis combined with the trance is especially affective in getting children over the fear of the needle. And as the following classroom recording proves, it can also be used with an adult:

ELMAN: Is there anybody in this room who would like to have an area on his body anesthetized to a degree where, from now on, you will never feel an injection again? You will never even know that you're getting an injection while it's being done. Anyone who dreads an injection terribly, and would like to have a Magic Spot on his body? . . . Come on up . . . Those of you who won't come up are going to be awfully sorry because this is a chance to get something which is fantastically good. This Magic Spot is amazing . . .

[to subject] Can you raise your sleeve a little bit? Now here's the greatest device for children. As far as that goes, it works on adults just as well as children, because I have an

adult right here. Now, watch this . . . I want
you to open your eyes wide, please. I'm going
to pull your eyes shut. All you have to do is
to pretend that you can't open your eyes and
keep on pretending you can't open your eyes—
so much so that when you try to open your
eyes they just won't open . . . Now let me see
you try to open them while you're pretending
. . . That's right . . . Now stay like that and
keep on pretending you can't open your eyes,
and the most amazing thing is going to happen.
You're going to have a Magic Spot put on your
arm. Once this Magic Spot is put on you,
never again will you have to feel an injection.
You'll know that the doctor is working there,
but nothing will disturb, nothing will bother
you. You'll never have any discomfort from
an injection, either before, during or afterwards . . . Now, who is in the habit of giving
a lot of injections, because I want this injection given in the usual way, once I've given
her the Magic Spot . . . Now, watch, I take this
area and I paint a Magic Spot with alcohol,
like that. Now, whenever an injection is given
in that area—she'll be able to point it out to
the doctor—nothing will be felt at all except
that she'll know you're working there . . .
She'll feel absolutely nothing . . . Now, doctor
. . . you'll see she won't even feel when you're
doing it. [Injection is given with a number
twenty needle.] Now, isn't that beautiful? . . .
[to patient] You've already had your injection and you know you didn't feel a thing.
From now on you will always be able to have
injections this easily. After a while, that
Magic Spot I painted on your arm will no
longer be visible to you or anyone else—except
for one important thing—you will know exactly where it is so that any time you must
receive an injection, you will be able to point
out the exact area to your doctor. If you wish,
you will be able to watch him giving you the

injection, and it won't bother you a bit . . . All right, open your eyes . . . What did you feel?

PATIENT: Nothing.

ELMAN: Now gentlemen, I want you to see how this works the next time the patient requires an injection. So we're going to pretend this same patient has come to your office for another visit. You tell the patient that you must give her another injection, and that as she already knows, it won't bother her at all. You ask her to show you where her Magic Spot is.

PATIENT: Right there, doctor.

ELMAN: All right, doctor. Here's another needle. Go ahead and give the patient an injection in the usual manner. You merely cleanse the area with alcohol as usual, and go ahead with your injection . . . Young lady, I want you to watch the doctor while he is giving you this second injection . . . [Doctor gives injection.] What did you feel?

PATIENT: Nothing.

ELMAN: And doctor, when you dismiss your patient, just make the statement that all is well, and that next time she needs an injection, it will again be just as easy . . . [to patient]   That bleeding will stop now. It's bled enough and now it will stop.

PATIENT: Did it stop?

ELMAN: Sure it stopped.

PATIENT: I'm going to remember that spot. It's going to come in handy.

DOCTOR: The trouble I have with these kids is that they won't listen to you to start with.

ELMAN: If they won't listen to you, then you've got to give the injection the hard way. If I can promise a child, "Look, if I give you a Magic Spot so that you never have to feel an injection

again, wouldn't you like that?"—then I have
no trouble with them. But you must get their
attention long enough to get this point across.
Our pediatricians who are working with a tremendous number of children—that's all they
do all day long—they tell us that the Magic
Spot is one of the most valuable things they
know. The mothers and fathers of these children come in later and ask for Magic Spots for
themselves. When the child comes back for
the next visit he usually says, "Right there,
doctor. There's my Magic Spot."

DOCTOR: Is this waking hypnosis?

ELMAN: This is a combination of the trance state and
waking hypnosis, developed by Doctor Earl
Farrell of Cincinnati, a pediatrician . . . You
use eye-closure to start with—then give the
injection. The next time the child may watch
the injection. And they'll be able to watch
and won't feel a thing. They lose all their
fear of an injection.

DOCTOR: That's the next visit you let them watch?

ELMAN: Yes. However, suppose you have a patient
who requires injections in several different
places. Give him a Magic Spot in each place.
Give the first injection with the eyes closed.
Then have him open his eyes and watch you
give the other injections. Sometimes when
you've given the first injection with the eyes
closed, the child will say, "You didn't give me
the injection." The doctor says "Yes, I did.
There's where I gave it to you."

DOCTOR: How about an external abdominal examination? Can we use waking hypnosis for that?

ELMAN: Yes. You'll find that when you use this "relax-
ing-agent" approach, they just automatically
relax. They have no control over it at all.
Their critical faculty is bypassed completely
. . . You'll find that you've already got the

anesthesia . . . If you want to make an external examination instead of an internal examination and you want the stomach muscles to be relaxed, this is a good technique. If you find, by any chance, a muscle or two is not as completely relaxed as you want it to be, just say, "In about ten seconds the relaxing agent will reach that area and even those muscles will relax."

DOCTOR: I would like to know a few phrases I can say in using hypnosis . . . For instance, we know the one, "Want it to happen and it will happen."

ELMAN: No, you wouldn't use that in waking hypnosis.

DOCTOR: What do you say then?

ELMAN: You do what we did here.

DOCTOR: I mean on complete strangers.

ELMAN: You would still say to the stranger, "Now I'm going to anesthetize this area so that you won't feel a thing—and this gadget that I have to put down your throat—you just won't mind it at all once we get this anesthesia in there.

DOCTOR: And you can do that with headaches, too?

ELMAN: I wouldn't try to remove a headache by waking hypnosis. Use the trance state for removing headaches. You'll get better results. I would use Waking Hypnosis the way I've indicated, and then widen your use of it as you go along as you learn to use it more and more. But don't try to use waking hypnosis to the detriment of the trance state. In other words, don't use it as an "instead-of" measure. It's just one more tool . . .

DOCTOR: How much anesthesia can you achieve with a child?

ELMAN: In waking hypnosis?

DOCTOR: No, in the trance—in the pretend game.

ELMAN:	You get a perfect anesthesia—the equal of any chemical anesthesia, just as you do with an adult in somnambulism. You've got to give the suggestion, "Now you won't feel anything. I'll be working there, but it won't bother you a bit." Those things you must get over.
DOCTOR:	With patients with acute back strains or cancer of the back or the sacro-iliac joints, could I have used some suggestions to relieve the muscle spasms?
ELMAN:	Yes, but for this type of difficulty too, our doctors get better results with the trance state. We think we only have control over certain muscles and certain organs of our bodies, but as a matter of fact, we have control over much more of our bodies than we think. It was possible for example, for me to say to that lady who received the injection, "It will stop bleeding," and it did. Because I knew if she didn't look at it, it would stop bleeding. She didn't look at it and it stopped bleeding . . . Now to get back to the muscle spasm the doctor asked about, first I would have used the trance state to let the patient feel the relaxation because the patient can feel it better when he lets himself go into deep somnambulism. Once in deep somnambulism, I would have swabbed the area with some type of lubricant and said, "I'm going to make sure that this area, particularly where the muscle spasm has occurred —that this area is relaxed. Now, you won't have to do a thing about this, but when I swab it, just stay relaxed and the relaxing agent will do the rest," and you would have locked his mind around the idea that the muscle was going to relax. And the inner control which we exercise—as she exercises inner control over bleeding, but doesn't know it—the inner control which we exercise over those interior muscles, would have manifested itself, and the muscle spasm would have been relieved . . .

Much as we think we know about the human body from our anatomy studies, we still can't look inside the human mind to see how it works. I've had doctors who've said that they believe that some illness is caused by emotion. Others say most illness is caused by emotion. I don't think most doctors would accept this hypothesis and I'm sure that I wouldn't ... but all neurotic conditions are caused by emotions, and perhaps some physical ones. Certainly it explains why we have control over bleeding. Our dentists say to their patients after an extraction, "That bleeding will stop when it reaches the top of the socket," and the bleeding stops as suggested. Physicians also have given their patients suggestions to control bleeding when indicated . . . We have much more control than we think we have, and that's what makes it possible for doctors to use suggestion in the manner indicated . . . Remember this, that with hypnosis you will never mask a symptom. You can alleviate a symptom but you can never mask a symptom. And if there is any pathology revealed by that symptom, it will be alleviated and eased, but it will not disappear.

DOCTOR: In other words, a ruptured disc would not be masked?

ELMAN: Of course it wouldn't. You couldn't mask a symptom. The patient would say, "My back feels a lot better, but it still hurts in there, doctor." And then before long it would be hurting as much as ever. So, you can alleviate it but not mask it . . . Here's a doctor who's already used hypnosis on four cancer patients. He can't mask a cancer. They know they have pain, but he has certainly given these patients a lot of relief. Isn't that right, doctor?

DOCTOR: Yes. They're not even taking aspirin.

                         *   *   *

Despite the fact that waking hypnosis can be used in every branch of medicine, I think its greatest value is in deep surgery, in alleviating the distress and worry of the patient before the operation. There are very few patients who face an operation without anxiety. Every one of these patients is wide open to waking hypnosis and to waking suggestion. Make your suggestions in such a confident, assured manner that you can see visible evidence of the disappearance of the unpleasant anxiety signs. Keep it up until you know the patient is ready to face the operation in the proper spirit. Lock the patient's mind around the idea that recovery will be swift and sure—that the operation is not an extraordinary one, but that it is done every day of the year in countless hospitals and that patients always recover from it fast. And then use waking hypnosis to remove postoperative discomfort.

I often advise doctors to get the patient into the hypnotic trance for presurgical visits or for preanesthesia visits. However, when pressed for time, you can do without the trance. I am not saying you should forego the trance. But I am saying that if there is any doubt of success in your mind, or if you don't have time enough to go for the trance state, use the waking hypnotic state and lock the mind of the patient around the idea that recovery will be swift and sure, and that patients always recover from such surgery fast. Lock the patient's mind around the idea that there will be no postoperative discomfort. You can counteract all the things that are worrying the patient.

If by any chance the patient indicates that he has the thought that he will not recover from the operation, cancel the surgery, or cancel your part of it at any rate, if possible. This case history will show you how important the preoperative attitude is:

Some years ago, a surgeon came to class and said: "I think I saved a life with waking hypnosis this past week. I was called in to do a prostatectomy on a man about seventy-six years of age. I was told that he was a cardiac case and that he couldn't take much anesthesia, if any. I've been in the habit of making preoperative visits, and I thought I should see that he was in the right mental state before I proceeded to do the operation with as little anesthesia as possible. I went up to see him and introduced myself as the man who would be in charge of the surgery. I started locking his mind around the idea that recovery would be swift and sure, and all that sort of thing.

"Suddenly he looked up at me and said, 'You know, doctor, I'm seventy-six years old. I'm an old man and I've lived a long time. I'm a cardiac case. So tomorrow I'll die on the table.'

"I told him that, as of that moment, the operation was cancelled. I said I would never operate on anybody in the world who thought he was going to die on the operating table, that I'd never had that happen, and certainly wasn't going to start with him. He looked relieved, but he kept repeating that he was a cardiac patient and couldn't live through the operation.

"I told him, 'You're seventy-six years old. I've done this operation on men in their eighties, and they're now in their nineties and just as healthy as they could possibly be. You're only seventy-six and you're thinking of dying because of a simple operation like a prostatectomy. You think you can't have anesthesia. That's what I came up here to show you. Since you don't have surgery scheduled for the morning any more I'll show you what you missed. I'm going to show you the anesthesia I would have used.'

"And then I got him into the trance state and anesthetized his entire body. He took the suggestion like a drowning man clutching at a straw and he had complete anesthesia. Then I had him open his eyes, and I made tests over his entire body. He couldn't feel anything. Then I had him close his eyes again, brought him out of the state and he looked up at me and said, 'You know doctor, with you for my surgeon, I believe I could get well.'

"After firmly locking his mind around the idea of easy recovery, I went ahead with the surgery. He has made a perfectly magnificent recovery, and I believe I saved a life. I had encountered the will to die and that man would have died on the operating table if not for waking hypnosis."

A physician once told me about a simple operation he had arranged to perform on a young man. The patient was taken into the operating room prepared for surgery. Suddenly, the anesthetist—who hadn't yet done anything to the patient—looked up and exclaimed, "My God, he's dead!" Every type of investigation was made, including an autopsy, and they could find no cause of death. Yet the man was dead.

He had occupied a semi-private room and the investigation revealed that just before he was taken down to the operating room he had turned to the patient in the other bed and said, "I'm never coming out of that operating room alive." What had caused his death was the will to die.

Doctors should beware of even casual remarks made by patients. Sometimes these seemingly casual remarks may be fatal. We have heard doctors report that they've been able to change the will to die to the will to live with waking hypnosis. They were alert enough to realize that suggestion was needed. Others have failed to do what was needed and have lost patients as a result. Here is a case history that illustrates both possibilities in surgery:

A student of mine, attached to a Catholic hospital, encountered the will to die when he was called in to do surgery on one of the nuns working at the institution. He made a preoperative visit, and during the conversation, she said, "You know, doctor, ever since I was a little girl, I've had the notion that some day I would die on the operating table, and I suppose this is it."

The doctor immediately began a program of waking hypnosis, locking her mind around the idea that recovery would be swift and sure, that as long as she'd been in the hospital she had never known of a mortality for this particular type of operation. Finally she said to him, "You know, doctor, I just know I'm going to recover with you for my surgeon. You can go ahead with the surgery." He performed the operation, and she recovered in a minimum of time.

About six months later, the patient had to have minor surgery done. The doctor didn't know the operation was scheduled. It was done at a different hospital by a different physician in another city. There was nothing dangerous, or even serious, about the surgery. She died in the operating room.

We are born with the will to live. The law of self-preservation is the primary law of our lives. It is fundamental. Yet, there are two types of people who do not possess the instinct of self-preservation at normal level. They are the suicidal depressive and the manic depressive. But even with people suffering from these two kinds of depression, the will to die appears to be a mere warp in the straight line of self-preservation. It is sometimes possible to straight-

en this warp with the means put at our disposal by psychotherapy and hypnosis. Every doctor who knows how to use
hypnosis is capable of changing the will to die into the will
to live in normal patients. Psychiatrists report it is worth
a try even with psychotic depressives; with nonpsychotics,
then, the chances of success are overwhelming.

One more aspect of waking hypnosis deserves mention
here. I spoke earlier of superstition, which is a manifestation
of unintentional hypnosis—a form of waking hypnosis. There
are other such manifestations. In one of my classes, a doctor told me this story:

During World War II, he worked as an anesthetist in a
station where casualties were brought in after battle. He
was working with nitrous oxide and the day had been a
very busy and trying one. He noticed that the nitrous oxide
tank was getting low but later, in the excitement, he failed
to notice that it was completely used up. When he finally
realized this, he drew the surgeon aside and said, "My God,
that nitrous oxide tank must have been empty for the past
hour or so. What are we going to do?"

The surgeon answered, "There is nothing we can do
now. We will have to keep on working just as we have been.
These men have been getting perfect anesthesia. They think
they are anesthetized, and consequently they are. Keep on
doing what you're doing and don't say a word." And they
completed their work in this manner. I would say this was
a combination of unintentional hypnosis, waking hypnosis in
its usual sense and somnambulism gained in the waking
state, without the use of the trance.

Chapter 12

SOMNAMBULISM AND THE COMPOUNDING

OF SUGGESTION

BEFORE we go into the deepening phases of hypnosis, I would like to explain the difference between light and deep hypnosis, and how to recognize each. Some people—a small percentage—spontaneously go into deep hypnosis without even seeming to enter the light state. They become immediately somnambulistic. What follows applies only to those people who do *not* go into somnambulism spontaneously.

When you are intentionally going after somnambulism and you do it by the mtehods which I advocate, the patient enters the light state of hypnosis by what I call the relaxation technique. I get the light hypnosis when the body is *physically* relaxed and then proceed to get the deep state of hypnosis by relaxing the patient's *mind*. I have found by long experimentation and intense study how mental relaxation is accomplished.

The closest I can come to describing mental relaxation is to have you think of yourself an instant before you fall asleep. Momentarily, before sleep actually comes, the mind becomes a complete blank, and then you drift off to sleep. In my opinion, when the mind is almost completely inactive, mental relaxation is achieved. In that instant when nothing disturbs, nothing bothers, and the mind is a complete blank, we have mental relaxation, occurring quite naturally every day of our lives, just before we fall asleep. I find that when I can induce the same state by suggestion I have succeeded in getting the patient mentally relaxed. Now, the difference between light and deep hypnosis is simply this:

When the patient is physically relaxed we get light hypnosis. When the patient is both mentally and physically relaxed we get the state of somnambulism. First, I make sure that the patient is physically relaxed. I proceed to

increase this relaxation until I can suggest that the mind
become relaxed as well as the body. If the patient is uncomfortable, distracted, fearful, etc., he can't possibly relax
mentally, because disconcerting messages are going to the
brain. When there is no message to the brain except one
of contentment, the brain has no need to be active with
disturbing thoughts, and is therefore ready for suggestions
of a welcome nature.

The suggestion for deeper physical relaxation is welcome, and the suggestion that the mind relax—that all is
well—is also welcome. A suggestion that there will be no
active, conscious thoughts, that the mind will momentarily
be blank, is usually readily acceptable. By this method, I
find that I can achieve deep somnambulism with almost
every subject with whom I work. The only time I don't get
the deep hypnosis is when fear is present, preventing relaxation. My students have found that by following these techniques they are able to get a very high percentage of success
in inducing the deep state known as somnambulism (and
other states which will be described as we go further).

In order to have you understand the techniques used,
I am going to give you an excerpt from our fifth session,
which is entitled "The Compounding of Suggestion." You
will understand the term "Compounding of Suggestion" if
you study this class lecture carefully:

Let us examine greater depths in hypnosis and what
makes possible these greater depths. If you have been working with somnambulism, the chances are that you have come
across certain difficulties, and yet have had success with
some patients. A patient might come into your office and
get physical relaxation quite easily. The patient will not
only relax his body but his mind. He presents no problem.
When you have physical relaxation only, you have light
hypnosis. You get deep hypnosis when the patient is also
mentally relaxed. How do you achieve this state of mind?
By having the patient relax sufficiently so that for a frag-
mentary instant, or even longer, you can cause the mind to
become blank concerning a specific thing, thereby causing
amnesia. It does not matter what that specific thing is.

The suggestion I prefer to give the patient in order to
bring on amnesia is that he will not remember numbers.
I have a patient count backwards from one hundred, and

relax more and more as he recites each number. As he relaxes further and further, the numbers gently fade from his mind, and when questioned, he has "numerical amnesia." The mind is blank concerning one specific thing—numbers. It is only when you are able to produce amnesia that you have the somnambulistic state.

The inexperienced operator, however, may succeed with one patient, then try the same procedure on the next patient and the same thing will *apparently* happen, but without the desired results. You may, for example, have two prospective mothers who are ready to deliver and each will get the physical relaxation, and each will appear to get the mental relaxation. Yet one patient will feel nothing during delivery; when you deliver the second one, you think you have the same state and that she will feel nothing, but you have to give her assistance from the first contraction.

You have hit two entirely different states that look exactly alike unless you know hypnosis. The two states look exactly alike from the outside but completely different from the inside. In only one does the patient lose the numbers completely and thereby get amnesia. That's true somnambulism.

In the other state—"artificial somnambulism"—the patient gets aphasia, an *unwillingness* to talk, rather than *inability* to remember. This is the case with the second expectant mother. She will start counting one hundred, ninety-nine, ninety-eight . . . and then will stop talking and you think that the numbers are gone from her mind. But they are not. I would hate to have anything painful done to me while in artificial somnambulism, because it would hurt like the very devil.

The student must work to produce amnesia, and if for any reason this isn't achieved he must know that he doesn't have the perfect state, and therefore must not go ahead with painful procedures. Doctor after doctor has constantly confused the artificial with the real. The artificial can be detected by certain tests which will be described later.

In true somnambulism, a woman can smile during delivery—from the time the contractions begin until the actual delivery. I have seen the episiotomy repaired and the patient maintain the smile on her face.

Then what is the value of the artificial state, if any? The state is sometimes erroneously called the medium trance. The medium trance has no value except this: Few people go into true somnambulism without *passing through* artificial somnambulism. In other words, in order to go from the light state to the deep state, they go through this artifiicial state in which the numbers are still remembered, but there is an unwillingness to say them. It is the gateway to true somnambulism.

There are four true states of hypnosis in addition to the waking state which should be of interest to you. They are: (1) the light or superficial; (2) the somnambulistic; (3) the coma (the Esdaile state, which you will learn about later); (4) hypnosis attached to sleep—the greatest depth of all, which I call hypnosleep.

In order to use hypnosis properly, it is necessary to understand and be able to produce, when necessary, any of these four states. Each of them has its place in medicine.

Most doctors prefer to treat patients in the somnambulistic state, for it is easy to induce and the patient is less critical of suggestions given to him. Suggestions go into his mind deeper and remain longer than in the light state. For example, in the light state of hypnosis you can achieve a mild analgesia; many patients can be given complete anesthesia in somnambulism. Anesthesia, whether it is obtained in waking hypnosis or the trance, is proof of deep hypnosis. The light state would scarcely make a dent in the pain threshold of an arthritic victim, but if that same patient is placed in the somnambulistic state and given proper suggestions, he can be given relief from his discomfort for hours, days, weeks and, in rare cases, even longer.

After you practice the instructions which follow you will be able to do things with hypnosis that you never dreamed possible. You'll be able to use hypnosis on a scientific level. Let's begin first by showing you the hypnotic process. Watch how simple the instructions are and how easy they are to follow. Then you will learn as you go along, *why* these particular instructions are given:

ELMAN: [to patient] Take a long deep breath and
                close your eyes. Now relax those muscles
                around the eyes to the point where they won't

work. Then test them and make sure they
won't work . . . Test them hard . . . That's
right . . . Now let that feeling of relaxation
go right down to your toes . . . Now we'll do
that over again, and the next time I have you
open and close your eyes, that relaxation will
be twice as great as it is now—and let it be
. . . Now, open your eyes—really relax—close
your eyes again . . . That's it . . . The next
time you do this you'll be able to relax even
more than you have relaxed . . . Open your
eyes . . . Now close your eyes . . . Now I'm
going to lift your hand and drop it. I want
it to be as limp as a dishrag . . . If you've
followed instructions, that relaxation will have
gone down to your toes. And when I lift your
hand it will just plop down—let it plop down
. . . That's right . . . Now physically you have
all the relaxation we need. We want your
mind to be just as relaxed as your body is,
so I want you to start counting from one hundred backwards, when I tell you to. Each
time you say a number, double your relaxation.
By the time you get down to ninety-eight,
you'll be so relaxed, the numbers won't be
there. Start from one hundred and watch
them disappear before you get to ninety-eight
. . . Double your relaxation and watch them
start fading . . . Now watch them disappear
. . . Now they'll be gone . . . Isn't that a nice
feeling? Are they all gone? Let them disappear . . . Are they all gone? That's right . . .
[addressing doctors] Now this is the very important part. We must make those numbers
disappear if she wants real help at delivery
time. In working with your patients for delivery or for any other cause, if they still have
the numbers, you cannot help them to any
great extent. That's why I made sure she
made those numbers disappear—for once having made those numbers disappear, notice the
beautiful things that happen instantly. See

how relaxed she is.   And [to patient] the feeling within is pretty good, isn't that right?

PATIENT: Yes.

ELMAN: Now, I will stroke your right hand, and watch the anesthesia come in.   Your hand is going to get so numb.   I'll stroke it three times.   One . . . two . . . three . . . How's your hand?

PATIENT: It feels cold.

ELMAN: All right, that means the anesthesia is starting. When I have you open your eyes, that anesthesia is going to get ten times as strong . . . Open your eyes . . . How is your hand now?

PATIENT: It feels funny.

ELMAN: [to doctors]   This is somnambulism with the eyes wide open, for we have retained the somnambulistic state with the eyes wide open.   If we want to have that anesthesia get stronger we can have her do almost anything and any act she goes through—any suggestion she follows—will make that anesthesia stronger.   For example [to patient] raise your left hand and drop it . . . What happened to your right hand when you did that?

PATIENT: It feels funnier.

ELMAN: Funnier than before, is that right?

PATIENT: Yes.

ELMAN: Now put your head back and bring it forward . . . How's your right hand?   [to doctors]   By this time it's so numb that she probably won't feel anything.   In order to let you see the depth of anesthesia we obtain, I'm going to be working on that right hand and she won't even feel what I'm doing.   In fact, to prove that she won't feel what I'm doing, I'm going to have her close her eyes while I work on it . . . [to patient]   Then I want you, with your eyes closed—after I work on your hand—I want you to try to locate where I worked on it . . . Now try to find, without opening your eyes, where I touched you. [to doctors] Notice how far she's missing it. She's about seven inches away . . . That's pretty good anesthesia when you're about seven inches away from allis clamps closed to the third notch . . . Let her tell us how little she felt. [to patient] I want you to open your eyes, and that anesthesia will be stronger than ever, but I want you to tell us what you felt.

PATIENT: Nothing.

ELMAN: Now, let's start over again and explain why we're doing this and why we did exactly as we did. [to patient] When I next talk to you and have you close your eyes, you'll be in exactly the same state as you were before. That is, the numbers will have disappeared and you'll be completely relaxed. [to doctors] For over fifty years I have been studying the subject of hypnosis, and in my early studies, I came across a book by Doctor H. Bernheim. In this book he states that when a patient came to him for the first visit, he hypnotized the patient and he went into a light state of hypnosis. A week later, when the patient returned for the second visit, he went into the same state. This happened for four successive weeks. But on the fifth visit, the doctor noticed that the patient went into a much deeper state identifiable by the fact that the patient developed amnesia within the state, or suggestions for amnesia would be readily accepted. He called this state somnambulism. It was the same state which the Marquis de Pusuygur had described. It occurred to me that if the patient had returned day after day instead of week after week, the somnambulism could have been achieved in five days instead of five weeks. Then the thought occurred that he could have made these visits an hour apart and he would then have gotten the somnambulism in five hours instead of five weeks. Continuing along these lines, I wondered if the state could not be produced even faster. I experimented and found that I could produce the somnambulistic state by hypnotizing a person repeatedly, in a much shorter interval. I was able to achieve, in three minutes, what it took Doctor Bernheim five weeks to accomplish. I call this method the repeated induction technique. [It was used in the excerpt from the class session which you have just read.] Here again, is the repeated induction method of achieving the deep state of somnambulism. [addressing patient] Close your eyes. Relax every muscle so that the eye muscles just won't work . . . Now test them. [to doctors] This is the first visit. [to patient] In a moment, I'm going to have you open and close your eyes and you'll be more relaxed than before . . . Close your eyes. [to doctors] Now we have given the second visit. Already we have the benefit of a posthypnotic suggestion, for while in the hypnotic state I am suggesting to her that the next time she opens and closes her eyes she will be more relaxed than ever. [to patient] Now, open and close your eyes. [to doctors] And now we have a patient who is more relaxed than ever. This is the third visit. Three visits plus two posthypnotic suggestions are certainly the equivalent of five visits to Doctor Bernheim. Now we're ready to test for the somnambulism. If she has followed orders up to this point we should be able to give her a suggestion for amnesia, or she should be able to develop amnesia within the state itself if she has really reached the somnambulistic state. We have determined upon a test which has this peculiar faculty: if it does not indicate that the somnambulism is there, it tends to *produce* somnambulism. In other words, the

very test suggests somnambulism. [to patient]
I want you to relax your mind as you've relaxed your body. Start counting from one
hundred backwards. Each time you say a
number double your relaxation. By the time
you get down to ninety-eight, there won't be
any more numbers, you'll be so relaxed . . .
Now start from one hundred and make that
happen . . . Are the numbers gone?

PATIENT: Yes.

ELMAN: [to doctors]   You remember, I stroked her
hand three times and said, "Anesthesia will
come into that hand," and I think it's still
there.   [to patient]   How's your hand?

PATIENT: Pretty numb.

ELMAN: I'll stroke it and it will be very numb. One
. . . two . . . three [to doctors]   Remember
what I did.   After I got the numbness started
I said, "When I have you open your eyes, that
numbness is going to be about ten times
stronger than it is now." [to patient] Now
open your eyes.   How's your hand?

PATIENT: Numb.

ELMAN: [to doctors]   Now what have I done?   I've
compounded the anesthesia.   I have her in the
somnambulistic state with the eyes wide open.
Now we want to increase that anesthesia.
Anything I do will increase it.   Watch.   Ask
her if she doesn't feel an increase in the anesthesia when I light this cigarette.   [to patient]
Watch me light this cigarette and then tell me
how that hand feels . . . How does your hand
feel?

PATIENT: Numb.

ELMAN: More numb than before?

PATIENT: Yes.

ELMAN: [to doctors]   Notice the desire for relaxation.
Any suggestion given can be employed to in-

crease relaxation. [to patient] Now you can close your eyes again. I'm taking away the anesthesia, and when you open your eyes you're going to feel better than you've felt all day, all evening, all month. And you're going to be in beautiful shape to be helped for your delivery. You will have that baby without feeling a solitary thing. Now open your eyes and notice how good you feel . . . How do you feel?

PATIENT: Fine.

ELMAN: [to doctors] Why was I able to get deeper anesthesia every time I gave a suggestion? Because suggestions can be compounded. The first one you give may be relatively weak. It becomes stronger, however, when you follow it with a second suggestion, even though the second one may be entirely different. You give suggestion one and that's weak. Then you give suggestion two and number one gets stronger. Then you give suggestion three and numbers one and two get stronger. Give suggestion four and one, two and three all get stronger. Give suggestion five, and one, two, three and four get stronger. *Always,* the first suggestion gets stronger. The progression extends back to the beginning.

*   *   *

Imagine a scene like this. I have a man and a girl in somnambulism. Near their chairs is a phonograph. I say to the girl, "The oddest thing is going to happen after I have you open your eyes. You're going to find that every time I pull my tie you're going to have an irresistible urge to turn that phonograph on."

Then I say to the man seated next to her, "And the oddest thing is going to happen with you. Every time anybody turns on that phonograph, you're going to have an irresistible urge to turn it off."

Now I have them open their eyes, but since I have a suggestion implanted, I still am maintaining the somnambulism. They're looking at me and I pull my tie, and very slowly, the girl turns and looks at the phonograph, but she does nothing about it. The man turns slowly and looks at her but that's all that happens. Then I pull my tie again, and this time, more quickly she looks at the phonograph, and more quickly the man looks at her. Now I pull my tie for the third time and she gets up slowly and deliberately and walks to the phonograph and turns it on, but just as deliberately the man follows her and turns it off.

Now, as they are halfway back to their seats I pull my tie and by this time, suggestion one is so strong that the girl races back to the phonograph and turns it on but the man races back to the phonograph to turn it off. And this is all happening as a result of the compounding of suggestion, a technique that can be applied in medicine and dentistry. I was using precisely this technique when I strengthened the anesthesia in the hand of the pregnant patient a short time. ago.

After some further demonstration, it will be the job of every doctor to do the following things: First, produce somnambulism by the repeated induction technique. Then, if you encounter artificial somnambulism, change it to true somnambulism by compounding suggestion. Once you have the somnambulism achieved in trance, you are to go after somnambulism with the eyes wide open. That means you must give a suggestion which holds over when the eyes are opened, at which time you must compound the suggestions until you have a depth of anesthesia that satisfies you as being medically or dentally useful. Now for another demonstration.

ELMAN: [to patient, who is in trance and somnambulistic] I'm going to stroke your hand and you're going to get some numbness in your hand . . . One . . . two . . . three . . . How's your hand?

PATIENT: I feel it coming.

ELMAN: When I have you open your eyes the numbness will increase ten times over . . . Open your eyes . . . [to doctors] This is somnambulism with the eyes wide open . . . [to patient] How's your hand?

PATIENT: I don't feel anything there.

ELMAN: Now we want that anesthesia to get ten times

	stronger. Tilt your head back and bring it forward, and notice what happens to your hand . . . How's your hand?
PATIENT:	Better yet.
ELMAN:	Do it again and that anesthesia will become so intense you won't be able to feel anything . . . How is it? Pretty numb now? . . . [to doctors] The same thing is true here. She won't feel a solitary thing in that hand, and I'm going to make the same tests and let you see that neither she nor the girl before her nor anybody else—once suggestions are compounded—can make a very good appraisal of where the test is made. That's how good the anesthesia is . . . [to patient] I'm going to be working on this hand. You'll know I'm working there but nothing will bother—nothing will disturb . . . Now, without opening your eyes try to locate where that test was made . . . [to doctors] Notice that, gentlemen. Every place but the right place. Now we want that anesthesia to be profound when she opens her eyes because I want to ask her a couple of questions about it . . . [to patient] Open your eyes, please . . . How's the hand? Pretty numb now? What did you feel of what I did?
PATIENT:	It didn't hurt.
ELMAN:	It didn't bother. Is that right?
PATIENT:	Yes.
ELMAN:	Was there any pressure there?
PATIENT:	Not enough to amount to pressure.
ELMAN:	[to doctors] You can remove the sense of pressure with many people with the depth of anesthesia you get by compounding. Those of you who need a very good grade of anesthesia will find that compounding enables you to get it . . . not only for deliveries, but for every type of work. Suppose we want to bring that

anesthesia some place else. Here's how you do it . . . [to patient] Put this hand right on top of your other hand. In about three seconds, that anesthesia will transfer to the other hand. You'll find that it's just shifted hands . . . How's the anesthesia in your right hand now?

PATIENT: It's there.

ELMAN: In other words, you can place the anesthesia anywhere . . . Put it in your toes, will you please. Touch your toes with your hand and just hold it there for a couple of seconds . . . How are your toes?

PATIENT: Numb.

ELMAN: Put that same anesthesia in your jaw and see what a good dental anesthesia you'll have . . . How's your jaw?

PATIENT: Real numb.

ELMAN: There's what I mean. You can move hypnotic anesthesia all around the body. If you have to work on both sides of the face . . . Watch, it's here now, and I want to bring it around to the other side, and there it is. How's the left side of your face?

PATIENT: Numb.

ELMAN: [to doctors] In other words, this is anesthesia you can work with. And what have I been doing? I've been compounding. Therefore, the anesthesia in her jaw will be stronger than the anesthesia she had in her hand since there have been about four or five compoundings since that time. I want you to see the depth of anesthesia we have here. Doctor, will you please test this patient for the anesthesia in her jaw? [Doctor makes test.] Excellent anesthesia—is that right? When you get anesthesia as good as that, it's pretty easy to work with . . . [to patient] What did you feel?

PATIENT: Enough to know he was in my mouth but not enough to bother.

ELMAN: [to doctors] Suppose we want all that anesthesia to disappear from every part of her body and have her feel wonderful, here's what we do . . . [to patient] Close your eyes. When I tell you to open your eyes, the anesthesia will disappear and you'll feel better than you've felt all day . . . Open your eyes . . . How do you feel?

PATIENT: Fine.

ELMAN: All the anesthesia gone?

PATIENT: Yes.

ELMAN: [to doctors] This is the thing that makes hypnosis work. From the beginning of hypnosis to its deepest state, it is all a matter of compounding. All you're doing at all times is developing a better state—a greater depth, and a greater anesthesia if it's anesthesia that you want. I want to show you something else about this. At no time do people in hypnosis lose awareness. Here is a little experiment to let you see that this patient in hypnosis has greater awareness than she could possibly have under ordinary circumstances. [to patient] Young lady, do you remember when you learned how to walk?

PATIENT: No.

ELMAN: Do you think anybody in this room remembers when he learned how to walk?

PATIENT: No.

ELMAN: Do you know that in the state in which we just had you we can let you see yourself learning how to walk? People have a funny idea about life. They think they forget things. Nobody ever forgets anything. Everything that we pass through in our lifetime makes an impression and we store it away. And when awareness is sufficiently increased so that we can pull that little remembrance out of its drawer—out of its hiding place—we get a very thrilling effect. If you asked all the people in this room, "Do you remember back to the time when you learned how to walk?" they'd say, "No." But every one of them does remember . . . [to doctors] Let me show you that concealed within this person is the memory of herself learning how to walk. She will see the people who were there—mother and dad, brothers and sisters if she had any. She'll be able to see them as she was learning how to walk . . . [to patient] Close your eyes. Make the numbers disappear, and you'll be right back in the state in which you were before . . . Numbers all gone? Make them disappear. You can do that right away.

PATIENT: They're all gone.

ELMAN: Fine. Now, here's what is going to happen. I'm going to open the drawer for you—or help you open the drawer in which is stored the memory of your learning how to walk. I'm going to snap my fingers and you will see an actual vision, an actual memory, of yourself learning to walk. And if it was an interior scene, you'll see the furniture that was there. You'll see the people who were there and how they were dressed, and you'll see yourself and how you were dressed. If it was an exterior scene, you'll be able to tell us what time of the year it was by the weather and not only will you be able to tell us what time of the year it was, but how you were dressed and how they were dressed, and what was said . . . Now, when I snap my fingers you will have that vision . . . When I snap them the second time you will open your eyes and tell us what you saw and the words that you heard spoken . . . All right now, here it is. [snaps fingers] Now when I snap my fingers again, you can tell us all that you saw. [snaps fingers] There it is. Now you can open your eyes . . . What did you see?

PATIENT: A couch.

ELMAN: And where were you?

PATIENT: In the middle of the floor.

ELMAN: Were you standing or sitting?

PATIENT: Sitting.

ELMAN: And what happened?

PATIENT: I walked to the couch.

ELMAN: What color was the couch?

PATIENT: Red.

ELMAN: And who was there beside you?

PATIENT: Mother.

ELMAN: How does she look?

PATIENT: A lot younger.

ELMAN: You noticed how she was dressed, didn't you?

PATIENT: No.

ELMAN: How were you dressed?

PATIENT: In a little yellow dress.

ELMAN: Now, in your mind's eye, take a look at your mother and tell us how she was dressed. Close your eyes and see her . . . There she is . . . How was she dressed?

PATIENT: A print dress with colors.

ELMAN: Is she helping you to walk or are you walking all by yourself?

PATIENT: By myself.

ELMAN: All right, you can open your eyes now. How does it feel to be able to see yourself learning to walk again?

PATIENT: It's a funny feeling.

ELMAN: It's a funny feeling to think that you have a

mind that good, isn't it? But remember, every person in this room would be able to do the very same thing . . . [to doctors] You can do it when you have the awareness brought on by the state the young lady is in. I'm going to remove the suggestions, but she'll still remember everything . . . [to patient] Close your eyes, please. When I have you open your eyes, you'll know that this is a very pleasant thing to be able to remember, and all the suggestions I gave you about this vision will be over, but you'll remember everything very clearly. And notice how good you feel . . . All right, you can open your eyes now . . . How do you feel?

PATIENT: Fine.

ELMAN: Can you see what I mean by increased awareness? I could also bring her back to the first remembrance she ever had when her intelligence formed, the first impression that was implanted after her memory formed. We'll go into that when we get to hypnoanalysis. This was to let you see that the state which we develop is one of keen awareness. It is not unconsciousness. It is not a state that you have to fear. This is a state in which the mind works so well and the law of self-preservation works so beautifully that no one could ever take advantage of you in the hypnotic state. That is why in the history of the world no harm or damage has been done by hypnosis. Unfortunately, there are books about this subject by authors who don't know how to explain these things, so they infest it with figments of their own imagination. People have infested hypnosis with a lot of false ideas. It is perhaps one of the most beautiful states that God has made possible to mankind, and this beautiful state contains nature's own anesthesia which He makes available to every one of us. But it has been abused sorely by people trying to make it voodoo, black magic. It's not.

When you're taught to look at hypnosis properly, you see it as a very beautiful, wonderful thing that God has made possible . . . [to patient] You've experienced it. Isn't it lovely?

PATIENT: Yes.

ELMAN: Here's a thing which has helped her to get rid of the nausea and vomiting of pregnancy. Here is something which makes it possible for her to remember when she was a baby, perhaps less than a year old. Should she not look upon it as a wonderful state?

There should be no fear with hypnosis. Even the wonderful states that you've seen tonight can be ruined by fear. Don't let fear enter. Don't let a nurse or doctor who doesn't know the semantics of hypnosis say the wrong thing in the presence of the patient. Think of an expectant mother's reactions when she hears a nurse exclaim, "My God, you're not going to let her have all her contractions and the delivery without any anesthesia at all, are you?" I have my doctor-students practice on each other and know everything that they're going to put their patients through. The reason so many misconceptions have crept into hypnosis is that thousands and thousands of well-intentioned people have studied hypnosis from the outside in instead of from the inside out. When you look upon hypnosis from the inside out, you know what is happening and you lose your fear of it. That's why I like the doctor to know what he's going to do to his patient; I want him to know what his patient is thinking and feeling. And when hypnotic anesthesia is given, how little he is feeling. I want my doctors to feel the anesthesia made possible by compounding suggestion and how beautifully the anesthesia develops.

In practicing this, bear in mind that you may encounter artificial somnambulism, which is almost impossible to work with. All you've got is light hypnosis. Now watch the method of turning artificial somnambulism into true somnambulism . . . [to a doctor serving as a patient, who had previously failed to achieve true somnambulism] I'm going to lift your hand and when I drop it, the lights will go out and the numbers will be all gone . . . Are the numbers gone?

PATIENT: Yes.

ELMAN: Now why did he fail before and why did he succeed this time? He was trying too hard to help and afraid he couldn't do it. He kept himself so worried that he didn't follow orders and therefore didn't relax properly. He'll tell you himself that that's what happened . . . [to patient] Doctor can you tell the difference between the way you are now relaxed and the way you were before?

PATIENT: Yes.

ELMAN: [to doctors] Let me show you again the technique I use when the numbers don't disappear. I lift his hand and say, "When I drop your hand the lights will go out and you won't see any more numbers . . . There you are . . . The lights are out and all the numbers are gone . . . That's how you change artificial to true somnambulism. In compounding anesthesia, all you need to begin with is a *little* anesthesia. But if you ask the patient how he feels after you have given an anesthesia suggestion, and he says, "Not much different," and then you compound—you can go on compounding to the end of time, and nothing times nothing equals nothing. He's got to have a little anesthesia to compound for greater anesthesia.
This doctor here has had some difficulty with this patient in compounding anesthesia. The patient acts as though not much is happening, but I believe he has ample anesthesia and I would suggest that you test him. Give him a

gentle dental test at first to be sure he has the anesthesia. [Dental test is given.]

DOCTOR: I have been testing for several seconds. What did you feel?

PATIENT: I could hardly feel anything, but I knew you were working there.

DOCTOR: I was breaking down tissue.

PATIENT: I didn't know that. I didn't feel anything. I didn't think I had anesthesia because I thought when a jaw has anesthesia it just feels frozen. It didn't feel like I thought it would. I didn't feel anything, although I could tell at the end that you were bearing down harder than at first, but it didn't bother.

*   *   *

When you change the artificial to true somnambulism, you can notice the way the person get increased relaxation as the true state comes along. There is a terrific difference. Patients describe this difference as a feeling of being more content; there are no conflicts once the numbers disappear. In somnambulism, suggestions become tremendously more effective and many more kinds of suggestions can be given. The truly somnambulistic patient is almost entirely uncritical of the suggestions that are given and will, to the extent of his capabilities and his needs, endeavor to accept them.

In the light state of hypnosis, the patient seems to be saying to the doctor, "I hope this works." Once he enters the deep state, however, the attitude of the patient seems to be, "I know this is going to work. This *must* work." And so it works. I believe if the doctor can understand the true reason why people accept suggestions better in somnambulism, he will be more adroit with hypnosis. Here, then, is the explanation:

You know already that hypnosis is a form of relaxation. As the patient relaxes more and more, deeper and deeper, a feeling of euphoria is brought on—a feeling of well-being, of contentment—which the patient has, perhaps, never before known. As this feeling increases, he gets a greater sense of confidence in himself and the doctor. In this euphoric state it seems to the patient that all is right with the world and that anything within human reason is possible. He therefore accepts at face value—without criticism—any suggestion that appears reasonable and pleasing to him.

Again, let me stress that in somnambulism you do not achieve a zombie-like state. The patient does not lose consciousness. Instead, he gains awareness. It has been estimated by various authorities on the subject that in somnambulism awareness of the patient is increased up to two thousand percent.

Take the young lady who was able to see herself learning how to walk again. Your awareness must be increased tremendously to be able to do this. I have a tenacious enough memory so that, without the aid of hypnosis, I can think back to incidents that occurred when I was three or four years old, but when I try to remember anything that happened when I was about a year old or less, I find it impossible. When awareness is sufficiently increased I can do it; so can you. And you see things buried that far back very clearly.

Note that the young woman in the demonstration was able to say that she had on a yellow dress. She was able to say that her mother was wearing a print dress that had colors in it. She actually saw these things in color.

You know what you have to do to achieve this state. Having advanced this far, you are at liberty to short-cut without fear of failing repeatedly or being fooled by artificial somnambulism. Endeavor to obtain the deep state within a minute.

But what do you do when you meet with resistance on the part of the patient? Don't try to produce the hypnotic state. Since hypnosis is a consent state, it is useless to carry on when resistance is there. In certain cases, a doctor can eliminate much of this resistance by saying to the patient, "Too bad. You don't want treatment the easy way. You'll have to have it the hard way." The patient usually becomes apologetic—afraid of the pain that may ensue if treatment is given the hard way—and will try to cooperate. With resistance gone you will be able to gain the state for many of these difficult patients.

If the patient continues to resist, quit trying. When someone fights me for more than a minute, I stop, noting to myself, "The patient doesn't seem to realize that I want to

help him.   If he doesn't realize that I want to help him, he
will have to undergo treatment the hard way."

This is the sensible attitude even in cases of delivery. If
the woman does not want to cooperate to the extent of relaxing in order to get the state in which painless delivery is
possible—if she insists on feeling the delivery—let her feel it.
There is nothing brutal in this attitude because if you let her
feel a contraction or two, she'll generally say, "Oh doctor,
help me to relax."   Then you'll find that you can get her into
the state, despite her tense frame of mind at such a time, and
can help her the rest of the way.

However, in the case of the rare patient who continues
to show conflict, resistance, fight, hypnosis is of little use
because it is a consent state.   Don't go on fighting back when
you're bound to be the loser.   Quit trying.   Use whatever
aids you've always used for your patients before you started
employing hypnosis.

Working with the patient with his eyes wide open in
deep hypnosis seems to be one of the things which the average doctor does not fully understand. The technique is to
give the patient a suggestion, while the eyes are closed, which
will stay in effect when the eyes are opened. An anesthetic
suggestion is the perfect device to keep the hypnosis riding.
It's a good medical way.   Then you can do all your work
with the eyes wide open.   It's a technique that is much to be
preferred for many people.

You can tell an amateur from a good hypnotic operator
by noticing whether he has learned to handle patients with
their eyes open.   If he can work with the eyes open, he knows
what he's doing.

One advantage of the eyes-open state is just this: no
one who walks into your office will know immediately that
you're using hypnosis.   You will not be worried about startling someone who has not been properly introduced to the
phenomenon.

Remember, this is not the same as waking hypnosis.
It's deep somnambulism with the eyes open, a completely
different state.   It's in this eyes-open state that you can say,
"I'm going to transfer the anesthesia from this hand to that
leg." You can say, "I'll snap my fingers and the anesthesia
will jump down to your toes."

You'll also notice that when you get this deep state there

isn't the tendency to come out of it that is present in the light state. A patient will only come out of it prematurely if something happens to frighten him or if you give him the wrong kind of suggestion. If you say, "That hurt, didn't it?" he will snap right out of the hypnosis. Don't do that. You should know the proper semantics to use by this time.

Open-eyed somnambulism has still further advantages. The patient can cooperate more fully with the doctor, pointing out troublesome areas, for example. The ophthalmologist obviously needs this state, as he works completely with the human eyes. The fact that the eyes can be kept wide open while the patient remains in deep somnambulism makes this the optimum state for him. Other medical and dental men find this state to be advantageous according to their requirements.

The doctor who treats his patients in this state is looked upon as a skillful practitioner, and for good reason. With proper technique, the patient has no realization that hypnosis has been used. He will not frighten uninitiated, perhaps superstitious, fellow patients. If questioned, he will usually say, "How could I have been hypnotized? I was wide awake and watched the doctor's entire treatment." Actually, you're always wide awake in hypnosis. You're never asleep, but most people are ignorant of this fact.

So that there's no possibility of confusion, be sure that you understand what a posthypnotic suggestion is. A posthypnotic suggestion is one given while the patient is in hypnosis to take effect after the patient is roused from the state. If you have been practicing the techniques described in this book, you have been working with posthypnotic suggestions from the beginning. When you give a health suggestion, it's posthypnotic. You say, "When I have you open your eyes, you're going to feel better than you've felt all day." You have been working constantly with posthypnotic suggestions applied to medicine and dentistry.

Chapter 13

THE ESDAILE STATE

THERE is a book by Doctor George Bankoff, a Fellow of the Royal College of Surgeons, entitled "The Conquest of Pain," and subtitled, "The Story of Anesthesia." In Doctor Bankoff's work is a report about a physician named Pien Chiao. Doctor Chiao, who lived about twenty-three centuries ago, claimed that two men visited him one day and he gave them a drink which reduced them to unconsciousness for three whole days.

Doctor Chiao penned this fantastic description of the incident: "Then I operated on them and explored the regions of the stomach and the heart. I then cut out the heart and stomach and exchanged them in these two persons. Such was the wonder of the drug that they uttered no sound, and in a few days I suffered them to return home, fully recovered."

Of course, knowing what we do about surgery, this is probably a tall tale. But the point is, his words show that physicians of his day took a great interest in anesthesia.

There is a tendency to look upon anesthesia as fairly modern. As a matter of fact, healers have been searching for good anesthesia since prehistoric times, and may have discovered it thousands of years ago.

In a papyrus known as the Ebers papyrus, accredited to 1600 B.C., is found a statement translated as follows: "Suggested as a useful treatment for the extraction of splinters: Cook the blood of worms and mix it in oil. Then kill a mole, cook it and drain it in oil, and follow it by mixing the dung of an ass in milk. Apply the paste with the proper incantations."

The "proper incantations," a favorite prescription in primitive medicine, amount to waking hypnosis.

Hypnosis was known and used under various names thousands and thousands of years ago. It has been called everything from Yar-Phoonk (in a Hindi dialect) to voodoo, magic, incantations. Before the days of Mesmer it was called

118

magnetism. Then its name was changed to mesmerism, then Braid came along and originated the words hypnosis and hypnotism (and tried to change the name to "monodeism" when he realized that hypnosis was not sleep, after all).

Opium and, in fact, derivatives of everything from poppies to Indian snakeroot found anesthetic employment during the development of modern medicine. But while chemical anesthesia was, and is, of vast importance in the history of healing, it does not have the advantages of mental anesthesia.

The first man of modern times to really rediscover this great power and put it to good use extensively was an English surgeon by the name of James Esdaile. He became interested in mesmerism before the word hypnosis was even known.

He went to India in 1845 and the work he did there with mesmerism is astounding even in the light of present knowledge. However, he failed to realize that it was the power of suggestion with which he was working. All he knew was that if he followed Mesmer's techniques and applied them diligently, he could achieve a better state of mesmerism than Mesmer himself had ever known. It took him a long time to develop this remarkable state. According to reports which I have read, it would take him an hour and a half or more in many instances.

It is worth noting that these were the days before modern anesthesia and the patients on whom he worked needed something which would alleviate pain; they reached desperately for the state that Esdaile attempted to create.

In this state, he was able to perform remarkable feats of surgery. It is said on good authority that he did every type of surgery known at the time—including amputations, abdominal surgery and various types of suturing for assorted wounds. Some books report that he did over three hundred deep abdominal surgical procedures in this state which was then completely unknown in medicine.

Mortality in surgery in Esdaile's day was fifty percent. Esdaile was able to reduce this mortality rate to eight percent by the use of his techniques, and his patients recovered more quickly and easily than the average surgical cases of his day.

He came back to England thrilled with his discovery,

eager to show the surgeons at home a method by which to reduce mortality and make surgery painless. In his lectures he tried to produce the state before audiences of medical men. He didn't realize that their very resistance would prevent them from entering the state. Doctors ridiculed him, calling him fake, charlatan and quack. Nevertheless, he opened a hospital in London, where he continued the work he had done in India.

There was only one man in England who believed in Esdaile's techniques. This was a doctor by the name of John Elliotson. Elliotson came to his hospital and watched Esdaile work about an hour and a half to achieve the necessary state on a patient, and then perform painless surgery. Elliotson became his staunchest supporter.

As a result, Doctor Elliotson, who was a professor of Practical Medicine in the University of London, was forced to resign his professorship. Esdaile was soon forced to close his hospital.

No doctors were able to duplicate Esdaile's feats. Incredulous as they were, many of them attempted to duplicate what Esdaile said was possible, but none of them knew how. All they succeeded in getting was a mild analgesia—nothing practical for surgery. In my estimation, all they got was light hypnosis. They didn't know how to correct their mistakes, and they certainly wouldn't ask Esdaile. In fact, they wouldn't even discuss their experiments among themselves. Nobody wanted anybody else to know he was working towards this wonderful thing and trying to duplicate the "charlatan's" success. Esdaile's career was ruined and so was Elliotson's. They died bitterly disappointed men.

Now we must turn for a moment to the stage operator and his work with thousands of hypnotized people. Every once in a while, such an entertainer would encounter a remarkable thing which he called the hypnotic coma because the people who entered this state *appeared* to be in a coma. They didn't move, they didn't speak, they simply didn't respond to anything. They would take no suggestions of any kind, including the one to come out of the state.

The stage operator was well aware of the fact that subjects in somnambulism could accept or reject suggestions as they chose. If the subjects didn't accept certain suggestions which he offered them in somnambulism, he either ignored them and worked with others or gave them suggestions they would take so that he could continue with his demonstration.

However, the coma subjects would accept no suggestion of any kind no matter how pleasing or reasonable the stage operator believed them to be. These coma subjects presented a problem because they not only did not participate in the action but, sitting there in the coma state, they distracted the audience. They were a nuisance.

The operator had to devise ways of getting rid of these people. How could he do it since they would not get up and walk off the stage? To carry them off would be disastrous. Moreover he had no way of knowing before hypnosis which of the subjects would go into the coma state. He was forced to develop techniques to meet the situation, and he eventually found several different ways of getting problem subjects out of the coma state. Sometimes these methods could be quite lengthy.

The stage operator was often embarrassed because the audience would become alarmed when subjects went into hypnotic coma. Therefore, when a stage operator finally succeeded in devising ways of bringing subjects out of hypnotic coma, he kept the information from his rivals. He never realized, of course, that he had inadvertently stumbled into the Esdaile state. If he had realized it, what could he do with it? When he succeeded in rousing the coma subjects he encountered, he was so glad to get rid of them that he dismissed them peremptorily.

It was necessary for me, like every other stage operator, to devise ways of rousing coma subjects. After rousing such a subject (by the trial-and-error method of simply working until I did rouse him) instead of dismissing him, I asked questions. I wanted to know why such people reacted differently to hypnosis than the average subject. From what they told me—*and they all told me the same thing*—I was finally able to devise a technique to bring coma subjects out of the state instantaneously.

By asking questions of these subjects, I quickly learned that the coma state was one of euphoria and that the subject merely didn't want to be disturbed. That was the reason he wouldn't come out of it. He had never had such a pleasant experience and he didn't want his enjoyment to be interrupted.

Upon learning this, it was easy enough to devise a sure-fire technique. All you had to do was to say to the subject who was in the coma state that if he didn't obey your instructions and rouse himself, he could never be hypnotized again. This was so effective that the subjects roused themselves instantly, and thereupon the coma no longer presented a problem.

When I first began teaching, I believed, like most students of the subject, that the coma could only be produced accidently, never on purpose. I didn't recognize that this was the Esdaile state. But by various tests I had made, I knew that the patients were completely anesthetized, just as Esdaile had claimed they would be. I also knew that they were completely immobilized. You couldn't get them to raise an arm or a leg. You couldn't induce them to open their eyes. The people who went into the hypnotic coma became catatonic.

If you lifted the leg of a subject, for example, it would stay in any position you put it into and would remain there indefinitely. It didn't matter how awkward a position you put it into. There was no rigidity in the limb; it felt just like wax and when you moved a leg it felt just as though you were moving wax, except that it remained in whatever position you moved it to.

Here is what Esdaile said of a patient in the coma state: "I extended her arm at a right angle to her body, in which position, or any other, it remained fixed till moved again, and her sister-in-law pricked her hand unheeded. I awoke her with considerable difficulty. The headache was quite gone, and she felt, and looked, greatly refreshed.

"The balance between the flexor and extensor muscles is so perfect, that any new position given to the head, trunk, or extremities, by an external force, is easily received, and steadily maintained. This passive energy of the muscular system, permitting the body to be moulded into almost as great a variety of attitudes as if it were a figure of wax or lead, is the distinguishing characteristic."

This confirms the fact that the patient in the hypnotic coma becomes catatonic, and is automatically anesthetized without suggestion.

The most maligned phase of hypnosis is the completely misnamed and misunderstood hypnotic coma. Esdaile refers to it as the mesmeric coma and again as somnambulism, confusing the two states. It has been misunderstood and mishandled by so many people because they never thoroughly investigated the state. Doctors all over the world were warned by textbooks and teachers that the hypnotic coma occurred accidentally in about one out of fifteen thousand patients, and that if they encountered or accidentally produced the coma, it was just one of those unfortunate incidents in medicine. The textbooks warned doctors to beware of it, stating that the doctor might be unable to rouse the patient from the state. Some of the books go on to say, "If a patient goes into coma, let him alone, and the coma will turn into natural sleep from which the patient will waken normally in from fifteen minutes to eight hours."

Books making this declaration (and you can find such a statement in hundreds of them) prove that their authors know little or nothing about the state. Their conjectures are entirely erroneous.

In the first place, few people, if any, find it possible to fall asleep in the hypnotic state. The statement that the coma will change to natural sleep is false. The patient will rouse himself if left alone for an indefinite period, but if interviewed and asked the question, "Were you asleep at any time?" will invariably say something like, "No, I was just so completely relaxed that I didn't want to be disturbed."

But doctors have looked upon the hypnotic coma as dangerous, and when they have encountered it, they have not paused to investigate. They have just let it completely alone, not realizing it could be of value to them.

You will find many people today who believe that hypnosis is dangerous because of the possibility that a subject will go into the hypnotic coma. At a demonstration, you occasionally will hear people in the audience saying, "What will happen if you can't wake him up?" They don't realize that no one in the world has ever been in hypnosis who hasn't come out of it.

Like everyone else, I believed at first that the coma occurred accidentally only and that there was no way of obtaining it intentionally. I had been teaching doctors how to rouse patients from the coma because I felt that if they used my technique they would run into the coma in far more than one in fifteen thousand cases. Therefore, I found it necessary to teach them the rapid method I had found for bringing patients out of the coma. To show you how effective this was, I would like to relate an incident that occurred in Fair Lawn, New Jersey, a number of years ago.

A stage operator had come to town to give a demonstration, and someone in the audience went into the coma. The people sitting around this person began to be violently upset. The stage operator came down off the stage and assured the audience that there was no cause for alarm, that he could rouse the person quite easily. He then proceeded to use his usual techniques, but the subject didn't respond.

The stage operator continued to assure the audience that he would rouse the subject if given sufficient time. In the minutes that followed, the audience became agitated because none of his techniques seemed to work. One of my doctors happened to be in the audience. He walked up to the stage operator, and said, "I can rouse him instantly. I am a doctor."

The operator said, "He doesn't need a doctor. What do you know about hypnosis?"

"I've studied the subject," the doctor replied, "and I wish you would let me try."

"Go ahead," the operator said. "After you've given up, I'll continue."

The doctor walked up to the subject, whispered a few words into his ear, and the subject roused himself immediately.

This story appeared in newspapers all over the country, and a great deal of credit was given to the doctor. I took pride in the fact that he was one of my students.

Another incident also showed how effective my rousing technique is. One of my doctors and his wife were in a restaurant with another physician and his wife. The doctor-student began to talk about my rapid methods of induction and how effective they are. The other doctor said, "Try it on my wife."

My doctor hypnotized her, and she immediately went into the coma state, whereupon her husband became alarmed and said, "I've studied hypnosis, and I've been told to beware of the coma. You can't bring them out of it and you have to let them sleep it off. I can't let her sleep it off here. I'm going to try to bring her out of it." He thereupon tried, uunsuccessfully. My doctor then whispered a few words into the lady's ear, and she came out of the state immediately.

For many years, doctors attending my classes had been told about the coma and how to rouse a patient from it. But because it was not known that the coma could be produced intentionally at any time, the students seldom got a chance to observe the state in class. I was teaching a class in Baltimore, when one of the doctors said to me, "I have a patient who goes so deeply into somnambulism that I believe with a little coaxing from you, we could get him into the coma state. I would like to see the hypnotic coma."

I told him I would try. I felt that if I did my utmost to produce a coma and didn't succeed, it would prove that the coma couldn't be achieved intentionally. I had no idea that it was the Esdaile state.

The following week, the doctor brought the patient to class and asked me to work with him. I told him, "You get him into somnambulism. Then I'll go on from there." And so he put his patient into the somnambulistic state.

As I remember, I spoke to the patient more or less like this: "I know how relaxed you are, but even in your relaxed state I'll bet you sense in your own mind that there is a state of relaxation below the one you're in right now. Can you sense that?

The patient answered, "Yes."

I continued, "You know that you can clench your fist and make it tighter and tighter and tighter—and you might call that the height of tension. You can relax that same fist until you can't relax it any more. You might call that the basement of relaxation. I'm going to try to take you down to the basement.

"To get down to floor A, you have to relax twice as much as you have relaxed already. To get down to floor B, you have to relax twice as much as you did at floor A, and to get down to C, you have to relax twice as much as you did at floor B. But when you reach floor C, that is the basement of relaxation, and at that point you will give off signs by which I will be able to tell that you are at the basement. You don't know what these signs are, and I'm not going to tell you what they are, but every person who has ever been at the basement of relaxation gave off those signs . . . Let's get started.

"You will ride down to floor A on an imaginary elevator and you will use that same elevator to get down to the basement of relaxation. You are on that elevator now. When I snap my fingers, that elevator will start down. If you relax twice as much as you have relaxed already you will be down at floor A. Tell me when you are at floor A by saying the letter A out loud."

In about thirty seconds, he murmured "A" in an almost indistinguishable voice. I followed a similar procedure, taking him down to floor B. It was almost impossible for him to say the letter B out loud, but he formed the sound with his lips. When he reached floor C, he was unable to speak, and not a muscle moved.

The depth of relaxation was astounding. Then, without a word of suggestion, we proceeded to give him the first test for the coma state—that is, a test for general anesthesia. The doctors tested him in various ways and the anesthesia was profound.

Remember, not a word of suggestion had been given to produce hypnotic anesthesia. It occurred automatically.

The second test we made was to order him to lift his leg. He didn't respond. There was a quiver in his leg, suggesting that he was trying very hard to move it, and then he apparently gave up trying. The third test was made on a smaller group of muscles, those around his eyes. The suggestion was given that he open his eyes. He didn't follow this suggestion either. I then lifted his arm and found it to be completely catatonic. It stayed in whatever position we put it into. The doctors put him into various positions, and no matter what position he was put into, he stayed that way.

To my knowledge, this was the first intentional coma recorded since Esdaile's time. Now that we had produced the coma, the doctors suggested that we leave the patient in this state for a while so that they could experiment. They wanted to see the reactions of a patient in the coma state.

One of the many experiments they performed was to put a lighted match between the patient's forefinger and thumb, closing the two digits tightly around the lighted match. When the flame reached the end of the match, the patient's fingers moved imperceptibly and the match fell to the floor. We did this repeatedly, always with the same results. We could never see the fingers move, yet at just the right moment the match fell to the floor.

We spent several hours making tests. Then we decided it was time to rouse the patient since it was almost 2:00 A.M. I had taught these doctors how to rouse a coma patient, but they decided, for experimental purposes, to try other ways. The doctors came up with a number of suggestions. They gave him simple suggestions that it was time to go home, that his family was waiting for him, etc. Nothing happened.

Then someone said, "We're all going home and we'll leave you here by yourself unless you open your eyes this minute." Nothing happened.

Then someone shouted, "Better wake up and get out of here! There's a fire!" Nothing happened.

Finally the doctors decided to rouse the patient by the method they had been taught. After he was aroused—without difficulty—the doctors decided to spend some more time questioning him. They wanted to find out about his reactions in the state. One of the things they asked was about the lighted match. He said, "When I thought it might burn me, I dropped the match. I didn't even worry about the match burning the doctor's carpet because I knew you were all here, and someone would put it out."

He volunteered the information that he had heard and understood everything that went on around him during the time he was in the coma state, and was able to tell us exactly what had transpired.

Thereupon, someone said, to him, "If you heard and understood everything that was going on, when someone shouted, 'Fire, let's get out of here,' why didn't you budge?" He answered, "Because I knew there was no fire. I heard you all whispering that you were going to pretend there was a fire and that you would shout the word fire to alarm me. I heard you discussing every test you planned to make and I knew at all times exactly what was going on around me. I had no reason to be alarmed. If there was a fire, why didn't anyone leave the room?"

It had been a thrilling experience for the doctors, to say nothing of the teacher. I couldn't help wishing the experiment could be duplicated in every class. The patient had entered the coma state with a minimum of coaxing after he had reached somnambulism.

The following day as we were driving to Philadelphia for our next class, my wife pointed out that he didn't seem to be any deeper in somnambulism than many doctors who attend our classes. "If you could do it once," she asked, "why couldn't you do it again with others?"

I said, "What happened last night was a complete accident. I hit that one in fifteen thousand, and it just wouldn't happen like that again. I couldn't be that lucky."

My wife said, "I don't think it was luck. At least, it's worth trying."

We arrived in Philadelphia, conducted the class as usual, and at the conclusion of the session I told the doctors what had happened in Baltimore the night before. I asked them if they would like to see the technique I used to produce intentional coma. Perhaps there were other people who would react the same way as last night's patient had.

The doctors were quite excited about the prospect, so I asked for a volunteer. I used the same technique I had used in Baltimore, and much to my astonishment, produced a second coma.

I had soon produced seven comas in seven consecutive classes. From then on I decided that this must be a definite part of my course. Whether we would be successful in every class didn't matter. The doctors should know that it was possible.

I guess I was lucky that first seven times because the eighth time I tried it I met with failure. I asked for another volunteer, and this time I succeeded.

In subsequent classes, I would fail every once in a while and would have to ask for a second volunteer, sometimes even a third. This was time-consuming. By now the doctors had heard that the coma could be produced intentionally, and they weren't satisfied until they saw it.

At one of these classes, I proceeded in my usual way to ask for a volunteer, but two ladies came forward. I decided that I might save time by trying with two people at once. In this way I would increase my chances of getting the coma. As it happened, both women went into the coma simultaneously. From then on I asked for two or more volunteers, and after a while, I was producing comas in four and five people simultaneously.

One of the facts we verified was that the time varied as to when each person would go into the coma. One patient would go into it after just a few moments of suggestion; but another wouldn't go into the coma for a few minutes more. I could never get them to go into the coma at the same time, even though they all did eventually.

Now we were able to produce hypnotic coma at will but we didn't have the slightest idea how it could be used medically. The patients were immobilized and didn't respond to suggestions once they reached the coma. What could a doctor do with a patient like that? Much experimentation was done with the coma in our classes. The patients were interviewed by doctors after being brought out of the state, and it soon became apparent that many misconceptions regarding the coma had crept into the literature.

Rather than being a state which is to be avoided, we found that patients described it as "the best state of hypnosis there is. It's wonderful. I don't know when I was so beautifully relaxed." The doctors began trying to induce the coma state in themselves. When they succeeded, they were equally enthusiastic about it. In Philadelphia one Sunday afternoon, a doctor in class went into the coma three times to let his colleagues study it. More doctors tried it. All reported on it in glowing terms.

The explanation doctors and patients give is that the coma brings with it a complete and entire euphoria. Rather than allow themselves to be disturbed, when anyone gave them a pain impulse, they completely disregarded it, thereby giving themselves complete general anesthesia.

Many doctors and patients reported that they could not even feel pressure in the state; others reported that they could feel something was being done to them, but didn't care. Some of them realized that in the state they were actually catatonic, and when told about it, ventured, "I was so comfortable, I guess it didn't matter much to me what position I was in. I just didn't want to be taken out of that wonderful state of well-being."

Some denied having been catatonic, apparently blotting that portion of the experiment from their memories.

We often observed this little side light: Patient after patient and doctor after doctor, upon being brought out of the state, volunteered the information that there came a time during the coma when they wished everybody in the room would stop talking, particularly the operator.

We learned that despite the euphoria in the coma state, if something should happen to alarm a patient, he is quick to rouse himself and go into any necessary action. *He is not helpless.*

We have produced literally thousands of comas in class for our students, and over the years have had the opportunity to compare the enthusiastic reports of doctors and patients who have been in the state. Every report is fundamentally the same: Patients and doctors love it. Not one unpleasant incident has been reported.

Prior to our own research, nothing at all had been done to find out why nature makes this euphoric state possible. We have told our many students to do research work in it: "Produce the coma in patients in an attempt to learn how nature intended it to be used. It seems to be nature's own anesthesia which has been made available to mankind since the beginning of time. The more research work you do, the more the world will be benefitted. Use it in every way possible. Let's find out just how valuable it is and if it is a technique which every doctor can use."

Doctors have asked, "Couldn't a psychotic or a pre-psychotic patient use the coma state as a retreat from reality?" My answer to that is that psychotic or prepsychotic patients don't need hypnosis to retreat from reality. They find their own means of doing it. Thousands of psychotic patients who have never experienced hypnosis to their knowledge, or even know the word, have retreated from reality.

Many psychiatrists use the Esdaile state in their work and are highly enthusiastic about it. Not one has reported unfavorably on it.

Some years ago, a number of doctors began using the coma state in arthritis and cancer cases to relieve intractible pain, and reported splendid success with it. Other doctors say it is quite useful in postoperative procedures, particularly when they want the patient to be immobilized in a particular position for an extended period without postoperative discomfort.

We finally learned another splendid use for the coma state. One of the doctors in class announced to his colleagues,

"This week I did two nose and throat operations on patients in the coma state, and I am of the firm opinion that the coma state is ideal for surgery. Imagine, in this state, without a word from me, the patients anesthetized themselves. No chemical anesthesia whatever was required. It is true that the patient won't take physical suggestions in the coma state as he does in somnambulism, but you have a patient who takes the surgery just as if he'd had a general anesthesia. It is remarkable for surgery, and I intend to do more operations using this state as time goes on."

When other doctors heard about his success, they tried the coma state for surgery, too. Obstetricians tried it for deliveries, and soon enthusiastic reports had come in from over one hundred doctors. The reports confirmed my suspicion: we had stumbled onto the Esdaile state.

As the reports continued coming in, I learned that one doctor did a complete hysterectomy in the coma state without any chemical anesthesia. Another doctor reported doing a radical breast resection the same way. Compound fractures were reduced in the coma state without chemical anesthesia; brain surgery, heart surgery and appendectomies were likewise reported.

In Newark, New Jersey, one day a doctor in class reported that he had used the coma for a delivery. Some of the doctors remarked, "Are you sure it wasn't somnambulism?" The doctor answered, "I have delivered women in somnambulism and I know the difference. This was the coma state. It was the most beautiful delivery I have ever seen. The patient maintained a smile during all of her contractions, during the episiotomy, delivery and repair. The only time she came out of the coma was at the instant the baby was born. She was so anxious to see her baby that she brought herself out. When she was satisfied, she went right back into the coma for the rest of the procedure. I tell you it was beautiful."

Soon, doctor after doctor reported handling deliveries in the coma state. Those who were not successful would say to me, "Maybe I didn't condition my patients properly. Couldn't we see how you would prepare a patient for delivery in the coma state." I asked them to bring their expectant mothers to class to prepare them for later delivery. Pretty soon the doctors were bringing pregnant women to class in great numbers in order to take advantage of my conditioning techniques. In each class, we spend a session preparing pregnant women for delivery. I have worked with as many as 102 pregnant women at one time, and 97 of the 102 went into the coma state. This figure is not presented as a boast but to show the percentage of success that may be expected.

This is the way to prepare a patient for surgery (or delivery) in the coma state of hypnosis:

The first thing you must do is to get the patient into somnambulism. Then explain that there is a basement to relaxation—a bottom floor—and you want to take the patient down to this bottom floor. Take him down to floor A, and you will find he is able to voice the letter A quite plainly. Tell him that in order to get down to floor B, he will have to relax twice as much as he did at floor A. When he gets to floor B, he may find difficulty in saying the letter B out loud, but tell him to do his utmost to say it out loud. Some patients will fail to be able to do it. This is a good sign.

Now, using the same procedure, take him down to floor C, at which point he should not be able to move his lips sufficiently to form the letter C.

When you are sure he is at floor C, without giving suggestions of any kind for anesthesia, take a pair of allis clamps or towel clips, and make a test for anesthesia. Don't use a word of suggestion for this If it is necessary to give suggestions for hypnotic anesthesia, you don't have the coma state.

When the patient has passed the test for anesthesia, he is ready for test number two.

Ask him to try to move a large group of muscles such as an arm or leg. If he is unable to move the big muscles; he is ready for the third test.

This should involve a small group of muscles such as those around the eyes. Ask him to try to open his eyes. If he does, he is not in the coma state, and you must take him down a flight further, until the eye muscles will not work.

In somnambulism when the patient tries to open his eyes you will see a movement of the muscles even though the eyes don't open. But in the true coma state, those tiny muscles don't work at all, and you see no movement whatever.

Your fourth test should be for catatonia. Realize that catatonia can be obtained in the lightest state of hypnosis.

Therefore, it means nothing unless it is the fourth test you make in the coma state. When a patient passes all of these four tests *in the exact order given,* you may be sure you have the true hypnotic coma, and can proceed from there. In your test for catatonia, no suggestions should be given. The catatonia must arrive by itself, without suggestions of any kind.

Never go on to a further test until the patient has passed the first one. Don't make test two until the patient has definitely passed test one; don't make test three until the patient has passed tests one and two, and so on.

When you obtain the Esdaile state, you will notice that the patient is truly incapable of taking a "physical" suggestion. When he is asked to raise his arm, the muscles may quiver. Then movement ceases. We have found that many patients, after coming out of the coma, are certain in their own minds that they followed the suggestions of the operator, and did raise the arm as requested. Remember, they can hear and understand every word you say.

In the true state of coma, though the patient's physical activities are immobilized—he truly cannot follow physical suggestions much as he might wish to do so—he is quite capable of taking "mental suggestions"—in which there is no physical movement. Our doctors have proved this in various ways. They have taken patients suffering from headaches, dysmenorrhea, and many other functional symptoms, put them into the coma state and given them suggestions for the relief of these symptoms. The patients did not have these symptoms at the time of induction. The suggestions were given as post-hypnotics, for the relief of these symptoms, quite successfully.

We have also talked to patients who have delivered babies while in this state, or have had major surgery done. These patients, in all cases, reported that while they were perhaps incapable of muscular effort, they were certainly able to take suggestions that did not involve movement. For example, surgical patients informed us that they would have appreciated a few remarks from the surgeon to the effect that the operation was proceeding nicely, and that the patient was doing well. The mothers who delivered babies in this state also assured us that a comforting word from the doctor would have been appreciated.

When physical cooperation is required—for example,

when moving the patient from cart to delivery table—have the patient come up to floor B to give the necessary cooperation; then have the patient go down again and stay down until such time as physical cooperation is needed again.

If you run into an accidental coma, the easiest way to rouse the patient is to whisper confidentially in the patient's ear, "If you don't open your eyes when I tell you to, you can never have this state again." This is an insidious suggestion because the patient wants to be able to reach that state again and again, and so he will promptly come out of it.

If, however, you are working with the coma and you use the technique described herein, when patients are down at the basement of relaxation, and you can't get them to open their eyes just tell them to come up to floor B, and they will be able to open their eyes quite easily. Bear these facts in mind when you produce the coma, and you will be delighted with your results.

It is important to know that in the coma state, the patient still retains the power of selectivity. In other words, he may accept or reject a suggestion as he sees fit, except suggestions for physical activity. If he does take a suggestion for physical activity he must terminate the state to do so.

In the many experiments we have conducted with patients in the coma state, we made every effort to give improper posthypnotic suggestions in order to test reaction. In every case the patient reacted like any other hypnotized subject. He either stayed in the state and later did not carry out the posthypnotic suggestion, or he instantly roused himself from the coma with the statement, "I would rather not do that."

Much research work remains to be done with the coma. It is up to medical and dental men to do that research. Please understand that we do not claim this is the best method for producing the hypnotic coma. It is merely the *first* method developed for producing it. Perhaps you may be able to perfect a better technique. One of our students has been working on a faster one:

I had been teaching in Tulsa, Oklahoma, and the following year I come back to conduct two more classes. As usual, old students showed up. One of them, a dentist by the name of Norval R. Smith, called me into the hall during intermission, and said, "Mr. Elman, may I speak with you privately for a minute? Either I have discovered something rather important or else I'm making an awful mistake, and I want your opinion on it. I'd been getting somnambulism in quite a number of my patients, but every once in a while I would fail because I couldn't get the patients to lose the numbers. I've been using the coma state whenever possible, and if I couldn't get somnambulism I figured there was no sense in trying to get the coma. One day, just for an experiment, I thought to myself, I'm not even going to ask the patients to lose the numbers . I'm just going to get the physical relaxation and see if I can take them down to the coma, bypassing the somnambulistic state entirely."

I smiled and said, "Of course, it didn't work."

He answered, "On the contrary, Mr. Elman. It worked beautifully. All I do is get the physical relaxation; then I take them down three flights, and they give off all four signs of the coma, and when I work on them, I have dental anesthesia without any suggestions having been given for it. Am I making a mistake, or am I not getting the Esdaile state you talk so much about?"

I didn't know how to answer him because I didn't know if what he said was possible. I told him, "Dr. Smith, if what you say works for you, it should work for all my doctors. I'm going to have a couple of hundred doctors try it and I'll give you a report on what they say."

About four weeks later I was able to tell Doctor Smith that I had reports from at least a hundred doctors who, using this technique, were successful in achieving the coma state.

I feel that Doctor Smith's discovery is extremely important, for it means that now a doctor can take a patient down to the coma in about five minutes. Try it for yourselves and see how easily you produce the state in which Doctor Esdaile did over three hundred deep abdominal surgical procedures. I am grateful to Doctor Smith for making this technique available.

Chapter 14

CONDITIONING FOR HYPNOTIC DELIVERY AND SURGERY

NOT very long ago, a medical report contained the statement that only twenty-five percent of expectant mothers can be aided by hypnotic delivery The experience of our doctors has shown that every woman who enters the delivery room can be helped, to some degree at least, by hypnosis, and in many of them complete freedom from discomfort can be obtained.

Some doctors report success in over ninety percent of their cases. Not every doctor has this high percentage of success but a surprisingly large number of them do. I was given a report recently by an obstetrician who stated that he never uses anything for delivery except hypnosis. He is one of the most popular obstetricians in his area and his services are constantly in demand.

Too many doctors do not realize the importance of semantics in preparing a patient for hypnotic delivery. I teach my doctors to give the patient a talk similar to the one that follows before they even attempt hypnosis for an expectant mother. This talk may be given at any time. It is not necessary to condition the patient during the first few months of pregnancy. I believe the ideal time for conditioning the patient is any time after the fourth month. Never use the word hypnosis in the presence of patients because this state is not yet properly understood by the public. It is my sincere hope that this book will help correct the misconceptions so many people have regarding the true value of hypnosis. I do not use the word hypnosis in speaking to patients, and I don't think you should. Just call it the Esdaile state. Patients expect—and want—a doctor to use esoteric, impressive terms, and this one is made to order for use in talking to them about an unfamiliar state without introducing fear or a feeling of mystery into your explanation. Here is the kind of talk I suggest giving expectant mothers:

"You are here for a very important purpose—so that you

can have your baby without feeling a thing, so that you can have your baby with a great big smile, so that you won't feel any discomfort, and the delivery of your baby will be a wonderful experience for you. I would not have had you come here for this purpose if I didn't know that all this is possible, and for your benefit.

"But first there are some things I want to discuss with you. There is one thing that can prevent your having a pain-free delivery despite the work that we do with you today. Only one thing—a thing called fear. Any kind of fear, no matter how small, can prevent you from achieving what you want at the time of delivery.

"You know, of course, that you will be given every possible aid for a pain-free delivery. You should have nothing to worry about. The only thing that should be on your mind is the fact that in a little while you will be seeing the wonderful baby you've been waiting for. Don't let little worries and annoyances interfere with this grand experience.

"When the time comes, you will have been conditioned for a pain-free delivery and will be in fine shape for it. Suppose it is now time for delivery and you are at the hospital, and you suddenly begin wondering if everything is all right at home, whether the baby sitter knows what to feed the children or whether there's sufficient food in the refrigerator.

"I am sure you realize this sort of worry is needless, and yet such thoughts can keep you from getting the state necessary for a pain-free delivery. The sort of worry that might occur to you could also be something like, 'I wonder how we're going to pay all the bills.' Or, 'I forgot to pay the gas bill. I hope they won't turn off the gas.' These are little worries. They are really unimportant compared to the great event that is about to take place. Your children at home will be well cared for. Your husband will take care of the necessary details at home. You have only one thing to do, only one thing to think about: having your baby as quickly and easily as possible. And you can do it!

"At the time of delivery you must be absolutely free of fear and worry if you want to have your baby easily. There should be only one thought in your mind—that in a little while you're going to see your baby, the baby you've been waiting for. We will have perfect results if you follow some simple instructions, and keep fear and worry out.

"If on the day of delivery, anything unpleasant has occurred, just say to yourself, 'That's not important now. I can straighten everything out when my baby comes. There's nothing so important as my baby right now, and that's all I'm going to think about.'

"I want you to know that if anything is troubling you, you should tell me about it. I'll do my best to help. My nurse or secretary can get a message to your husband or baby sitter if necessary. We will all be working together to make the delivery of your baby a memorable experience for you.

"Is it possible that you won't get this state that we're going to work for now? I don't know. That's up to you. If you regard this as a joke, you won't have it. If you sit there in your seat and say to yourself, 'No, I won't do what the doctor says,' you won't have it. What *do* you have to do? Just follow instructions, and believe me, these instructions are so simple even a baby could follow them.

"All you have to do is follow my instructions and you will be helped from that point on. Now let's be sure you're comfortable. Please get rid of anything in your hands or in your lap. Put your purse and gloves on the floor under your chair. Get rid of your wraps. Nothing should be in your hands or in your lap.

"If you are chewing gum, please take the gum out of your mouth. You can't relax all the muscles in your body properly when you're chewing gum. And I want you to be as relaxed and comfortable as possible.

"Incidentally, if you feel the need to use the bathroom, please do so right now. We can wait. You can't relax when nature is calling, and we don't want our procedure interrupted. Are you comfortable in your chair?

"All right, we will now get started. Please follow my instructions and you will have a wonderful experience ahead of you."

*   *   *

Now the doctor can begin preparing the patient for hypnotic delivery. And it should be noted that a busy obstetrician can do this with a whole roomful of women; he doesn't have to work with each patient alone. The first thing you must do is to get the patients into somnambulism. Make sure that you have true somnambulism or the instructions that follow will be ineffective. It is only in true somnambulism that patients will accept these suggestions. I emphasize this point because it is so important for success. Make sure that you are not working with artificial somnambulism. It must be true somnambulism if you want your patients to enjoy pain-free delivery.

Assuming that you now have a given patient in true somnambulism, keep her that way and address her as follows:

"I want to tell you about the benefits of relaxation. You know very well that if you were tense and I had to give you an injection, you'd feel the entrance of that needle very sharply because of the fact that you were tense, wouldn't you? But suppose you were relaxed like this. You wouldn't be able to feel the injection at all just because of the fact that you were absolutely and utterly relaxed. You can reach such a state of relaxation that you have no discomfort at all at delivery time. It is in this state, when you are physically and mentally relaxed that it is so easy to have a baby. It's in this state that the contractions, instead of being unpleasant, become very pleasant.

"The average mother-to-be has heard talk from friends, or relatives perhaps, that having a baby is a horrible ordeal. So she looks forward to what she has heard described as labor and labor pains and hard labor. There's no such thing as labor or labor pains or hard labor. There's no such thing associated with the birth of a baby. All those terms are false names that keep a mother's attitude in exactly the wrong state.

"But we can change that to the right attitude by having you know just what does happen when a baby is born. Nature has a method of making the birth of your baby possible by contractions. Each contraction you have helps push the baby a little bit forward so that the baby can be born very easily.

"Now, you do have contractions. But you don't have labor and you don't have labor pains or hard labor. All you have are these contractions. And the odd thing about these contractions is that if you look forward to them pleasantly and know that they are going to be something nice to have, you won't mind them at all. You'll know you're having contractions, but you'll only feel them in a pleasant way. Here's what will happen. When you have the first contraction, I want you to let me know and I'll tell you what to do from that point on. Then when you're at the place of delivery, I want you to close your eyes just as you have them

closed now and relax completely, just as you are relaxed now.
I'll be there to help you with the birth of your baby, but
until I get there I want you to relax as you're relaxed now,
and then the birth will be so easy for you.

"One of the wonderful things this relaxation will do is
to shorten the delivery period tremendously. It will shorten
it miraculously. You'll be so delighted, because with each
contraction, the contractions will get so pleasant [Doctor is
at this point compounding suggestions.] that with about
the third or fourth contraction you have you'll actually begin
smiling and looking forward to the next one as you say, 'I'm
that much nearer the birth of my baby. Now that that contraction is over I'm that much closer to the birth of my
baby.' With each contraction you'll have that thought, and
it will keep a smile on your face all the time, and you'll feel
so good all the time the baby is being delivered. Then, after
the baby is delivered, you'll see the baby instantly. You'll
see your baby the second it is born because you'll be wide
awake during the entire delivery.

"Remember that this relaxation that you're having now
is going to be used in addition to all the aids that medical
science has invented to make the birth of a baby easy for a
mother. So this is going to be a wonderful plus to everything
else that you will have to make that birth of the baby easy.

"After the baby is born, you'll feel so good. You'll be
able to use the telephone—call your friends—a few minutes
after the birth of your baby because you'll be just as strong
then as you are now. Your strength will be complete; your
feeling of well-being will be complete and you'll recover so
much more quickly than you ordinarily would. Then, if
you want to nurse your baby, this relaxation will make it
possible for you to do it so very, very easily.

"I want you to practice relaxation. I want you to practice just what you're doing now. Learn how to relax at
home, so that when your baby comes you'll be all ready for
it, and feeling so wonderful on the day of delivery, and feeling so wonderful during delivery and after delivery. Notice
how that feeling of relaxation holds on and makes you say
to yourself, 'Motherhood is going to be a glorious adventure
for me. I'm going to love every minute of it.' "

*   *   *

At the conclusion of this conditioning talk, of course, your patients are, still in somnambulism, and this assures them of a relatively pain-free delivery. However, if they want to achieve an *absolutely* pain-free delivery, now take them down to the basement of relaxation for the purpose of achieving the Esdaile state. This is the best state for achieving a pain-free delivery. If you have done deliveries in somnambulism and have been well satisfied with them, you are going to be delighted with the success you have with the Esdaile state. Follow the instructions for achieving the Esdaile state previously given. Observe these instructions closely and you will have excellent results in many cases.

Let me warn you, however, that even after following the instructions precisely, if fears are generated in any manner —by unfortunate remarks made by nurses, assistants or other doctors who happen to be present—the Esdaile state will be lost. Remember that your patients hear and understand everything that is going on. Therefore, your nurses and assistants should be trained in the proper handling of hypnotic deliveries. If you have guest doctors attending a delivery and they are not well versed in the semantics of hypnosis, insist for the benefit of your patient that they keep quiet during the entire procedure.

You will notice that all we have talked about here is delivery and yet this chapter is headed "Conditioning for Hypnotic Delivery and Surgery." The reason is simply that the state necessary for surgery is exactly the same as for delivery—the Esdaile state. Your procedure throughout should be the same, except that for surgery your conditioning talk will obviously have to be somewhat different. Instead of talking about contractions, delivery and babies, you will be talking about the surgery. Make it clear to the patient that surgery presents no problems, that he is in good shape to undergo the operation or you wouldn't be doing it, that if he relaxes properly the surgery will be easy for him to take and will proceed rapidly, and that recovery will be swift and sure. And of course, that after the surgery is accomplished he will be in better health than previously, since the entire aim of everything you're doing is to improve his health.

Chapter 15

HYPNOSIS IN DENTISTRY

ONE OF the first students I ever had was an oral surgeon of marked ability. He had studied with me for just a few weeks when he began to report oral surgery done with hypnosis as the only anesthesia. He was adept in the use of nitrous oxide, but told me he seldom had to use it any more; and when he did use it, it was in limited amounts. Instead, he reported that he was using "the best anesthesia in the world—and the safest—hypnotic anesthesia."

Here are this doctor's words, recorded after he had studied hypnosis for only three weeks:

"I had a patient in the office and was going to remove a horizontally impacted third molar—an operation that usually takes a while. I gave the usual suggestion for anesthesia and made the initial incision. Then an incision over the ridge and an incision down. I chiseled the bone and removed the tooth. I roused the patient and asked her if she felt anything at all. She asked me when I was going to take out the tooth. It had already been taken out. I did the suturing afterwards. She felt nothing and was happy about the whole thing."

Another doctor who saw this work being done added the comment, "I don't think the doctor mentioned that salivation was down to a minimum and blood flow was negligible."

Continuing, the oral surgeon said, "During the suturing process, I gave her the suggestion that she open her mouth wide and couldn't close it. I suggested that she would have no postoperative discomfort. When I roused her I asked her how she felt. She said, 'Fine.'" I am quoting this report to let you know how quickly a good student can put hypnosis to work for extensive dental procedure.

Dentists use hypnosis primarily for analgesia and anesthesia. They use it for extensive surgical procedures. Hypnotic anesthesia can be obtained instantaneously if you know how to do it. Too many dentists are under the impression that it takes a long time to attain a usable anesthesia by the hypnotic process. They have become accustomed to old-fashioned techniques and they don't realize modern professional techniques are available. They don't believe instantaneous anesthesia is possible.

I have heard dentists say, before they became acquainted with modern techniques, "I took a course in hypnosis. The doctor who taught me even came to my office to work with my patients; and it takes three or four conditioning visits before the patient can be treated by hypnosis."

This is utter nonsense. An unconditioned patient can be given hypnotic anesthesia faster than it can be obtained with novocaine or xylocaine.

There are certain situations in dentistry in which hypnosis is indicated; and in my estimation, far greater than its value as an anesthetic is its value in correcting these situations.

Bruxism—the gnashing of teeth at night or in the daytime—is sufficient to cause destruction of the mouth structure. If you ask the average dentist if he has ever been able to treat a case of bruxism successfully he will say, "No. It can't be done." He will explain that he builds up the mouth structure again with the full knowledge that later on the same patient will be troubled with the same condition, and further rehabilitation work will be necessary. He will admit that he has never been able to correct the condition permanently.

Certainly the correction of bruxism is well within the dentist's province, for it directly concerns the teeth and the mouth structure and damage done to the teeth and the mouth structure. This is the type of problem that can be helped by hypnosis; I have talked to thousands of dentists about it and not one of them has ever said that he had turned a case of bruxism over to a psychiatrist.

If hypnoanalysis is used in these cases, the dentist may be able to correct the condition permanently by locating the cause. However, most dentists shy away from the use of hypnoanalysis as if it were poison instead of another tool. The following case histories show how bruxism is corrected through the use of hypnoanalysis by an adept dentist. Not many dentists yet use hypnoanalysis, but those who do find it extremely valuable. Judge for yourself:

"Mrs. T.—age 55: Diagnosed by a psysician as tic dou-loureux. I believe the trouble was due to temporomandib-ular joint referred pain. Under hypnoanalysis, it developed that thirty years ago, while standing on the corner of Holly-wood and Vine, she first bruxated. She was waiting for her husband, to whom she had been married for three months. Already she knew that he was seeing other women and that her marriage was doomed . . . No recurrence of the pain in two years—elapsed time, twenty minutes."

"Mrs. R.—age 35: Severe case of bruxism with lower anteriors worn off halfway down to the gingiva. Under hypnoanalysis, it developed that she first ground her teeth as a teen-ager when her father, of whom she was extremely fond, became ill. Habit had persisted over the years when any member of the family became ill. Half-hour session."

These reports were sent to me by J. Stadden Miller, DDS, a student in California.

Occasionally a dentist will bring a patient to class whom he has been unable to handle. I would like to give you an instance.

A dentist told me he had a teen-age patient who really wasn't a patient. He had been treating this girl's family for years, and she had been brought to him repeatedly for treat-ment, but he had never been able to do five minutes' work on her. Considerable work was necessary; the patient had several decayed teeth, crooked teeth, etc. But the prospect of letting the dentist put instruments in her mouth caused such panic that correction was impossible.

The dentist brought this patient and her parents to class in the hope that we could find out what the difficulty was and be able to pave the way for the dental work to be done. She sat in that meeting room between her parents, quietly watch-ing us work with other patients. Then, suddenly, she began to cry. My wife took her out of the room and tried to calm her down. The girl volunteered the information that she was crying because soon it would be her turn to be worked with and she was frightened. When my wife assured her there was no reason for her to be afraid because all that would be done was to talk with her, she said, "I don't believe that. Somehow, they'll fool me and start putting dental instru-ments into my mouth, and I don't want that no matter what."

My wife explained to her that we didn't make promises

we didn't keep and that no dental work of any kind would be done in that room; no dental instrument would be put into her mouth unless she herself asked for it, and that at any time, in the midst of the interview, she herself could terminate it. She asked my wife to stay by her side while the interview was going on. They returned to the room and the young lady offered to come up for hypnoanalysis.

Hypnoanalysis revealed that when she was about five years old one of her kindergarten classmates told her she had just been to the dentist and gave her the gory details. She said the dentist had fooled her by telling her that nothing would be done, and that he then put a big knife into her mouth and cut her gums. She also added how terribly it hurt.

This classmate had so terrified her that she decided she would never allow that to happen to her.

Now we had the cause of her panic, but our work wasn't quite done. Under hypnosis we convinced this girl that no one was going to fool her, that some dental work could be done without hurting her, etc. I was delighted when the dentist returned to class the following week and told us that this young lady had been to his office, and he had done the first dental work for her that she had ever had done. There were no tears, no hysterics, and she was actually looking forward to the time when the decayed teeth would be removed and her appearance improved. This is another way in which the dentist can use hypnosis: to relieve panic and fear.

What about the patient who complains that the upper denture burns but not the lower denture? According to the dentist there should be no difference; he has done everything in his power to fit both dentures correctly, and yet the patient insists he can wear the lower denture, but not the upper. These patients often go from dentist to dentist seeking help and registering the same complaint with each of them. Hypnosis can help these patients. And speaking of dentures, here's a case that came to light in one of our midwest classes:

A female patient in her fifties, was brought to class by her dentist. The problem was her dentures—both upper and lower; they hurt. The dentist who brought her to class was the last of several dentists she had been to with this same problem. She said, "All the dentists I have been to have told me the dentures are perfect and that I should be able to wear them without any difficulty. In fact, I had more than one set made, but that didn't help either. It's easy for the dentist to say they fit perfectly; all I know is that they hurt so badly I just can't wear them."

Hypnoanalysis revealed that this lady had been happily married for over twenty-five years. When her teeth started troubling her and the dentist suggested dentures, she discussed this with her husband. He said to her, "I'm sure that's a good idea because for the past several years your teeth have been getting worse and worse, and it will be nice when you get those dentures to see that your smile is as lovely as it used to be."

And so she had the dentures made. She had been wearing them comfortably for about a week when her husband died of a heart attack. It was the morning of the funeral and when she was dressed she started to put in her dentures and this sad thought flashed into her mind, "He'll never see that lovely smile. Now that he's gone I have no one to smile for. I certainly don't need dentures any more." Despite this thought, she did wear the dentures and by the time she returned from the funeral the pain in her mouth was unbearable. From that time on she was unable to wear the dentures without pain.

After the hypnoanalysis we discussed our findings with her quite thoroughly and she said, "Yes, I remember feeling that way. Nothing seemed worthwhile without him. It's three years since that happened and I realize, of course, that life must go on. He wouldn't want me to go around with an unattractive smile, or with a sore mouth, either, for that matter. I never realized the connection until now." From then on she was able to wear the dentures in complete comfort.

Because there are other illustrations of dental cases in this book, I think the illustrations given above will be sufficient to convince the average dentist that hypnosis has far more uses than dental anesthesia alone. The cases cited are not exceptional. Dentists are constantly confronted by patients who have neurotic dental problems. In preparing this chapter, I wrote to my dental students, asking them to report interesting dental problems they have been able to solve through hypnotic techniques. Here are a few of the many reports I have received:

Report 1: "The thing which amazes me is the ability of so many people to produce a hypnotic hemostasis [by means of hypnosis]. Before being aware of the use of this, I had many calls at night regarding postoperative bleeding. This has been cut to a very few and often I can suggest that the bleeding will be stopped with relaxation. One university student gained such complete hemostasis that I had to suggest that he allow some bleeding in the socket after extraction of an upper central incisor. When he let the bleeding go, only a ring of blood at the gingival margin occurred, and the bone in the socket showed no bleeding. Later, when I asked him to, he produced the usual bleeding from the apex of the socket. It is very gratifying to be able to hand a patient a mirror and let him see his new bridge or denture which has been placed directly after extraction, and know that there will be no unsightly bleeding. Recovery also seems more prompt and less eventful."

Report 2: "A woman patient, for whom I had inserted an immediate upper denture about a year ago, brought her son in for an appointment. She was not wearing the denture, and explained that she was pregnant and the denture caused her to gag. I put her into somnambulism and gave her the appropriate posthypnotic suggestions. The entire procedure took less than fifteen minutes. The result reported on subsequent visits was entirely satisfactory."

Report 3: "I was having difficulty with two orthodontic cases where the patients would, through bruxism, break the ligating wires before the next appointment. Through hypnotic suggestion, this was discontinued, with much more rapid progress as a consequence."

Report 4: "We use hypnosis in one form or other in so many ways it is hard to pin-point them. First of all, we use it to keep control of our own self, to stay relaxed so we can handle the problems we see. We dispell fears of our patients so that instead of dreading to come to see us, they look forward to it. We control postoperative bleeding, pain, swelling, and [we] promote healing with suggestion. We remove teeth without our patients even knowing they are out in probably 85 to 90 percent of our cases, and administer local anesthesia via injection with probably a like percentage of our patients not even knowing we have a needle in our office. With our children we use our 'magic sleepy medicine.' "

Report 5: "I had started a large session of surgery on the lower jaw of a patient. We were taking out several teeth and doing an alveolectomy, and our chemical anesthesia failed. We were able, with the use of somnambulism only, to get sufficient anesthesia to complete the required surgery and to teach the patient to be relaxed and less nervous for future work."

Report 6: "An eleven-year-old girl had knocked out two front teeth in a swimming pool accident. I didn't see the patient until some four hours after the accident. After preliminary examination at the patient's home, I brought the two teeth to my office and did root canals upon them preparing them for reimplantation, putting orthodontic bands on the teeth, and then brought the patient to the office to continue the procedure. This was now some six to eight hours after the accident. A normal blood supply to an accident area gives the best possible chance of healing, and this also applies to reimplantation of teeth. The vasoconstrictor in the chemical anesthesia reduces the blood supply in an area for from four to six hours, and therefore I did not want to use chemical anesthesia. I put the patient into the somnambulistic state. The patient cried out in protest of the currettement of the socket and the force necessary to force the reimplanted teeth to place in the socket. Afterwards the patient was quite placid and we were able to complete the ligation of these teeth to an archwire and the orthodontic bands which had been placed on the devital teeth and on the teeth on either side. The patient recalls little discomfort at the time of reimplantation. I feel that without the use of the vasoconstrictor in the chemical anesthesia, I have had a better chance of succeeding with the implantation of these teeth. It was also possible for me to avoid injecting already very painfully bruised tissue, ordinarily a very uncomfortable sensation."

Chapter 16

STUTTERING

THERE is no such thing as a congenital stutter. A stutter or stammer must be precipitated. Over the years, many doctors have brought stutterers to class in the hope that through various techniques we would be able to help them. It is pitiful to see a youngster trying to speak and only able to utter a word after extreme effort, but it is equally distressing to meet a woman in her thirties or forties who has the same problem as the little boy or girl.

Everytime I see one of these patients, I feel a pang, recalling my first meeting with a stutterer when my father hypnotized a young girl in her teens and stopped her from stuttering. Then when the hypnosis was over, she stuttered as badly as ever. I used to wonder why the problems of these people couldn't be permanently corrected. I don't remember the first time I ever used hypnoanalysis to help a stuttering patient but, admittedly, there have been many times when I have been unable to give them permanent relief. Nevertheless, it is pleasant to remember the many who have been helped considerably.

When a stutterer comes to a doctor's office, the usual procedure is to examine the patient carefully, and when the doctor finds he can do nothing to help the stutterer, he sends him to a speech therapist. The speech therapist works diligently with the patient, and in a number of cases finally succeeds in helping him to some extent. But the number of failures is depressing.

It is my firm belief that every stutter has a basic, investigable cause. Over the years, I have tried to get doctors to change their attitude towards stutterers and treat the *cause* rather than the *effect*. I recall one instance in particular. A doctor came to me and said, "I have a patient who is extremely ambitious. He wants to attend law school, but no law school will accept him because he stutters so badly that he can scarcely speak a word without effort. I've tried

149

to help him and so have speech therapists, all without success. Is there any way that hypnosis might do the job?"

I told him that the only way to help the boy would be to find out the reason for the stutter by means of hypnoanalysis. If we could locate the cause perhaps we would be able to treat him effectively. Perhaps we could even give him normal speech. The doctor, not being very familiar with hypnoanalysis, hesitated to attempt it himself, but asked me to work with him.

I explained that one session of hypnoanalysis might perhaps locate the cause but even if it did, it might not necessarily remove the stutter. Once the cause was located it would be necessary to see that whatever inner conflicts the boy had were resolved completely or else we couldn't expect to give him permanent help. Hypnoanalysis is not a one-shot therapy; exploration must continue until these inner conflicts are resolved, and this sometimes requires extensive treatment. The doctor said, "Would you undertake the first hypnoanalysis?" I told him I would be glad to, but that he would do well to attempt for himself some of the techniques I had taught him. Weeks passed and he did not bring the patient to class. Then, finally, he surprised me by reporting that he had done the first hypnoanalysis by himself after all, and that he had been quite successful with it.

I said, "Keep working with him and you may be able to help him a great deal more than you thought possible."

The following fall I was pleased when the doctor reported to me, "The boy has been accepted by a law school and he is without a stutter."

During the next winter I continued to get reports. The boy was now at the head of his classes, and I have learned that he is now a successful attorney. This sort of case makes me feel that encouraging doctors to use hypnoanalysis is worth my every effort.

A psychiatrist in Chicago went so far as to tell me he considered hypnoanalysis as the crown jewel of hypnosis. Many psychiatrists realize that hypnoanalysis is the key to the solving of many emotional problems, but although I have taught thousands of doctors how to use hypnoanalysis, comparatively few of them are adept at it and I think I know the reason for this.

Too many of them are unwilling to devote the necessary

time to it or are unwilling to probe deeply into the human mind. I have known doctors who, for practice, will take the time to regress a patient to an early age to see reactions that are not of a startling nature; they like the idea that they can take a patient back to the time when he was two or three years old and let him see again how the toys under the Christmas tree looked. This is interesting to see and, the doctor feels, harmless. The same doctor will make no attempt to delve into what might have made the same patient stutter. Yet I agree with the psychiatrist acquaintance in Chicago that eventually hypnoanalysis will be recognized as a valid and useful therapeutic technique which can be used by every doctor in solving emotional difficulties. Psychiatrists are trained to resolve inner conflicts. When they resolve these conflicts they feel that the patient is well on the road to recovery. Hypnoanalysis enables the therapist to locate the sources of inner conflicts, and is the best technique I know for getting at the root causes quickly. It saves months and months of work. I wish I could make every doctor see hypnoanalysis the way that the psychiatrist sees it.

Talking about root causes and inner conflicts, what are those of a stutter and related speech difficulties? In a moment, I will relate a few instances which show typical causes —which in most cases are not related to pathology. Actually, I don't know of any stutter that was created by pathology, although I am well aware that medical researchers suspect a functional disorder in certain cases of such speech defects. Studies have been made at Johns-Hopkins and other medical centers of the effects of specific dyslexia, a constitutional language disability. This syndrome, sometimes called strephosymbolia, primarily affects reading and writing ability, but is likely to occur in children who were slow to learn how to talk, and whose family histories included stuttering, among other difficulties. It has nothing to do with intelligence. Rather, it seems to stem from an organic weakness of a section of the brain controlling the differentiation of left and right. Dyslexics have trouble telling a "b" from a "d" or the word "saw" from the word "was." Some authorities doubt the existence of pathological dyslexia, however, feeling that it is a syndrome of some psychiatric block. I mention it here only to show that I realize the *possibility* of a pathological stutter, from this or several other causes. Having said so,

I must repeat that I know of no stutter of which the cause was proved to involve pathology. Now let's examine examples of emotional causes. Doing hypnoanalysis to locate the course of a stutter, we found this case history:

Trying to get answers from the patient was extremely difficult because he stuttered so badly. I regressed him to the age of five and learned that he stuttered at that age. I took him back to the age of four and found that the stutter was full-blown even at that early age. When I finally got him back to about two years of age, he related an unusual incident. There was a lumber yard near his home and he wandered into it because it seemed like a good place to play. He saw two men fighting. The argument developed into blows. It became a terrific battle. Finally one of the men was knocked to the ground and when he managed to get up he grabbed an axe that was lying nearby and struck his assailant, knocking him to the ground—and then chopped his head off.

The child was terrified. He ran home to his mother. He was afraid that the murderer had seen him, would follow him, would perhaps do the same thing to him. When his mother asked him what was wrong, he had reached a point in his life where he didn't want to talk, or couldn't talk. That was how the stutter began.

I discovered an analogous, though not horrifying, instance when I did hypnoanalysis on a young man and regressed him to the age of two, to find that his stutter began when he accidentally pulled a tablecloth off the dining room table. The table had a lot of dishes on it. His mother came storming into the room and he knew he was in trouble. He tried to talk his way out of it but the words wouldn't come. I remember saying to myself, "That is certainly not sufficient reason to start a stutter." So I decided to take him back to the time when he was about a year old.

It was his father's birthday, and his mother had baked a beautiful cake for her husband. The little boy climbed on a chair to get a closer look at the cake, holding on to the tablecloth as he climbed. The cake came tumbling down and spattered all over the floor. His mother, hearing the crash, came storming into the room, and when she saw what had happened she scolded the baby severely for spoiling his father's birthday celebration. This incident at age one didn't, by itself, cause the stutter, but when a similar incident took place a year later the stutter was precipitated. The boy had reached a point where he was obliged to talk but didn't know what to say, and the reason was clear. When the first incident occurred, the baby was distressed because he knew he had done something naughty and his mother was angry. When the same thing happened a year later, he not only knew that he had done something naughty and that his mother was angry, but at a level below conscious awareness he was reliving the incident which had upset him one year before. Even a minor trauma can, like suggestion, be compounded by repetition. Every stutter has its beginning in a situation in which the victim reaches a point where he doesn't want to talk and yet is obliged to.

Let me give you another example of how a traumatic situation causes a stutter to begin. A woman patient was brought to class. She was in her fifties, and claimed she had stuttered since she was a baby. Trying to correct a stutter half a century old didn't strike me as an easy task, and I thought surely this patient would require a great deal of hypnotic therapy before she could be helped on a permanent basis.

Before hypnoanalysis, I usually ask the patient a lot of questions. Interrogation revealed that she believed her stutter to have begun at an early age, when she had been troubled by convulsions. When asked what caused the stutter, she said it must have been started by an awful scare she had as a baby. She didn't remember what the scare was. When asked if the scare might have also been the cause of the convulsions, she didn't know but she didn't think so. I didn't think so either. Nevertheless, the fact that she could answer without hypnoanalysis that the stutter and the convulsions both appeared at approximately the same time set me to wondering. This is what the hypnoanalysis revealed:

At the age of about two, while she was ill in bed, she heard her mother and father quarreling. The child had never heard them argue so violently before. When the fight had grown intense, the father threatened to kill the mother and also the little girl. He started toward the bed where the child was lying ill. The mother ran to protect the screaming child, while the child herself tried to talk but couldn't because of her terror. She went into convulsions.

The father calmed down and the child soon recovered from the convulsions. But from that time on, every time her father approached her she became terrified and couldn't talk. Her stutter had begun.

It would seem from the case histories I am citing that all stutters begin at an early age. This is not true. You will find many people who think that they have stuttered all their lives, but when hypnoanalysis is done you find that the stutter didn't begin until they were eight or ten years of age, or older. I have even run into cases in which the stutter didn't begin until the patient was of high school age. Yet all these people will say they do not remember a time when they didn't stutter. Perhaps it is painful for them to remember when (and coincidentally how) the stutter began, so they employ the defense mechanism of blotting the memory out.

One young college student who was brought to class had a very pronounced stutter. He was one of those patients who claimed he had stuttered all his life and couldn't remember a time when he hadn't. During hypnoanalysis, it was revealed that when he was five years old he didn't stutter. When he was six years old he didn't stutter, and even at the age of eight he didn't stutter. But when he was nine years old he did. We learned that his playmates had tied him to a tree one day, binding him securely with a rope around his neck. Then they piled wood on the ground around the tree and started a fire. At first, he thought it was a game, but when the fire started he began to yell for them to set him free. Apparently, the kids got scared and ran off, leaving the boy helpless. Luckily, a passerby saw him, stamped out the fire and released him. By this time the rope had abraded his neck. He ran home. When his mother saw him she was very upset by the appearance of his neck, but he was afraid to tell her what had happened. He thought she might punish him or—worse—speak to the parents of the boys who had hurt him. If this happened, he thought, they might try to do it to him again for telling. He had reached a point where he didn't want to talk.

There have been cases—fortunately rare ones—in which only partial help has been possible because only partial causes have been found. And a cause must be understood to be treated. In one such case, a psychiatrist found that one of his patients had begun stuttering in early childhood, after being frightened away from the entrance of a cave he had begun exploring. Even in hypnoanalysis, the patient could not bring back the memory of what had terrified him. This obstacle does not hinder the therapist in most cases, however.

Here is the transcript of an actual hypnoanalysis on a stuttering patient; note the technique used to determine the root cause:

ELMAN: Do you know when you started stammering?

PATIENT: [Stammering] Well, no. I believe I did all my life.

ELMAN: It seems to you that you did all your life?

PATIENT: That's right.

ELMAN: And yet your common sense tells you that nobody is born with a stammer . . . So it must have originated somehow. And if we can find out why it happened, we might be able to help you cope with the cause and get rid of the stammer entirely. When do you stammer most?

PATIENT: Especially when I'm excited.

ELMAN: Then the stutter gets awfully bad, is that it?

PATIENT: Yes, sir. I'm worse now than I've been in a long time.

ELMAN: Are you going through some trying times at present?

PATIENT: No, sir.

ELMAN: Is everything all right at home? Family all right?

PATIENT: Yes, sir.

ELMAN: And you're doing all right? Business is all right, or your work, whatever it is?

PATIENT: Yes.

ELMAN: What do you do for a living?

PATIENT: I'm an operating engineer.

ELMAN: And do you find that your stammering interferes with your work?

PATIENT: No, sir.

ELMAN: You've taken a line of work where the stammering does not interfere . . . We've got a pretty good indication that you have a severe stammer and if I'm going to help you I have to give you some simple instructions. If I meet with resistance I'm unable to help you, so if you will try to work with me, maybe I can help, and if you try, maybe together we can get some place . . . [Places patient in somnambulism.] . . . That's good cooperation. When you're relaxed like this, you can live through any part of your life. Most people believe that they are unable to recall incidents of long ago. This is not so. Everything that has ever happened to us is registered in our minds and can be brought forth. So, I would like to take you back to the time when you were a boy to find out if the stammer or the stutter, whatever you want to call it, was there when you were small . . . Tell me this, did you celebrate Christmas in your home when you were a little kid?

PATIENT: No, sir.

ELMAN: There was no Christmas tree or anything like that?

PATIENT: No.

ELMAN: Did you have birthday parties when you were a little kid?

PATIENT: No.

ELMAN: But you did go to school . . . is that right?

PATIENT: Sure.

ELMAN: All right, I'm going to take you back to the first grade in school because I want to talk to that little kid in the first grade. Did you go to kindergarten? Maybe I'll take you back to kindergarten.

PATIENT: Yes.

ELMAN: All right, I'm going to take you back to kindergarten, and when I lift your hand and drop it, don't try to remember, because that's what defeats us all the time . . . Just say to yourself, "It's going to be there and I'd like it to be there," so when I lift your hand and drop it, it will be when you were in kindergarten and you'll see yourself in kindergarten as clearly as when you were there the first time. And I'm going to talk to you in kindergarten. Stay completely relaxed when I lift your hand and drop it and watch it happen . . . That's it . . . There you are . . . You're in kindergarten . . . Do you like kindergarten?

PATIENT: Yes, sir.

ELMAN: Take a look around kindergarten. Do you get along with the kids all right?

PATIENT: Yes, sir.

ELMAN: Do you get along with the teacher?

PATIENT: Yes, sir.

ELMAN: Do you like the teacher?

PATIENT: Yes, sir.

ELMAN: Tell me this, you're in kindergarten and everything is clear—do you have fun in kindergarten?

PATIENT: Yes, sir.

ELMAN: And do you ever stutter or stammer?

PATIENT: Yẹs, sir.

ELMAN: You do. So this means you started to stammer or stutter before you went to kindergarten . . . We're going to take you back now to before you started kindergarten, and you'll be doing something that you haven't thought of ever since the time you did it, but it will be something that you like to do. I'll be talking to you and you'll be a little boy just three years old . . . There you are . . . What are you doing?

PATIENT: Playing in the back yard.

ELMAN: What are you playing with?

PATIENT: Some dirt.

ELMAN: You're about three years old, aren't you?

PATIENT: Yes, sir.

ELMAN: Do you ever stammer? [Patient doesn't answer.]
             Maybe you don't know what that means. Do
             you ever stutter? Do you ever have trouble in
             talking?

PATIENT: Yes, sir.

ELMAN: When I lift your hand and drop it, it will be the
             first day you ever had trouble with talking. And
             you'll know what caused it when I lift and drop
             your hand . . . Stay relaxed and you'll have it
             . . There you are . . . What's been happening to-
             day that makes a little boy have trouble talking?

PATIENT: My father came home. Mommy says he's drunk.
             [Starts to cry.]

ELMAN: What happened? Tell me, because this may stop
             you from stammering forever if we get all this
             out and we want all this out. So, what did your
             daddy do? You can tell me.

PATIENT: He beat me.

ELMAN: Why did he beat you?

PATIENT: 'Cause I must have done something he didn't
             want me to do.

ELMAN: What did you do?

PATIENT: I don't know.

ELMAN: When I lift your hand and drop it you'll know
             why it was he beat you. [Note the compound-
             ing of suggestion.] . . . and what you did, if you
             did anything. Stay relaxed and you'll know.
             What did you do.

PATIENT: We had some little wood chickens and I drowned
             them.

ELMAN: You drowned them?

PATIENT: Yes.

ELMAN: You said "wood chickens."

PATIENT: No. Little chickens.

ELMAN: Did you do it accidentally?

PATIENT: No. I just did it on purpose.

ELMAN: You did it on purpose? You drowned them? Now, there must have been a reason why a little boy would pick on those chickens, and maybe we can find out. Maybe there was a little resentment against them, or something, or somebody. Was there anybody you didn't like at this time?

PATIENT: No, sir.

ELMAN: Did you like daddy all right?

PATIENT: Yes, sir.

ELMAN: Did you like mother all right?

PATIENT: Yes, sir.

ELMAN: Brothers and sisters?

PATIENT: Yes, sir.

ELMAN: Did you like the little chickens?

PATIENT: Yes, sir.

ELMAN: Did you take them out of the house to drown them?

PATIENT: They were out in the yard.

ELMAN: You be out in the yard when I lift your hand. It will be before the chickens are drowned and then you can tell me whether it's on purpose or not. And maybe you don't even know whether it was on purpose or not. And maybe you'll find out now. Because it will be just before they were drowned . . . What are you doing, playing with the chickens, are you?

PATIENT: No, they're ducks.

ELMAN: See, now we find out more. Take a look at the ducks. Do you like these little ducks?

PATIENT: Yes, sir.

ELMAN: You do like them. Well, what are you doing with them if they're ducks?

PATIENT: I'm putting them in the tub of water.

ELMAN: Putting them in a tub of water?

PATIENT: Yes, sir.

ELMAN: Well, isn't that all right for ducks, to go in water?

PATIENT: Yes, sir.

ELMAN: Do you have any idea of what you want to do with the ducks?

PATIENT: I want to watch them swim.

ELMAN: Now you're watching them swim. Is there any idea on your part to do anything harmful to the ducks?

PATIENT: No, sir.

ELMAN: Then what happens to these ducks?

PATIENT: They all drowned.

ELMAN: In the water?

PATIENT: Yes.

ELMAN: How did they drown?

PATIENT: Because they couldn't swim.

ELMAN: Well, ducks naturally swim. Take a look at them again. Are they ducks or are they chickens? If they're ducks, they'd naturally swim.

PATIENT: They're chickens.

ELMAN: Chickens can't swim. But ducks can swim.

PATIENT: Yes, sir.

ELMAN: What made you think for a while that they were ducks? You called them ducks a little while ago.

PATIENT: I don't really know. I just thought that they could swim.

ELMAN: I see. Then you really didn't want to hurt these chickens, did you?

PATIENT: No, sir.

ELMAN: So that this would be just a little mistake that a little boy made. Is that it?

PATIENT: Yes, sir.

ELMAN: And because he made this little mistake his daddy came home and beat him for it and now because he doesn't know what to say to daddy —he tries to talk and explain . . .

PATIENT: He wouldn't—he wouldn't—he wouldn't—

ELMAN: You'll be able to talk without stammering when I snap my fingers. [Snaps fingers.] . . .

PATIENT: He would never let me cry.

ELMAN: He wouldn't let you cry?

PATIENT: No, sir.

ELMAN: I see. And that's repression—unable to cry. Did he give you any reason why he wouldn't let you cry?

PATIENT: He said he would beat me harder if I cried.

ELMAN: So you were afraid to cry. And that stammer represents that concealed cry. Is that what it is?

PATIENT: I don't know, sir.

ELMAN: Well, now let me tell you. I want you to notice how close a stammer is to a sob. It's awfully close, isn't it? And it's that stifled sob every time you stammer. Did you ever realize that?

PATIENT: Yes, sir.

ELMAN: In other words, you've known this all along, is that right?

PATIENT: Yes, sir.

ELMAN: You've known that it's because he wouldn't let you cry that you stammer?

PATIENT: Yes, sir.

ELMAN: Well, you can get rid of that cry now. That is, you can cry if you want to. If you feel like crying you can just let loose, because you're a big man now, and if you feel like crying, you can let it all out, because this is the emotion you felt as a little kid, and if it comes out now it will do you a lot of good. If you feel like crying, let it go . . . [Patient sobs for prolonged period.] Let it all out and you won't stammer any more just on account of it. Get rid of that emotion that's been pent up inside of you for so many years. Let it all out. Just let it come out good . . . [Patient goes on crying. Elman addresses attending doctors.] I've never known a stammer or a stutter that didn't involve some emotional situation. He'll get that out of his system and then you'll see how well he talks. There will be no stammer there at all. And if his father had let him do it when he was a kid he wouldn't stammer. But this was a misunderstanding of a parent and a child . . . [Patient's sobbing has subsided. Elman addresses patient.] It felt kind of good to get that out of your system, didn't it?

PATIENT: Yes, sir.

ELMAN: Let all that pent up emotion come right out . . . [to doctors] This has been concealed in him— and he was about three years old when this thing happened . . . [to patient] How old are you?

PATIENT: Fifty years old . . . I'm forty-nine now.

ELMAN: [to doctors] That's forty-seven years—forty-six years—of repressed emotion, and what that will do to a person! It's probably meant a lot of difference in his living conditions, in his life—in the way he's made his living—in the way he's gotten along with people . . . And if his dad had just let him cry it out when he was a little kid, he would have been just as normal a youngster as anyone in the world. When he wants to cry, his dad says, "I'll beat you all the more if you cry." So, afraid to cry . . . every time he wants to cry, there's a stammer. Every time he has an emotion it's in the form of a stammer.

    Maybe I'm making it sound too easy. I'm not trying to indicate that after one such session he needs no more . . . There's not a person that I work with ever in hypnoanalysis who couldn't stand more than one session. And this is not advanced to you as a panacea or elixir. It's not advanced to you as a cure-all, but as a technique of getting at the cause of these conditions . . . [to patient] I'll bet you feel a lot better.

PATIENT: Yes, sir. I sure do.

ELMAN: And there's no stammer there now, is there?

PATIENT: No, sir.

ELMAN: Do you think there ever will be?

PATIENT: No, sir.

ELMAN: If there ever is—if there ever shows the slightest sign of a tendency to a stammer—I want you to think instantly of those chickens and your father beating you. Think of it instantly, and it will be like a mental flash—and the minute you do, say, "I'm not going to stammer just because my daddy wouldn't let me cry." After all, there was no venom in what you did as a child, was there?

PATIENT: No, sir.

ELMAN: You didn't mean to go out and kill those chickens, but this was a natural mistake that any little child might make. You wanted to see the little birds swim You didn't know they couldn't, and when they drowned you were, I suppose, just as heartbroken as anybody about it, but your father wouldn't let you explain He just beat you for it.

PATIENT: Yes, sir.

ELMAN: I don't think you'll stutter or stammer any more, what do you think?

PATIENT: No, sir. I don't think I will any more either.

ELMAN: And if you do . . . [to patient's doctor] Doctor, if he shows any tendency toward a recurrence of the stammer, take him back and do this over again, and each time you do it you'll find he gets tremendous help out of it. I think that you've probably got a complete removal of the stammer by what we've let him do today. I can't swear to it. Sometimes we get these sensational recoveries that look like magic, and sometimes we don't. But I'm not trying to get a sensational recovery in any case that I work on. So many doctors tell me, "I haven't got the time for hypnoanalysis." I think any doctor should be willing to spend the length of time I spend with these patients in order to correct situations like this.

* * *

Incidentally, I have found again and again that the victim of one neurotic ailment is apt to be the victim of more neurotic ailments. The point I am trying to make is that just because the patient loses the stutter, you haven't necessarily solved all the patient's neurotic problems. That is why I make the statement that all these patients can benefit from further work by the doctor. Internal conflicts must be resolved entirely if the patient is to be helped completely.

The man in medicine best trained to resolve inner conflicts is the psychiatrist, and if the doctor in any other branch of medicine finds that he is unable to resolve those inner conflicts permanently, in my estimation, he should turn the patient over to the psychiatrist.

*   *   *

In dealing with a stutter, follow these instructions. First, remember that every stutter has a beginning. Take the stutterer back to the traumatic situation that caused the stutter, and let him relive it in an abreaction or by seeing the same thing happen to another person on an imaginary television screen. In many instances, patients gain insight about the true cause of the first stutter and are helped permanently. What happens if you don't get back to the cause of the stutter? The most you'll be able to do is to give the patient temporary help. If the cause remains within him, the stutter will return.

Sometimes a doctor will get back to what he thinks is the true cause and the patient will apparently be helped. Then the stutter returns. The doctor should know from this that he has not found all the disturbing material, and will have to probe further to get out all of the true cause before he can permanently help the stutterer. This explanation not only applies to stuttering but to every neurotic problem; if the help is temporary, the true cause has not been exposed and further work is indicated.

A technique is demonstrated in hypnoanalysis which has been found vastly beneficial in many types of neurotic disturbances. We know that emotional illnesses are caused by repressions. A person lives through a situation with which he cannot cope. He is not prepared for it by experience or training. The memory of the incident is horrifying. He represses all thoughts of the traumatic situation. Sometimes he even succeeds in putting it below the level of consciousness, so that eventually it becomes truly a part of the unconscious material of his mind.

This does not mean he is not affected by it. On the contrary, this very repression of traumatic experiences will most certainly continue to do damage at the conscious level. In many cases, we are able to bring repressions from below the level of conscious awareness to a place where they are known and recognized at a conscious level. We then make sure the repression is not allowed to retire into the unconscious again. Note how this technique was demonstrated in the foregoing case of the stuttering man.

Too many people believe hypnoanalysis is a "one-shot" therapy. Nothing could be further from the truth. Doctors are inclined to believe that if they can't get permanent results with one application of hypnoanalysis, the therapy won't work on that particular patient. This is not evidenced from our experience.

Not long ago, a doctor in one of my classes asked if I would work with his son, a stuttering boy. The boy's family was most cooperative. We worked with the youngster but got nowhere. When the boy showed signs of tiring, we gave him some superficial suggestions to rid him of his stutter temporarily at least and to increase his confidence.

Two weeks later we were told that the boy spoke without a stutter for about ten days and then the affliction returned. Again we worked with the child. This time we began to get the answer to the stuttering problem, but certainly didn't complete the therapy.

Again the child showed improvement, but by this time the father and mother were showing disappointment that a miracle had not taken place in two sessions. My class in that particular city came to an end, and there was no opportunity to go on giving the boy the additional help he needed. I advised the doctor to continue the program of hypnoanalysis with one of my students. Because of his disappointment, however, I do not believe he did so. And yet his boy might have been helped permanently.

That same doctor would probably be provoked if one of his patients took only two teaspoonfuls of a prescription and then took no more because the two teaspoonfuls did not cure him permanently. Why people expect the techniques of hypnosis to work like magic is beyond my understanding.

The question might be asked, "If the father was a student of yours, why didn't he complete the hypnoanalysis himself?" Possibly because the child was reaching a stage in life where ambivalence towards his parents was beginning to be manifested. The father might find resistance within the child, though another operator might find none. Still, such a situation should not be allowed to stand in the way of helping a child.

Always remember this: The severity of the traumatic event accounts for the severity of the stutter; find the cause, treat it, and the effect will automatically be alleviated.

Chapter 17

OBESITY

WHEN the doctor is confronted with an obesity problem, he usually puts the patient on a diet, supplemented by proper medications, and a warning about the possible medical consequences of overweight. Some patients will stay on the diet and absorb the medications (and warnings) until the necessary poundage is lost. Then they part company with the doctor. A year or two later, they are back to see the same doctor about the same problem "They're as fat as ever," the doctor says to himself. "They just don't seem to have any sense about food intake." There are also patients who say they want to lose weight, but won't or can't stay on the diet prescribed by the doctor. Under the doctor's care they don't lose an ounce; in fact, they gain weight while they are supposed to be losing it. Compulsive eaters aren't necessarily gluttons. They are often people who are searching for security. This search takes them back to the time when oral satisfaction represented complete security—when mother fed and took care of them. They eat, and continue to eat, because eating gives them the sense of security which allays a fear lurking below the level of conscious awareness.

With every patient, the fear has a different cause, but it is really the same *kind* of fear. In effect, all such fears are similar. However, this does not mean that the same diet-medication-warning treatment will work with every patient, nor does it mean that hypnosis should be used simply to give every patient hunger-allaying suggestions. A hypnotic diet, without the removal of causative fear, may provide only temporary help. The doctors who recognize the problem are remarkably successful with obesity cases, and some of them actually specialize in obesity problems. Excessive overweight is often caused by strong emotional conflicts, which can be resolved—like those associated with stuttering —by an approach utilizing hypnoanalysis.

I want you to read part of an actual transcript of one such hypnoanalysis. The patient in question was slender

until she was fourteen years of age, and then suddenly started to gain weight:

ELMAN: [After regressing patient to early childhood]
            You're in the fiirst grade. I want you, mentally,
            to stand up in your seat there in the first grade
            and look across the room at the kid furthest
            away from you. Is that a boy or a girl?

PATIENT: A boy.

ELMAN: What's his name?

PATIENT: John.

ELMAN: Now your awareness is increasing. I'm going
            to ask you a few questions while you're in the
            first grade. I'm coming up to your seat now and
            I'm saying to you, "You're six years old. Are
            you a fat little girl?"

PATIENT: No . . . [The patient is now taken through suc-
            cessive school levels, and it is found that she
            was slender until she reached the eighth grade.
            The transcript is resumed at this level.]

ELMAN: Now, when I lift your hand and drop it, you'll
            be in the eighth grade. There you are. Tell me,
            you're about fourteen years old now. Take a
            look at yourself. How's your weight?

PATIENT: A little heavy.

ELMAN: You're in the eighth grade and you're beginning
            to be a little bit heavy. When I lift your hand,
            it will be vacation time, and it will be just before
            school starts for the eighth grade . . . You know,
            school is starting in just another few days. Will
            you be glad to get back to school?

PATIENT: Yes.

ELMAN: Tell me, did you like this summer? Did you have
            a nice summer?

PATIENT: I had scarlet fever.

ELMAN: You were pretty sick with scarlet fever, were
            you?

PATIENT: Yes.

ELMAN: Did you at any time have thoughts that were unpleasant while you were sick with scarlet fever?

PATIENT: Yes. I was afraid I wouldn't get well, and if I did, I worried about the aftereffects.

ELMAN: We've got the whole reason there, haven't we? Why a little girl would feel the need for security.

PATIENT: Yes.

ELMAN: Now we know the whole reason as to why you got fat, don't we?

PATIENT: Yes.

ELMAN: You were a slender little girl. Then you saw yourself at the end of summer vacation, and you saw a little girl who was just getting over scarlet fever. And then you saw that little girl in the eighth grade, and she was beginning to get fat; already showing the need for security. The morbid thoughts that you must have had about what would be the aftereffects, was that it?

PATIENT: Yes.

ELMAN: And so that little girl in her search for security found the natural outlet of more food and more food because that gave her satisfaction. It made her feel secure. The security she knew as an infant when she didn't have to worry about the future. Is that so?

PATIENT: Yes.

ELMAN: Now we've found the cause, and you don't have to worry about scarlet fever any more, do you?

PATIENT: No.

* * *

Every neurotic problem has a beginning, and obesity is most often a neurotic problem. The cause-finding technique, illustrated above and used in obesity as it is in stuttering and similar difficulties, is called pinpointing the start of a neurosis. After all, the patient wasn't fat up to the eighth grade, but in the eighth grade we find she was beginning to get a little heavier. Something must have caused it. What?

The summer before the eighth grade started, she had scarlet fever. The severe illness frightened her. Would she ever get well? And if she did what would be the aftereffects? She certainly experienced enough fear to cause a child to search for security. And she found that security in the oral satisfaction she knew as an infant, when life was at its sweetest and she knew no problems, when she was safe in her mother's arms and well fed. She began to overeat to recapture that feeling of security she once knew. Like alcoholics and drug addicts, overeaters develop a tolerance for the object of their craving. More and more food is needed to achieve a given degree of satisfaction. Now it takes an immense amount of food to give this patient her feeling of security. The result: obesity.

Did she ever realize this at a conscious level? Of course not. She knew that she had had scarlet fever, and she would have been able to tell you that she was terribly scared by it. But she did not relate the scarlet fever to her obesity. She had no idea that food represented an escape from the fright engendered by her illness. Now she understands her problem. She doesn't have to worry about the effects of scarlet fever any more; a vicious habit pattern is all that remains of her search for security, and hypnoanalysis enables her to break up that habit pattern.

Her doctor subsequently reported that under medical supervision, she lost over one hundred pounds, and has maintained normal weight ever since.

I said before that fears in such cases are all of the same kind. To illustrate this, let me recount another case in which fear caused an overweight problem. The patient was a woman in her fifties. Her doctor told me that she had been a patient for many years. She had always been slender until she had undergone a hysterectomy; after that, she started putting on weight at an alarming rate. Now she was in desperate need of help because no matter how hard she tried, she couldn't stay on the diet prescribed for her.

After getting this information, I began the hypnoanalysis. Every fact mentioned by the doctor was verified, and now I started to probe for the cause of her difficulty. I took her back to the visit she had made to her doctor before the operation. She told me everything the doctor had said at the examination, reliving the experience vividly. She said the doctor told her she had a large fibroid tumor—perhaps more than one—and that surgery was indicated. Hearing the word tumor, she became frightened and asked the doctor if it might be malignant. She remembered very clearly his telling her that they couldn't tell for sure about such things until surgery was done, but that in his opinion it was most certainly not malignant.

I brought her mentally to the period just after the surgery had been accomplished. Despite her doctor's assurances before and after the operation that there had been no malignancy, she could not get out of her mind the idea that she might have cancer. I asked her why she felt that way, and she said she wasn't sure, but that she thought a question asked by the doctor during the preoperative examination planted the disturbing thought. I asked her, "What was that question?"

She said, "He asked me if there had been any loss of weight recently. Well, it so happened that I was on a diet at the time in an attempt to take off a few pounds. As the doctor told you, I was never heavy, but I thought losing about five pounds might give me a better figure, and that's why I went on this diet. It worked very well, too, because I had lost a couple of pounds. But when the doctor asked me if I had lost any weight I wasn't sure whether I had lost it because of the diet or because of the tumor."

She just couldn't get that thought out of her mind, and when she recovered from the surgery, she began to overeat in an effort to gain weight—to make sure that no malignancy was present. This fear, operating at an unconscious level, caused her to overeat, gaining weight until she was a very fat woman.

The doctor helped me to eliminate the thought of cancer. Once the hypnoanalysis unearthed the cancer phobia, with the doctor's further help, she was able to stay on a diet and get down to normal weight. Since the tendency to eat too much is a reaching for security, you must combat it by pinpointing a concrete fear that brought on the eating response.

A doctor brought his young daughter to class some time ago. She was in her early teens, and had an excess weight of about forty-five pounds. Interrogation before the hypnosis established the fact that she had been slender until she spent a summer at camp with a lot of other youngsters.

After she came back, she began to put on extra poundage. She continued to gain weight, for she was now eating more than she usually did. When her father tried to bring her down to normal weight, she didn't stay on the diet but continued to gain weight. By the time I saw her, she was extremely fat.

Upon putting her into deep hypnosis, we learned that she had had several terrifying experiences at summer camp. The first episode was the capsizing of a boat in which she and several companions were sailing. She was very frightened because she did not know how to swim. The children nearly drowned before they were rescued, and of course she longed to be safely at home.

The next incident took place while she and a group of other children were playing hide and seek. She was hiding behind a car, and a dog happened to be there. The dog found a poisonous snake, and kept bothering the reptile, keeping it away from the children. Her grandfather killed the snake, and then he beat the dog because the dog was not supposed to be there. She was very upset. She felt that the snake could have bitten any one of them. In both cases the child was made panicky by fear and she longed for the security which she found at home in her mother's arms. However, when she got home, her father was sick, and she was temporarily denied the security she thought she would find at home.

These three happenings were the cause of her excessive eating. She was unconsciously searching for security, and the only way she could find it was in oral satisfaction.

Another obese patient was brought to class by her doctor. With hypnoanalysis and under the doctor's careful supervision, she lost eighty pounds. Then the same doctor brought her back to another class a year later. "She stayed on the diet beautifully," he explained—"until she lost eighty pounds, just half of what she should lose. Why shouldn't we be able to help her all the way?"

This doctor, like so many others, had assumed that one session of hypnoanalysis was all that was necessary. After the single session, he had merely supervised her diet, without giving her further help.

Since there had to be a reason for her behavior, we put the patient into hypnoanalysis again. Once in deep somnambulism she exclaimed, "I don't want to lose the other eighty pounds. My doctor says that when I lose that eighty pounds I'll be in good enough physical condition to stand surgery, and I'm scared to death of surgery."

Obviously, the patient was so frightened of an operation, which the doctor had told her she must have, that she was determined not to lose the other eighty pounds. Fear is the disorder requiring treatment. Locate the fear, remove it, and under good medical supervision the excessive weight problem can be solved.

A fat patient will sometimes tell the doctor, "I don't know why I'm fat. I eat so little." Put such a patient into hypnoanalysis and take him through a typical twenty-four hours to find out every morsel of food eaten that day. You'll be surprised to find how much the patient who "scarcely eats anything" eats.

One doctor asked for my advice about an obese patient who was at least fifty pounds overweight as a result of compulsive eating. "Should we put her on a hypnotic diet?" he asked.

I told him that putting her on a hypnotic diet at this point might not do much good. Of course, she would lose a lot of weight and be delighted with the results, but a year later she would be back again as fat as ever. The only way to help her would be to find out why she was searching for security.

The doctor agreed to my suggestion, and hypnoanalysis revealed that when the patient was a little girl she was in an automobile accident. She was taken to the hospital where the doctors went into consultation within her hearing. The girl, wavering in and out of consciousness, heard them discussing whether amputation of her legs would be necessary. One of the doctors said, "Maybe we can save those legs," but another doctor remarked, "It looks pretty hopeless."

It was unfortunate that the girl heard those remarks. Now she was put into anesthesia for necessary surgical procedures. Amputation was deemed unnecessary, but when she recovered consciousness she was still anesthetized and couldn't feel her legs. She thought that she had lost them, that they had really been amputated. When she was given assurance that she still had her legs she didn't believe it until feeling returned. Though she completely recovered from the accident, from that time on she was a compulsive eater, searching for security.

When we recovered these facts in hypnoanalysis, she made an astounding statement: "Now I know why I have closets full of shoes in my home. I can never pass a shoe store without buying shoes. I don't think I'll have to do that any more."

I am happy to relate that she too, lost considerable weight as a result of the hypnoanalysis, and kept her weight down to within normal limits.

Almost every time we use hypnoanalysis for an obese patient, we find the same basis for the trouble. It is almost always the result of mental trauma. If the trauma is a minor one, there is a weight increase of only thirty or forty pounds. But if there is a major one, the weight increase is absolutely astounding.

We have seen patients in the four-hundred-pound class. The fattest person who was ever brought to class was certainly in this category. He wouldn't let me perform hypnoanalysis on him although he professed that he wanted help. He resisted every effort to hypnotize him and when the class was called to a close, he mentioned how terrible he felt that he couldn't be helped.

As usual after our class sessions, my wife and I went out to eat. We had only been seated in the restaurant a few minutes when in came the fat man. He may have seen us; I do not know. He struggled into a seat several tables from us. It must have been close to midnight, and we thought he was going to have a cup of coffee and perhaps a snack before retiring, as so many people do. Since we were doing exactly that, the assumption seemed natural.

Imagine our amazement when we saw the waitress, without consulting him, bring him a platter of turkey, mashed potatoes, peas, salad and bread and butter. He finished all of this plus several slices of bread and butter. Then he repeated the entire order. After that the waitress brought him whipped cream cake and a cup of coffee. He finished this, and she brought him a second order of whipped cream cake and coffee. He ate it all with gusto.

We intentionally dawdled, and after he left the restaurant I asked the waitress about him. "He's one of my steady customers," she explained. "He comes in every night at this time, and that's what he gets. I don't have to ask him what he wants."

He had just come from a classroom full of doctors who were discussing the dangers of obesity. His own doctor had said in front of him, "We must help this man before he suffers a heart attack from carrying that weight around." And immediately after hearing this statement, he had proceded to eat more than enough for two men. Here was a patient who didn't want help. He didn't know it, but he was unconsciously attempting to commit suicide. Such patients are extremely difficult to help.

When I hear about intractable obesity problems, I recall the doctor who said, "Mr. Elman, your next class will be attended by an extraordinary man. He's a psychiatrist who does remarkable work with the emotional problems of his patients, but he isn't able to solve his own." I was curious enough to ask for details, but my informant only answered, "Wait until you see him."

It was easy to recognize the man who couldn't solve his own emotional problems. He was at least 150 pounds overweight. Since he was not very tall, his girth was actually startling. He must have weighed more than 300 pounds. We had not had many class sessions before he asked if I would work with him to see if we couldn't determine the cause of his overweight. During hypnoanalysis he went into an abreaction that disclosed several traumatic episodes, and as he relived various experiences, he cried bitterly. I am not at liberty to disclose the details of this case, but we did find the reasons for his search for security, and he agreed that the findings were accurate. Nevertheless, I was unable to give him any real insight regarding the connection between this search and his weight problem. I don't think he benefitted from the hypnoanalysis. If this seems strange to say of a psychiatrist—a man trained to understand such connections—bear in mind that there are undoubtedly people who don't want their problems solved. They profess a desire for help and even seem to seek it, but when the help is offered, they refuse to take it. I am of the opinion that this unwillingness to get well is part of their illness.

When a person is only moderately overweight, trauma doesn't have to be the cause, and I think I should make this point very clear. I know a patient who is only ten or fifteen pounds overweight, and she tells a story that explains why. She says that when she was a child, every time she cried, her mother stuffed her mouth with food, and in that way kept her from crying. If she hurt herself, her mother gave her food; if she couldn't go to sleep at night, her mother gave her food. On all occasions when the child was in discomfort or unhappy, her mother stuffed her with food. The habit of eating during times of stress—not trauma but merely tension—became ingrained. This woman laughs about it today, but brings her own children up the same way. If these children become overweight, she will never realize that she was probably the cause of it, just as her mother was the cause in her own case. Many people may be overweight because of habit patterns developed in infancy and childhood.

There are certain pathological conditions which cause overweight. Every physician knows what they are, and checks these conditions when examining his patients. Such cases, of course, do not require hypnoanalysis as part of the treatment program. And even in cases involving emotional conflicts, a doctor sometimes can do an amazing job without the use of hypnoanalysis. If a doctor gives a patient sufficient incentive to lose weight, that person, despite strong emotional problems, will manage to stay on a diet. Here is a case history to illustrate the point:

A young married woman, who had been tremendously overweight for years, was now happier than she had ever been in her life. After ten years of marriage, she was pregnant for the first time and was looking forward to the birth of her baby. She had fitted up a beautiful nursery, prepared a layette, and when I saw her she could talk about nothing but the child that would soon be theirs. She carried to full term, but the baby was stillborn. She and her husband were heartbroken. She had been overweight for so many years that when she gained even more weight during pregnancy she was not disturbed. It seemed to her quite natural to put on weight during pregnancy. When it was over, she was too upset to give much thought to dieting. After her discharge from the hospital, her doctor told her the sad news that she would never be able to have a baby. In all probability she had had previous emotional problems; now she had an additional one, and the pattern of overeating, if it changed at all, became stronger. About two years later, she went to another doctor because she had a cold. During the interview, she mentioned the fact that nothing would make her happier than having a baby, but had resigned herself to the fact that this could never be. The doctor said, "Do you mind if I examine you to confirm that."

"It would probably be a waste of time," she told him, "because I've already been examined and told I could never have a baby. I lost the only one I ever carried. But I want a baby so badly. Go ahead, doctor, let's see what your examination shows."

After the examination he said, "I don't agree with the previous diagnosis. If you will lose at least seventy-five pounds, I promise you will have a baby."

This was such welcome news to her that she told the doctor, "I could starve myself if the reward were the baby I want. What do I do?"

He prescribed a diet, warning her that if she strayed from it there would be no baby. "You must eat the things I have prescribed," he cautioned her, "because you must maintain good health to have a healthy baby. You can be sure that the diet I have given you is good for you. Eat everything on it, but nothing else."

She followed his instructions implicitly, actually enjoying her diet, and every time something tempted her, she gleefully remarked, "That's not for me. I'm going to have a baby and I don't need that fattening stuff."

She lost eighty pounds, and she became pregnant. Of course, she and her husband were delighted. Now their task was to be sure that this baby was born in good health.

The doctor who had put her on the diet took care of her during pregnancy. He now put her on another diet, one that would maintain health but would not add weight. She delivered a healthy baby, and at this writing, she is a slender, happy mother. It is plain to see from this case history that the proper incentive can help even a person with great emotional problems to maintain a proper diet.

But this does not mean that hypnoanalysis can often be dispensed with. Some years ago, nationwide publicity was given to a professional hypnotic operator who said he had been tremendously successful with hypnotic diet in obesity cases, and the publicity actually contained some re-

markable statistics. The doctors in my classes asked me
why I hadn't taught them how to handle obesity problems
by the use of hypnotic suggestion.

As I explained to them, it is easy to put patients on
hypnotic diets, but in most cases as soon as the suggestions
wear off, they'll regain the weight they have lost. In the
final analysis, what good are the suggestions if they don't
give permanent results? Hypnotic suggestions will not enable the patient to solve his basic problem. He will lose
weight fast; of course he will. But later on, he will be as
fat as ever. I don't believe a doctor should use hypnotic
suggestions for this purpose until he has solved the basic
problem, learning why a patient has to eat so much, and
then treating the cause and not the effect.

The doctors insisted, however, that I teach them how
to put a patient on a hypnotic diet. I did so, and doctor
after doctor reported how successful he had been. Weight
losses were reported of thirty, forty or fifty pounds, or even
more. But the same doctor who had been so successful
would often report a year or two later that "Those obese
patients are as fat as ever. Hypnosis doesn't give permanent results."

Because of these reports, I refused to teach any more
doctors how to put a patient on a hypnotic diet. However,
a psychiatrist made me change my thinking. "Think of the
doctor who is in cardiology for example," he said. "His
patient must lose weight fast. If hypnosis will help his
patient lose weight fast, you have no right to demand slower
methods for lasting results. Even temporary help might be
vital to such a patient. And you don't have to be in cardiology to meet cases of this type. Give these doctors the
instructions they need."

After a great deal of reflection, I decided to make an
instructional recording on the subject. This, I felt, would
save doctors much valuable time if they were made to understand that hypnotic diet could not, by itself, constitute complete treatment. I gave a series of lectures on the subject,
asking the doctors to tape record every word said. Then I
asked them to allow their obese patients to hear the tapes
to see whether or not by listening to a recording they could
be placed on a hypnotic diet.

The tapes must have been effective, for soon doctors

began requesting that we make a phonograph record which could be given to obese patients to use at home. We made such a record. Then an interesting incident took place. An obstetrician came to class one night and explained that many women after delivery seem to gain an unusual amount of weight. She wanted to get these people down to normal size again and had therefore invited a group of her obese patients to a meeting with her so that she could discuss their obesity problems. A surprising number of patients showed up for that first meeting. She held a lengthy discussion of the disadvantages of extra poundage, after which she played the record for them, gave them a diet to follow and told them to come back one week later for a checkup.

An odd thing happened with these patients. They began to compete with each other to see who could lose the most weight in the shortest time. Moreover, the class which had originally started with seventeen obese patients grew to thirty-five at the second session. The doctor weighed each patient and found that every one of them had lost weight. She decided to call a third meeting, and this time so many patients showed up that she was obliged to divide the class into two groups. Finally, she had to have three groups.

She suggested in class that other doctors form classes in obesity, remarking that, "There are enough fat people for all of us." I repeated her story in all my classes. Soon doctors were treating obesity patients in groups, and this group therapy seems quite effective. The patients actually compete with each other, and it is impressive what competition does in accomplishing weight reduction.

I think I should mention at this point a California physician, Doctor Peter G. Lindner, who has been so successful with this sort of class instruction that he has written a book on obesity. The book is entitled "Mind Over Platter," and to learn interesting facts about obesity, I recommend that you read it.

Don't think because of what I have said that a recording will do the job alone. It must be supplemented by sound advice from the doctor and a diet prescribed by him, plus additional therapy, including hypnoanalysis, when indicated. The diet must be followed conscientiously. All the record will do is strengthen the patient's determination to stay on the diet.

To conclude this discussion of weight problems uncovered in hypnosis, I believe we should recount one case history which is the complete opposite of any thus far related:

A young lady was brought to class who was a pleasure to see. She was about sixteen years old, and beautiful. If there was any flaw in her appearance, it was that she was extremely slim—though not skinny. Her doctor said, "I'd like you to work with this girl. She's in deep trouble. She has an enormous appetite. It's unearthly. It's just an inordinate appetite, but after every meal she regurgitates everything she has eaten. We're worried about her and we can't find anything organic that makes her vomit. We think it's purely a functional symptom but at the same time we can't find out what this functional symptom represents. We're rather lost in the handling of her. I wonder if through hypnoanalysis we can find out what's causing the trouble."

The young lady accepted deep hypnosis quite readily and I attempted to pinpoint the start of the neurosis. I had her relive the events leading up to the first time she ever vomited, and it seemed to me I was going in the right direction. It started with the first prom she'd ever attended. She was fourteen years old, and a seventeen-year-old boy had asked her for the date. The girl was delighted. They went to the prom and she found out that he couldn't dance. This was a terrible disappointment to the fourteen-year-old. She had a miserable time. She had built the prom up in her mind as a tremendous event. Afterwards, he took her to a hamburger stand with the rest of the school crowd. As she ate her hamburger, she thought about how nauseating an evening it had been. In her own words, "I just couldn't stomach that boy." Her reaction was to vomit; that was the first time. I felt sure I was on the right track.

Now I took her to the second time she ever vomited to see if I could find a habit pattern. Sure enough, her second date was nauseating, too, and so was the third one. By this time I was convinced I had found the reason for her problem and that it could be solved easily. Preparing to do it, I asked her the preliminary question in deep hypnosis. "How would you like to get rid of that vomiting?"

She threw us all for a loop when she answered, "Oh no. I don't want to stop."

"Why don't you want to lose that vomiting habit?"

"Before I learned to vomit I was fat. Don't tell me that I should lose this vomiting habit, because if I don't vomit I'll get fat like I used to be and I don't want to be fat. I love to eat and I'd rather vomit than diet. Vomiting works wonders for me."

Of course, this case required further work. I included the incident here to show that in hypnoanalysis the patient doesn't let you get far off the track for very long. A patient with an awareness of two thousand percent or more above normal won't let you make (and hold onto) a mistake very easily. You can make a temporary error as I did, but when I make a mistake the thing that often puts me back on the right track is the awareness of the patient. It reveals itself in some such statement as, "No, I don't want to lose the vomiting habit."

In doing hypnoanalysis it is well to bear in mind that things are not always what they seem. Listen carefully to what a patient reveals about himself during this period of heightened awareness. And remember that a single session is not a cure. Uncovering a problem in obesity does not necessarily solve the problem. In every case I have mentioned, further work was indicated.

Chapter 18

PHOBIAS AND MORBID FEARS

ONE OF the most interesting experiences a doctor can have is the tracking down of a phobia. It is my contention that every phobia can be tracked to its originating source, and that bringing this source to the conscious attention of the patient in many cases helps the patient tremendously, and in some cases results in a complete correction. Unfortunately many doctors think that the cause of a phobia is difficult to determine and that investigation requires an interminable time. As a matter of fact, hypnoanalysis offers a rapid way to expose and resolve a phobia.

Of course, many individuals have phobias but don't recognize their difficulties as such. Some people will refuse to ride an escalator but will deny the existence of any phobia: "I just don't like escalators. It isn't a phobia; it's an idiosyncrasy." Similarly, fear of walking downstairs is labeled "just an eccentricity." We are all apt to rationalize actions which do not appear to be within the norm.

A phobia is an abnormal fear, a dread of any object or action. Chances are, if you search yourself honestly, you will find that you are the victim of one or more phobias. These fears are anything but unusual, though they may sometimes manifest themselves in unusual ways.

I can best illustrate from my own experience. I am afraid of riding in an airplane, though I flew a great deal, without any fear, until a particularly upsetting incident left the stamp of panic on me.

It happened when my oldest son got on a plane at LaGuardia field, bound for Florida. Many students were going to Florida and it was decided to accommodate these students in two flights. My wife and I were seeing our son off to school. We watched both planes take off, then wandered around the terminal for several minutes. As we were about to leave, we heard a loudspeaker report that one of the planes leaving for Miami had crashed. There was pandemonium in the terminal. We had failed to note the number of my son's flight and for the rest of the night we tried, without success, to find out whether he had boarded the doomed plane. Finally, all people who had no immediate business at the terminal were asked to leave and wait at their radios for further news. But there were no further details on the radio. When we were just about crazy with worry the phone rang. I was afraid to answer it. I lifted the receiver and heard my son's voice saying, "Hi, Dad. I'm at the airport in Florida. It was a wonderful trip."

Since that time I've always dreaded an airplane flight. I have a phobic fear of plane rides, though I force myself to fly when necessary. I believe a few sessions of hypnoanalysis under proper guidance would enable me to overcome this fear completely.

Let me tell you about some of the interesting phobias I have encountered in my teachings. If a few seem amusing to you, remember that they certainly were not amusing to their victims.

A doctor declared: "Mr. Elman, my wife is deathly afraid of cats. If we are walking down the street and happen to see a cat, she will insist that we cross the street. If she is walking by herself and happens to see one, she will go several blocks out of her way to keep from passing it. I believe if I ever made her approach a cat she would actually go into shock. You couldn't get her to touch one no matter what reward you offered her."

He said this before the class, and his wife laughed, but the laugh was one of embarrassment. However, she confirmed what he said, and the doctor asked, "Do you think we can determine the source of her unusual reactions?"

Before I started to work with her in hypnosis, I questioned her extensively:

"Did you ever have a cat for a pet?"

"Of course not—never in my life. I couldn't bear the thought of it."

"Did you ever have an unpleasant experience with a cat?"

"Not that I know of. I don't know why I can't stand them."

I continued to question her but could learn nothing that would establish a cause for the phobia. By this time the doctors were anxious to learn what hypnoanalysis would reveal. She accepted somnambulism quite readily, and I found her a most willing, cooperative subject. I was able to take her back to the time when she was a few years old and found that even at this very early age she was afraid of cats. It was necessary to regress her to the age of two before we could locate the source of the trouble.

Her parents had given her a little kitten for a present. The child loved the kitten so much that she took it to bed with her night after night. One morning she woke up and the kitten was cold and silent beside her. It was dead. Frightened by her first encounter with death and upset at the loss of her beloved pet, she was deathly afraid of cats from that time on. She first learned that the kitten was dead when she touched it, trying to get it to play as usual. She would never touch one again.

At subsequent class meetings her husband told me they were now able to walk down the street and see a cat without her showing any unpleasant reactions. No longer did they have to cross the street to avoid them. She could even walk down the street alone and pass a cat without betraying the slightest bit of emotion. However, when I asked her if she would like to have a cat for a pet, she answered, "Decidedly not. No, never."

"Would you be able to touch a cat without having an unpleasant reaction?"

"I believe I could do that all right, but I wouldn't want one for a pet.'"

Maybe you look upon this as a complete correction. I don't. I still believe further work was indicated.

We were conducting classes in a western city, meeting in a room which was several stories up from the lobby. On several occasions, before the session started, I would see a doctor climbing the stairs as I was coming out of the elavator.

I asked him one time, "Why don't you take the elevator?"

He answered, "I prefer the stairs."

I didn't question him further, but one night he came to me and said, "Maybe you wonder why I always walk up the stairs instead of taking the elevator. I have claustrophobia. I can't get into an elevator. It's too small and confining a space. I am never able to go into a confined space because I suffer torture when I do."

I asked him if he would like us to find out, by means of hypnoanalysis, the cause of his difficulty. We found the source in his early childhood. He was raised by his aunt, who used to punish him for minor misdeeds by making him stand in a corner. If he had done something really naughty, she would punish him by putting him into a dark closet and leaving him there for quite a while. This was all right with him; he was not scared at all at first. But one day when she locked him in the closet, she went out shopping and completely forgot about him. After quite a while, he tried to get out of the closet. When he couldn't, he shouted for his aunt. Nobody answered—she didn't come—and he went into a panic. Finally, his aunt came home to find a shrieking, terrified boy. She released him from the closet, but in a way she was too late; his claustrophobia had begun. It delighted me to see that after the hypnoanalysis, he took the elevator to our meeting rooms.

The number of phobias listed in dictionaries and medical texts is astounding—fear of water, of height, of depth, of birds, of darkness, etc., etc., etc. People in the music business still recall that one of their union leaders scarcely ever shook hands with people. It was said that he feared the contamination that might possibly result from germs being transferred in a handshake. The condition is called bacteriophobia, and is not as uncommon as you might think. The person who has this condition looks upon it as plain common sense, and would deny vehemently that it is a phobia. Yet phobias are all the more damaging because they are so common and because they go unrecognized.

Medical dictionaries list one definition of phobias as "morbid fears." If we regard these as phobias, I might easily think of countless examples. It is my contention that morbid fears are responsible for many neurotic aches and pains, and sometimes even for deaths.

These morbid fears may go undetected in cases where they exist below the level of conscious awareness. The doctors who most often come upon them and recognize them are men in the psychiatric field. When they resolve the inner conflicts promulgated by these morbid fears, they have the patient well on the road to recovery. I have heard psychiatrists in class, as I uncovered some of these fears, say, "It will be easy to go on from there with the information you've extracted."

We had been discussing phobias one night in class, and when the session was over a doctor came up to me and said, "Talking about phobias, how would you explain this? I can't walk down the street by myself. Walking down a street alone is absolutely frightening. For example, if I am making a house call and the patient lives just a short distance away, I don't walk. I drive. There is nothing wrong with my legs, no aches or pains. It's just that I can't walk down a street by myself. Yet if I walk with somebody, I am not disturbed at all."

He wouldn't undergo hypnoanalysis before his fellow students, but what he was learning in class seemed to help him. Before the course was over, he came to class one night and proudly announced, "I walked by myself today, for three whole blocks. And for the first time since I can remember, I enjoyed the walk. I stopped to window shop. I have never been able to do that. Believe me, it is a pleasure to be able to walk down the street by myself like other people. Thanks for your help."

Since I had not given him any specific help, I can only assume that, having seen the work we did in the classroom on similar problems, he applied the knowledge to himself and was thereby able to help himself.

One of the most common phobias is fear of the dark. Some people are afraid to enter a closet or a dark room. I remember investigating a case of enuresis, and finding that the problem was solved immediately when a fear of the dark was uncovered. The cause of the fear was determined to the child's satisfaction, and the bed-wetting ceased. Some phobias, however, can have far more serious consequences than a child's wetting of a bed. They can even affect pre- and postoperative prognoses.

Abnormally severe preoperative apprehension is some-times encountered in medical and dental practice. The patient goes through a trying ordeal. This is particularly true of children, yet many youngsters can be helped by hypnoanalysis. Children are easy to hypnotize. Get them into the somnambulistic state and simply ask them why they are afraid. Most of the time these youngsters will disclose the disturbing factor and the doctor can usually correct the condition quickly.

In the case which follows, you find a fear much deeper than the usual preoperative fear of a child. You have the morbid fear of death, produced by seeing a veterinarian put a dog to sleep permanently. From that time on morbid fear was present, penetrating deeper and deeper into his thoughts. Eventually he began to associate the anesthesia he had had in previous operations with the actions of the veterinarian, and became deathly afraid of doctors and any anesthesia.

He was ashamed to reveal his fears to anyone, particularly to his father, who was a doctor. He tried to repress his fear, but could not cope with it. Eventually he was almost in a panic state at the very thought of the operation which he knew would be necessary.

Operations done under such circumstances are traumatic events for the patients who undergo them and are responsible for slow recovery and much postoperative discomfort. Merely remove a child's tonsils while he is in a panic state, and you leave him with a morbid fear that conditions his actions all through life.

In the hypnoanalysis which follows, pay particular attention to the "thumb" or "finger" technique employed. In the case of the boy with the morbid fears, it was used to get him to reveal what he was ashamed to tell. It was known material, being intentionally withheld by the patient. It is important that you know how the case was explained to me before we worked with the boy. His father told me the boy had had four operations on his eyes. He had shown no unusual apprehension during any of these operations. A fifth operation had been performed for the removal of his tonsils, and at this time he had gone into a panic. Now another operation was deemed necessary on the boy's eyes, and his father was extremely worried. Five operations would upset anybody, but would not necessarily be responsible for morbid fears.

With this information, I began the hypnoanalysis. I investigated the first three operations to find if anything untoward had occurred during any of this surgery. The following excerpt begins with the investigation of the third operation:

ELMAN: When I snap my fingers it will be a week before your third operation . . . [snaps fingers] How old are you?

PATIENT: Seven.

ELMAN: And you're going to have your third operation. When are you going to have it?

PATIENT: July.

ELMAN: Let's take you right to the third operation now . . . [snaps fingers] They're dressing you for that third operation. How are they dressing you?

PATIENT: In sort of white pants.

ELMAN: Was there anything that disturbed you in that third operation?

PATIENT: No.

ELMAN: Now, it's just one week before the fourth operation. What grade are you in school?

PATIENT: Third grade.

ELMAN: Now tell me, what time of the year is it?

PATIENT: It's winter.

ELMAN: And are you in school now as I'm talking to you? Where are you in your mind?

PATIENT: At home.

ELMAN: I'm talking to you at home, and I'm saying to you, "You're going to have the fourth operation on your eyes, aren't you? And you're going to have it in about a week. Is that right? Tell me, how do you feel about this operation? Do you mind having it? You didn't mind having those other three, did you? Well, you're going to have the fourth operation." When I snap my fingers it will be just before the fourth operation. You'll be seeing how they dress you and everything . . . [snaps fingers] How are you being dressed?

PATIENT: White.

ELMAN: Same way?

PATIENT: Yes.

ELMAN: They're wheeling you into the operating room when I snap my fingers . . . [snaps fingers] Anything different about this operation so far?

PATIENT: No.

ELMAN: All right. Now you're in the operating room and what's the first thing that happens?

PATIENT: Sleep.

ELMAN: All right. How'd they do that?

PATIENT: They put a needle in my arm.

ELMAN: Did you mind that?

PATIENT: I liked that better than the ether.

ELMAN: They put this needle in your arm. Now what happens after they put the needle in your arm?

PATIENT: I sleep.

ELMAN: Do you go right to sleep? Let's see if you went right to sleep because this will be just about two minutes after they gave you the anesthesia and I'll know whether you're asleep or not by your answer. It's two minutes after they gave you the needle. Are you asleep? [Patient nods.] Are you worried about anything? [Patient shakes his head indicating 'no'.] When they finished the operation you were up in your hospital room, is that right?

PATIENT: Yes.

ELMAN: How do you feel coming out of the anesthesia?

PATIENT: Okay.

ELMAN: Do you hear anything? Anybody saying anything in the hospital room?

PATIENT: Yes.

ELMAN: Who's talking?

PATIENT: Mother.

ELMAN: What's she saying?

PATIENT: They're dressing me.

ELMAN: Putting your clothes on, you mean?

PATIENT: Yes.

ELMAN:	The idea being to take you home? Was that the idea?
PATIENT:	Yes.
ELMAN:	Was there anything about this dressing that alarmed you? Everything was quite in order? [Patient nods.] Let's go to the time when you had your tonsil operation, should we? You weren't afraid of anesthesia all the time you were having the eye operations, were you?
PATIENT:	No.
ELMAN:	All right, now we're going to just about the time when you're ready to have your tonsil operation . . . [snaps fingers] How old are you?
PATIENT:	Seven.
ELMAN:	Now it's going to be just about a day before your tonsil operation. When I snap my fingers, I want you to answer me just as if you're seven years old . . . [snaps fingers] You're going to have your tonsils out tomorrow. You don't mind it, do you?
PATIENT:	No.
ELMAN:	Not scared of it at all. Are you going to the hospital to have it done?
PATIENT:	Yes.
ELMAN:	All right. Now you're in the hospital and they're getting ready to take out your tonsils. When I snap my fingers . . . [snaps fingers] How do you feel about this operation on your tonsils?
PATIENT:	Okay.
ELMAN:	You aren't scared, are you?
PATIENT:	No.
ELMAN:	And you don't mind taking medicine to put you to sleep?
PATIENT:	No.
ELMAN:	Your parents are gone from the hospital . . . What are you thinking about after they go?
PATIENT:	I'm scared.

ELMAN: You are scared? You're scared because of the tonsils coming out, is that what you're scared about?

PATIENT: No.

ELMAN: Well then, you tell me, just what makes you scared. Maybe if you tell me what makes you scared I can get that scare out of you so that you'll never have it again.

PATIENT: Ether.

ELMAN: Afraid of the ether. What are you afraid of the ether about?

PATIENT: It smells awful.

ELMAN: Are you at the place where they're going to give you the ether now?

PATIENT: Yes.

ELMAN: Have you ever had ether before?
PATIENT: Yes.

ELMAN: And you're scared about the ether. This is stuff you never told me. What makes you scared about the ether?

PATIENT: The smell.

ELMAN: Is that the only thing? What else are you scared about? Just the smell? Look, there's more to it than that because just the smell of something doesn't scare anybody. For instance, if you smell vinegar, you don't get scared, do you? If you smell alcohol, you don't get scared, do you? If you had to smell some type of acid that smelled badly you wouldn't get scared, would you? But all of a sudden you're scared because of ether. Now, there's a reason for it, and I'll tell you what we're going to do to find out what that reason is. You're going to lose complete control of this thumb. You won't be able to move it. That thumb is going to represent your deep inside mind and that thumb is going to be controlled by your inside mind. The rest of you will be controlled by your outside mind, your conscious mind. If you tell me that the ether just scared you and there's something *else* to it, that finger will move because you can't keep it from moving. See what I mean? But when you tell me exactly what it *was* that scared you about the ether, then you'll find that finger won't move any more because that finger always tells me whether your outside mind is agreeing with your inside mind. You know what I mean by the concious mind and underneath the conscious? Do you know what I mean?

PATIENT: Yes.

ELMAN: All right. So, now you answer the questions. You've had ether before. How did you feel before when the ether was administered?

PATIENT: I didn't like it.

ELMAN: Well, let's take you to the time when they are giving the ether for this tonsil operation. There's more to it than the smell. Notice how the thumb is moving? What else is scaring you about it? You could feel that thumb moving, couldn't you? So that means there's more inside that you haven't told me. When you tell me the whole thing, that thumb won't move any more. So, tell me the whole thing, won't you?

PATIENT: I don't know.

ELMAN: The thumb says you do know. The thumb just said that you do know. Now, we've got to find out because you want to be helped, don't you? Of course, you do. So, there was something else. And you'll know what that something else was when I snap my fingers . . . [snaps fingers] What was it?

PATIENT: Doctors.

ELMAN: You were scared of all the doctors, was that it? You see, your thumb stayed pretty still that time. But there's still something else about the doctors or something, because every once in a while it's got that jump in it. See that? There's something else. Tell me what it is so that I can help you, won't you? What is it?

PATIENT: The tools.

ELMAN: The tools that they work with? Is that it? Did
            you get a chance to see all these tools in the
            hospital room, was that it? Was that at the eye
            operations that you saw them or just at the tonsil
            operation? When was it you saw all these tools?

PATIENT: At the tonsils.

ELMAN: In other words you were never scared during
            the eye operations, isn't that right? But you
            were scared at the tonsil operation. Is that what
            happened? You see, when you said yes the
            thumb stayed still, but if you'd said no you would
            have seen that thumb jump. Was it the tools,
            the instruments that the doctors had that scared
            you? [Patient does not answer.] You say they
            gave you ether. At what point did you start
            getting scared?

PATIENT: The ether.

ELMAN: Started with the ether. You didn't like the ether
            from the very start? Well, you'd had it before
            and you weren't scared. What made you scared
            this time?

PATIENT: The smell.

ELMAN: Well, you'd smelled ether before, hadn't you?

PATIENT: Yes.

ELMAN: And you never were scared of the smell before.
            This time you were scared of it. Why? You'll
            know when I snap my fingers . . . [snaps fingers.]
            Why?

PATIENT: It didn't smell good.

ELMAN: Had it smelled good for the other operations?
            . . . But this time it really smelled bad. What
            is it that is really scaring you? See that thumb
            moving? What is it that you're not telling me?
            You can feel it move, can't you? So you know
            that I know there's something else that has to
            come out. You're in the operating room for the
            tonsils, and this is the first time you were really

	scared. Now, when I snap my fingers you'll know what scared you . . . [snaps fingers.] What scared you? Did anybody say anything?
PATIENT:	No. Tools.
ELMAN:	It was the tools. What kind of tools scared you? Your thumb is begging you to tell just what did happen that scared you. Don't you know that if you tell this and once get it out of your mind you won't have that scare any more? And then you'll be able to look at operations as a person should look at them when they're necessary, without that terrible fear. You know what fear does to a person, don't you?
PATIENT:	No.
ELMAN:	Oh, yes you do. You know that it's made you scared of the eye operation that you ought to have. Hasn't it? Now, you want your eyes to be well, don't you? And if you once get rid of this fear . . . See that thumb jumping all over, saying, "Boy, I would like to tell. I would like to tell just what caused that fear because then it wouldn't be there any more." Do you want to tell me what caused that fear?
PATIENT:	I don't know what it was.
ELMAN:	Does your inside mind know what it was? What does your thumb keep saying that you should tell me?
PATIENT:	Medicines.
ELMAN:	Medicines during the operation?
PATIENT:	Medicines before.
ELMAN:	The anesthesia, is that what you mean? The thing that puts you to sleep, is that what you're thinking about? Those medicines? What is there about those medicines that scares you? And when did they scare you? Because I can't find any scare there. Oh, but look how that thumb is saying, "Yes there was plenty of scare." What was it?

PATIENT: I was afraid I wouldn't wake up.

ELMAN: See, that's what your thumb is saying, that's what you were thinking, wasn't it? In other words, it was the fear of death, was that it? Now, was that so hard to tell me? Don't you feel better for having gotten it out of your system? Because you know that fear wasn't justified. What gave you the idea that you might not wake up from the ether? Or that you might die from the ether? What gave you that idea?

PATIENT: Dog put to sleep.

ELMAN: Oh, you saw a dog put to sleep, did you? Oh, now, you see what the whole thing was. Don't you understand that? Don't you see where it all comes from?

PATIENT: I saw a veterinarian put a dog to sleep forever.

ELMAN: They don't do that to humans. There isn't a doctor in the world who would ever, ever, ever do a thing like that to anybody. You'd never meet a man like that in your whole lifetime. You can't imagine a person doing a thing like that to another person, can you? And yet you had a notion the ether was going to do that to you. You thought that's what they gave to the dog. That isn't what they gave to the dog at all. They wanted to put the dog out of its misery, painlessly. But they aren't allowed to do that with human beings. Do you see that? Is that fear all gone now? Look, the minute you told me that, notice how still the thumb stays. Whenever something like that gets on the inside of your mind and bothers you terribly, don't keep it inside. Let a person know what it is. You were ashamed to tell me. Afraid to tell me weren't you, at first? Because it might show that you weren't a man or something like that, or it wouldn't be manly. But you can be awfully manly and have fears. Don't you know that? And you never have to be afraid of the truth. You know that you're all over being scared be-

cause your finger said that and you said that and
we know that. And when you have the operation on your eyes, you're not going to be scared
any more, are you? You know that, don't you.
And you're never going to have the thought that
anybody is going to put you to sleep permanently. You won't ever have that thought again,
will you?

PATIENT: No, [sobbing] I'll be all right now.

                    *   *   *

The finger technique can often be valuable to the adroit
operator in hypnoanalysis. In recent years, the patient's reactions to this technique have become known as "ideomotor
responses," and they are also used to extract unknown material lurking below the level of conscious awareness. Here
are instructions for employing the finger technique.

Stroke the little finger or the thumb of the patient as
you tell him, "This finger is being put under the control
of your inside mind. In just a few seconds, when your inner
mind takes over, you won't be able to bend this finger no
matter how hard you try. You'll have no control of it consciously. You can go ahead and try to bend it but you'll
find it won't bend."

After testing to make sure the patient cannot will the
finger to bend, continue speaking as follows: "Just as I said,
that finger is now under the control of your inside mind—
the real you. The real you knows exactly what happened—
it can't lie to you because you know the truth of everything,
and that inside mind is the real you. If I should ask you
something and you don't tell me the entire truth, or if you
should tell me a falsehood, that finger under the control of
your inside mind will bend and I'll know there is something
more to the story than you are telling me."

The suggestion that the patient's finger will bend if he
isn't telling the truth or is hiding something, is an insidious
one. It gives him the impression that the movement of that
finger is beyond his control. In this way, when he tells a
lie, he gives himself away by moving the finger, thereby
keeping the operator on the right track. Should this occur,
the operator must then find another means of arriving at
the truth.

Be sure to make your statement casually, as if this were the most normal behavior pattern in the world, and in many cases you will get at the complete truth of the situation. As you work, watch the finger or thumb. The instant the patient varies from the truth or does not give a complete answer, his inside thoughts will speak out through spasmodic movements of the immobilized finger. Sometimes if the patient in hypnoanalysis begins to tell a protracted false-hood or gives misleading information, the finger will creep upward, not with spasmodic movement, but little by little and steadily, and the patient will not even know it has changed position.

The patient who bends his finger from the very outset, when you are first giving him the suggestion that it will not bend but that the finger will be under the control of his inner mind, is resisting from the outset. This patient knows that he is hiding something and prefers to keep it that way. On the other hand, the patient who accepts this suggestion and cannot will his finger to bend, but later bends it when he tells a lie, is not resisting. Actually he has accepted your suggestion that the finger will move when he lies, thus keeping you on the right track. The finger technique is a valuable tool for unearthing the causes for all sorts of phobias.

*   *   *

To treat a phobia, however, you must of course recognize it. Sometimes phobias are unrecognized even by the doctor. A doctor's wife was brought to class for hypnoanalysis. Her husband was at a loss to understand the cause of her ailments. Three dermatologists had diagnosed her condition as scleroderma. The effect of the illness was evident in a scalp condition which resulted in the loss of hair and eyebrows. This condition began prior to a stillborn delivery. In addition, the patient had suffered from rose fever since childhood. Hypnoanalysis revealed a deep-rooted morbid fear—a phobia. Here is an excerpt from the transcript of the hypnoanalysis:

ELMAN: I want to go to the time when you were a little girl in the first grade. School was enjoyable to you, wasn't it?

PATIENT: It wasn't in the first grade.

ELMAN: You didn't like the studies, or anything like that?

PATIENT: No, the teacher.

ELMAN: Did this affect you in any way? Did you feel
            so badly about school that it made you react in
            any way?

PATIENT: No. It never did.

ELMAN: In other words, you were able to handle that.
            What we're going to do now is to take you to
            the fourth grade. Where are you sitting in this
            room? Your memory gets better with every
            breath you take.

PATIENT: In the third row.

ELMAN: Tell me, have you ever had rose fever?

PATIENT: I think I did.

ELMAN: Now, we're going to take you back to the third
            grade. In the third grade you'll see it even more
            clearly than you did in the fourth grade. As I
            said, with every breath you take, your memory
            gets better. You can feel it getting better, can't
            you? Did you ever have rose fever while you
            were in the third grade? [Patient does not an-
            swer.] All right, we're going to take you back to
            the second grade. Tell me, you're in the second
            grade right now, did you ever have rose fever?

PATIENT: I don't think so.

ELMAN: Then something happened between the second
            and third grades that was an emotional involve-
            ment of some kind. Let's go to the end of the
            second grade. It's June now. You're about sev-
            en years old and you're not having rose fever
            now if you're in the second grade, are you?

PATIENT: No.

ELMAN: It's Christmas time and you're in the third grade.
            Has anything happened in the first part of this
            year that upset you in any way?

PATIENT: My aunt died.

ELMAN: What did your aunt represent in your life?

PATIENT: Very important.

ELMAN: The important person. Even when you think about it now you can feel as you felt when you were a child. Had your aunt been ill long?

PATIENT: She died in childbirth.

ELMAN: And this was the thing that upset you? And this was the time when the rose fever came on that year?

PATIENT: She liked roses.

ELMAN: And so that's what brought on the rose fever. Now, let's go a little beyond that. This rose fever—was it because you thought of her in connection with roses, was that it?

PATIENT: I'd never thought of it.

ELMAN: You never thought of it from that day to this. You never realized that there was any connection. Did you continue to grieve over her pretty much?

PATIENT: Yes.

ELMAN: And how did the rest of the family take it? They were grieving too, were they—pretty bad? Tell me, what did you find yourself doing?

PATIENT: It was a great loss and I cried a great deal.

ELMAN: How did you react to it? Did you find yourself crying by yourself and things like that?

PATIENT: I couldn't stop crying.

ELMAN: So that by the time the roses came along which she liked . . .

PATIENT: I've disliked roses ever since.

ELMAN: Now that you realize where the rose fever came from, I don't think you'll ever be troubled with it again . . . And now you will be able to handle the situation . . . Now I want you to remember the first day you ever found this skin condition, and you'll be able to tell me where you were and how you happened to notice it. What happened?

PATIENT: I remember when my hair was thin in a spot.

ELMAN: Where you had been pulling it?

PATIENT: Yes. And I remember sitting—I was outside. And I remember the coolness of my skin and scalp and it frightened me that the spot was so large.

ELMAN: When was this?

PATIENT: It was before I delivered.

ELMAN: Was there anything on your mind about the delivery? Were you worried about it?

PATIENT: Not that I know of.

ELMAN: Was anything upsetting you during this period?

PATIENT: Yes.

ELMAN: You tell me what was upsetting. What was it?

PATIENT: I was very tired. I had a year-old baby and a three-year-old and I was tired and we were moving.

ELMAN: Just too much for a young mother to take at that point. Was that it? Or what? Remember, you told me a very important thing—that your aunt died in childbirth. Remember that? Now you told me your baby was stillborn. Remember also that probably there was still a great love for your aunt. Is that correct?

PATIENT: Yes.

ELMAN: So now we put two factors together and find out that you were expecting to deliver and going through a very trying pregnancy because you were so worried and tired. Is that correct?

PATIENT: Yes. I had often said that I didn't think I could ever deliver. I felt guilty about that. I was talking to the neighbors and I would say I was too tired to deliver.

ELMAN: Then there was a terrific worry and a holding back.

PATIENT: It went ten months.

ELMAN: Afraid to deliver, in other words. Was that it?

PATIENT: I seemed to be.

ELMAN: And this dermatitis condition—did it develop during this time?

PATIENT: Just a raw spot. Very large.

ELMAN: You said the baby was stillborn?

PATIENT: Yes.

ELMAN: Did you expect that because of the trying pregnancy or for any reason?

PATIENT: No.

ELMAN: But you did feel that you were holding back during the pregnancy. Is that right?

PATIENT: I didn't know I did it at the time.

ELMAN: But you do now that you look back on it? I don't want to put words in your mouth, I want you to tell me what happened.

PATIENT: Well, I kept going back to the doctor when it was due. But I got so tired. But they thought I would deliver because the first one had been almost ten months. And then I had a dream.

ELMAN: What did you dream?

PATIENT: I dreamed that I was sitting in the waiting room and the doctor went by. I was hemorrhaging and I pleaded with him to do something and he had a tennis racket and shorts and he said, "I have to play tennis," and laughed. And I just knew that I needed help That's all there was to the dream.

ELMAN: Just wait—wait. I know that dream roused you. When I snap my fingers, you're going to realize what that dream meant—the significance of the dream in your life, and you'll be able to tell me when I snap my fingers . . . [snaps fingers] What did that dream mean to you? . . . You know.

PATIENT: I thought the doctor was not listening to me when I told him at my visits that I was tired.

ELMAN: And that you were begging him for help and he wasn't giving you help. The doctor was holding back. And that was the sum and substance of the dream. In other words, he was playing ball while you were going through this pregnancy and you were worried about it.

PATIENT: Yes.

ELMAN: Now, did your aunt's death occur in her third pregnancy?

PATIENT: The first.

ELMAN: Did you connect any situation of your aunt with your own? Did you feel as though you were going through what she had gone through?

PATIENT: It's hard for me to talk about that but each time before I would have a baby my mother would say, "It's an awful thing you're going through." It frightened me. [Patient begins to cry.]

ELMAN: Now we're getting to the real cause of this head condition. I'm sure. Because we can see how you would react to that. If it occurred each time you had a baby and—

PATIENT: She was with me when I delivered and helped me move.

ELMAN: If that ever occurs again it would be better if she isn't there.

PATIENT: Yes, I had thought of that.

ELMAN: You can already see that this thing—this dermatitis—just any form of it—shows that there's an emotional problem a person is trying to solve, and as the emotional problem becomes too big, apparently the patient doesn't know how to face it and the dermatitis begins. But we have uncovered the fact that you were so scared during this pregnancy because of that tired feeling, and because of the words that your mother said, and that at the previous deliveries you had held back —probably unconsciously—and the spot appeared before the birth. But after the baby arrived stillborn, tell us how that spot developed. Because I imagine after that it came on very strongly. Is that right?

PATIENT: Yes, it did.

ELMAN: Now you see what that indicates, don't you? What does it indicate? Don't let me tell you. You tell me what that scalp condition indicates. You ought to know.

PATIENT: After I lost the baby I just felt terrible, but I didn't want to show it because of the other two children. I put myself into as much as I could in every way and outwardly I couldn't show it.

ELMAN: But inwardly you were feeling pretty badly. Wouldn't you say that your holding back may have done damage? Did you feel that? In other words, what I'm getting at—this dermatitis condition—say it very bluntly—what does it represent? A sort of punishment for what happened?

PATIENT: I hadn't thought of it that way.

ELMAN: Well, is that the way you've been feeling about it?

PATIENT: I thought it was tied up with whatever prevented me from delivering. I thought it was hormones.

ELMAN: Mostly, strong emotional conditions are the precipitating factor. It could have been the feeling that in this terrible fright that you went through and then the holding back—also the fact that your aunt had died in childbirth, and now your baby was stillborn—it appeared to you that maybe the baby could have been saved if only you hadn't been so terribly tired. Although you didn't want to be responsible you felt perhaps you could have been responsible? Wasn't that the feeling? Was that the feeling you had?

PATIENT: Yes.

ELMAN: You wouldn't have done anything in the world to intentionally prevent that child from being born just as your other children were born, alive and healthy. But there was the feeling that maybe you had unconsciously or unwillingly been a contributing factor?

PATIENT: Yes.

ELMAN: Would you call it a guilt complex?

PATIENT: Yes.

ELMAN: That's the term I'm hitting at. You do feel that
            the dermatitis represents a guilt complex?

PATIENT: I do. And I also hoped that I could have gotten
            help. I mean that I felt I needed help from the
            doctor and I felt—

ELMAN: Did you ever consciously put these thoughts
            together?

PATIENT: No.

ELMAN: In your mind did you think, "I wonder if the
            birth of the baby and all of that had anything to
            do with this scalp condition?"

PATIENT: Oh, yes, I thought that all along.

ELMAN: Well, let me tell you how to get rid of that scalp
            condition permanently. In the first place, let me
            say this: We are not responsible for what hap-
            pens to us from external sources . . . For in-
            stance, if I happen to be the sort of person who
            gets scared to death because somebody comes at
            me with a gun, it's not my fault if I have heart
            failure, is it?

PATIENT: No.

ELMAN: Do you think a person is at fault whose aunt
            died in childbirth, and who is going through a
            terribly trying time because she's so tired and
            this pregnancy doesn't seem like the previous
            ones—all external influences. Do you see what
            I mean? Now the time comes when your own
            mother unwittingly points the pistol at you and
            says, "You're having a terrible time." And you
            know the fear that it brought on. It brought
            on the fear of the same thing happening to you
            as happened to your aunt—and it was there,
            wasn't it?

PATIENT: Yes.

ELMAN: So, can't you see, that there was no reason for a
            guilt complex within yourself? These things
            were externally caused. Can't you see that? The
            fear that the doctor wasn't helping you enough.
            That dream tells me—if it doesn't tell you, it

should—that you were begging for help. And the doctor seemed to say, "No, I'm going out and play tennis." Now, when you were over there you weren't hemorrhaging, but Freud said that every dream is a wish fulfillment.

PATIENT: I was—almost.

ELMAN: Yes. But look at the situation. In every dream a person has there is a wish fulfillment some place. In that dream you're asking for help— that was a wishful thing, wasn't it? You wanted help.

PATIENT: Yes.

ELMAN: What did you get instead of help? You got the impression he was going out to play tennis . . . Here was a terribly frightened woman who wasn't getting the right kind of encouragement to help her. It wasn't your fault. These were all external causes. Nevertheless, you would feel that maybe in some way you might have contributed—that you might have done something. And that, eating at your vitals, would cause the dermatitis. Do you see what I mean? You want to get rid of this feeling and you get the scalp condition. But you won't have to give it any more mechanical irritation because now that you know the cause—and the cause *is* completely revealed to you—you'll find that you have no desire to touch your scalp any more . . . Feels better already, doesn't it?

PATIENT: Yes.

ELMAN: And you know you're not going to have rose fever any more, because now that you know where it stems from, you can cope with it. You know that you don't have to hate roses any more . . . And now, when I have you open your eyes, just notice how good you feel . . . You'll remember every word that we've spoken . . . How do you feel?

PATIENT: I do feel better.

*   *   *

It will be worthwhile at this point to read a report by the patient's husband on the results of the hypnoanalysis recorded above. Though I had not had any opportunity to work with his wife again, he described a gratifying outcome of this single session:

"After one session of hypnoanalysis, the improvement has been very remarkable. The scar-like tissue which was once as big around as a silver dollar has now returned to normal except for a small groove which is about five millimeters wide. And hair has been growing and shows signs of completely filling in. The rose fever has improved one hundred percent. Now when roses are in bloom or whenever we have roses in a vase in the house she can enjoy them. I hope this will help to show many others the far-reaching beneficial effects hypnosis can have."

You have seen how morbid fear played an important part in the case histories you have just read. However, the examination of still another example will deepen your understanding of phobias and their results (which may be symptomatized by a wide range of disorders, including such disparate troubles as allergies and emotional exhaustion). A doctor brought a patient to class who was a sufferer from hayfever. He had told me beforehand that she was a victim of congenital syphilis and she was filled with emotional problems. As you will see, he also armed me with a number of other relevant facts. Then he asked me to work with her; the story she related in hypnoanalysis revealed fears implanted deeply in her mind, and these morbid fears, phobias by our working definition, had resulted in the hayfever. To avoid embarrassing the patient, we did not mention her congenital syphilis. The names of all patients and places have been altered in this case (as well as in all others related in this book). Here is the transcript of the hypnoanalysis:

ELMAN: Were you working when you were eighteen or were you just living at home?

PATIENT: I was just living at home. My mother had to go to a nursing home because of illness and my father's drinking, and our home was broken up.

ELMAN: Then this wasn't a very happy time for you, when you were eighteen.

PATIENT: Never, never. We were always afraid of my father.

ELMAN: Well, I want to ask you something when you were eighteen years of age. Don't talk about the illness the doctor was telling me about. Don't mention that at all. There's no necessity for it. But at eighteen, I want to find out if things at home—the high emotions and the unpleasantness that you knew—had they resulted in any illnesses for you other than that with which you were born?

PATIENT: Nothing—only nerves.

ELMAN: But they had resulted in strong emotionalism because of the tensions at home. Is that right? [Patient nods.] But when the hayfever season came along, you went right through it without having any signs of hayfever, isn't that right?

PATIENT: Yes.

ELMAN: Now let's go to the time of your first marriage. You're about nineteen, and you're getting married. Are you in love with this man that you're marrying?

PATIENT: I think I am.

ELMAN: Are you sure you're not just trying to get away from home?

PATIENT: I think I was trying to get away from home, too.

ELMAN: In other words, it was a combination of both. Now, you're married to him. Your first marriage—tell me, how are you getting along?

PATIENT: Everything is a disappointment to me.

ELMAN: In other words, it's jumping from the frying pan into the fire. Is that it?

PATIENT: Yes.

ELMAN: Have you had any emotional problems? Remember, you were just a bunch of nerves when you were eighteen. Now you're nineteen—you're married—things aren't as good as they were at home. Has it affected you in any way? Have you had any illnesses because of it, or are you able to bear up under it pretty well?

PATIENT: No—I almost had a nervous breakdown.

ELMAN: You got married, and immediately you got pregnant.

PATIENT: Ten months later exactly from the day I was married my first baby was born.

ELMAN: And were you happy with that first baby?

PATIENT: Very happy.

ELMAN: That compensated a little bit, did it, for the fact that you were unhappily married?

PATIENT: I was happy with my baby.

ELMAN: But not with your husband, is that right?

PATIENT: No. Very unhappy with him. He wasn't paying bills.

ELMAN: But you still stuck by him, and then you found yourself pregnant again. Tell me about the second pregnancy.

PATIENT: Well, I had gotten yellow jaundice suddenly when I was about two months pregnant, and I got awfully sick and I went to the hospital, and they didn't give me too much medicine. They said—they led me to believe that was the cause of my yellow jaundice—the medicine I was taking for that illness that I was born with. And then I was awfully nervous all the while that I carried him and short of breath. And I never got much sympathy from my husband because he drank a lot. And I had a fear of dying.

ELMAN: Yes, that's what I wanted you to tell me . . . When I snap my fingers, you'll tell me the first time you ever got this fear of death . . . [snaps fingers] When was it?

PATIENT: I felt the whole while I carried him that I wasn't going to live.

ELMAN: Because it was just about this time that it was revealed to you about the illness that you were born with, is that it?

PATIENT: No. I never knew anything about it until I was trying to get married and when they told me I didn't even know what the word meant . . . [Patient begins to cry.]

ELMAN: Yes, I know. Was it when you got that horrible shock—was that when you got that morbid fear of death?

PATIENT: Yes. I knew that my mother was awfully sick and they told me that was the reason for her illness, and I was afraid I would be crippled up the way she was and that I wouldn't live beyond maybe twenty-two or -three years old.

ELMAN: You didn't know what the word meant when they told you what the illness was?

PATIENT: No, I didn't.

ELMAN: Who told you? Was it your father or mother?

PATIENT: My father died before I was married.

ELMAN: Then who told you?

PATIENT: I think it was my oldest sister. She knew it. She was born with it and so was I. And she thought that I ought to know. I was treated for it but I thought I was anemic all the time.

ELMAN: But the results were good and you did get rid of this illness entirely, so you did have nothing to worry about there . . . Now, if a girl goes all through her formative years believing one thing and then gets the horrible shock that you got when you were just ready to get married—she doesn't even know the name of the illness, and all of a sudden she hears it and she's never heard it before—can you imagine all the many, many fears that would enter her mind. Here's something she's not responsible for. She had nothing to do with it, and she's being punished for something she knew nothing about. And that's exactly the feeling you had, wasn't it?

PATIENT: I was frightened to death after they told me what it was. My doctor told me. He tried to explain to me that I was all right.

ELMAN: There are a lot of doctors present, and every
           doctor here probably realizes the seriousness of
           this case. Do you think that any person in this
           room would have reacted any differently than
           you did? You know that if I had heard such
           a thing about myself, or if any doctor here had
           heard it about himself or herself, that every one
           of us would have been frightened to death. And
           that's where your morbid fear of death came
           in. Don't you see? This acted as a traumatic
           incident—a trauma—an emotional situation with
           which you could not cope. Do you understand?

PATIENT: Yes.

ELMAN: And when you heard that this thing was some-
           thing that could kill, wasn't it quite natural that
           you should have thought of death? But illnesses
           such as you had can be completely cured. Is
           that correct, doctor? Say it out loud so that
           she knows it.

DOCTOR: It certainly is true.

ELMAN: Now, in other words, once you got rid of the
           illness—and you did—you know that—you know
           there's no trace of it in you now. Once you got
           rid of the illness, you had not gotten rid of the
           trauma. Do you see what I mean? The shock.
           And so the morbid fear of death remained. And
           that fear of death has been with you every day
           since then, hasn't it?

PATIENT: Yes.

ELMAN: Did you know that even before you got here,
           your doctor told me that you had this morbid
           fear, and now you see how pronounced it was.
           You hadn't been sitting here more than a few
           minutes before you, yourself, came out with it.
           But remember, the disease is gone—the illness is
           gone—all that remained was the trauma, the
           shock, the situation with which you could not
           cope. But this situation no longer exists. Do
           you see what I mean? And since the situation
           no longer exists, there's nothing for you to cope

with . . . Except what? Except the shock that was given to you when you were a young girl. Now, talking it over when your awareness is about two thousand percent above normal, I think we put that fear in a completely different light, didn't we? This awareness lets you see that as a girl of nineteen you had every reason to be frightened, but there's no more reason for you to be frightened now than there is for any person in this room to be frightened. Do you see what I mean?

PATIENT: Yes.

ELMAN: You're not going to have those fears any more. And as a result, you're going to find, I believe, that you're going to live a much happier life. From this point on, you'll be able to put that fear into its proper place in your life. This was just a shock. It was a horrible shock. Nobody here would care to go through such a terrible situation. The only thing that wasn't gotten rid of was the shock and we're getting rid of the shock now by letting you see it again. Now let's go on a little bit. It may be that your fear is also the cause of the hayfever, I don't know. Let's find out if the hayfever is caused by the fear. I'm going to take you to the first time you ever had a hayfever attack. I'm going to take you right to it. This is your second marriage now and you have had two children during this marriage. How were the children two years ago?

PATIENT: Fine.

ELMAN: How were the children who were living with the aunt? How were they?

PATIENT: They were all right.

ELMAN: But there was worry about them?

PATIENT: Mark had an accident.

ELMAN: That's what I want to get at. Now we're getting at the cause, aren't we?

PATIENT: Well, now I am also recalling trouble that we had there in our neighborhood.

ELMAN: Yes. Now we're coming to that very time when
            you had the first attack of hayfever. I want you
            to tell me about the trouble you had in the neigh-
            borhood. If it's the type of thing you'd rather
            not talk about, you don't have to talk about it.
            So long as you know about it. Do you want to
            talk about it?

PATIENT: A person in the neighborhood tried to hurt my
            husband. Things are coming back to my mind
            —that and Mark's accident.

ELMAN: Yes, and that's when the hayfever first came up
            . . . So, we'll take you to the minute that the
            hayfever first came up and we'll find out whether
            it was Mark's accident or whether it was your
            husband with this bad person in the neighbor-
            hood. I'll snap my fingers, and it will be the
            first time you ever had a hayfever attack . . .
            [snaps fingers] Where are you? When is it?

PATIENT: I seem to be at home.

ELMAN: Where are you?

PATIENT: In the front room.

ELMAN: What's been happening?

PATIENT: All I can remember is Mark's accident.

ELMAN: Mark is your son and is one of the two boys not
            with you?

PATIENT: No, Mark is my baby. He is with me.

ELMAN: So when your little baby had the accident was
            when the first attack came on, is that it?

PATIENT: Yes. I mean, that's all I can think of.

ELMAN: Yes, because the two things are interwoven.
            What were you worried about with that accident?
            What kind of accident was it?

PATIENT: Well, I was going to go shopping and my older
            daughter was across the street. She had been
            playing with two relations of my husband.
            They were visiting from the country. They had
            taken Mark across the street and were waiting
            there by my car. I was locking the door and
            had started out and Mark started across to me

and I saw this car coming and I screamed and I hollered—it wasn't coming very fast—I just knew that Mark was going to get run over and killed. And then it hit him.

ELMAN: Was he hurt very badly?

PATIENT: No. But it frightened him.

ELMAN: Yes, but so were you. Because you can see by the very reliving of it how frightened you were. Can you see that that would cause any mother who had been through emotional strain such as your own, to manifest emotional symptoms after that? Because in addition to her own morbid fear of death now she had morbid fears regarding her child. And that was it, wasn't it?

PATIENT: Yes. I have a terrible love for my children. Some way, I always thought they were going to be taken from me or I would be taken from them.

ELMAN: You don't have to have any worries about that. Don't you see where that thought came from? A girl of nineteen, suddenly told that she was the possessor of something horrible, over which she had no control. But thanks to modern medicine she is able to get rid of the illness. She's not able to get rid of the fear, though, that took hold when she was told about the illness. Her morbid fears of death continued over the years and every day that went by she had those fears in her mind. Now she sees her child get injured by a car . . . I want to ask you something; if this happened to anybody in this room who had a background similar to your own, don't you think they would have reacted with an emotional illness of some kind?

PATIENT: I guess so.

ELMAN: Both times you were up against a situation with which you could not cope. You couldn't prevent the accident to Mark, could you? There was nothing you could do. You couldn't prevent this illness you had, which was no fault of your own. Each time, death was connected with those incidents. The thought of death was connected with Mark. Now, you were not only afraid for yourself, but for your children, too. Do you see what I mean?

PATIENT: Yes.

ELMAN: So what happened? You began to manifest the symptoms that have troubled you since. Isn't that correct? You know that to be so.

PATIENT: Yes.

ELMAN: Now that you know that's so, do you think there's any need for you to ever have hayfever again?

PATIENT: No.

ELMAN: Does this give you a new insight into the hayfever—something you never had before?

PATIENT: Yes.

ELMAN: You're going to find from this point on you won't have any hayfever because if we've done anything, we've certainly removed that first fear, haven't we? We've certainly removed that second fear because Mark's quite all right and so are your other children and things are going well. You have a husband who certainly loves you or he wouldn't be here tonight. You know that. Isn't that so?

PATIENT: Yes.

ELMAN: You're going to find that as a result of our talk tonight even those polyps you have, which have been characterized as allergic polyps, won't come back. You don't *need* the hayfever any more. You're not going to have the morbid fears of death. They're going to be erased completely. You're going to have normal fears that any person has, but they won't be morbid fears. There's no need for morbid fears . . . Instead of looking forward toward blackness, look forward toward light. I want your life from now on to be full of light and not thoughts of death. And

I don't think you'll have any hayfever at all . . .
[addressing physician] Doctor, would you give
us a report on this case as time goes by? [to
patient] You know you're going to be well, don't
you? All right, when I have you open your
eyes, you're just going to feel grand . . . All right,
open your eyes . . . How do you feel?

PATIENT: Fine.

ELMAN: I think you're going to be all right.

* * *

The prognosis expressed in the last line above is proving
accurate. The case histories in this and the foregoing chap-
ters exemplify an important principle: that physical difficulties—stuttering, obesity, allergies, etc.—as well as strictly
mental ones often have a basis in emotional conflicts. Such
conflicts may arise from insecurities, griefs, inability to cope
with given situations, out and out phobias. But they all
have this in common, that hypnosis can be employed as an
effective medical tool, to alleviate or correct them.

Chapter 19

ALLERGIES

IN transcripts of hypnoanalysis, it is impossible to show facial expressions, gestures, reactions, and extreme emotions displayed by patients. You might not know, for example, that the patient who was the victim of a congenital illness showed such extreme emotion that in the tape recording made at the time you can hear violent sobbing and the gasping for breath. I can assure you, however, that her reactions were not unusual for a patient going through an abreaction in hypnoanalysis.

As we examine the circumstances surrounding the emotional problems of this patient, we begin to wonder why her hayfever didn't show up during her childhood or first marriage. Certainly there were great problems in her late teens. But the hayfever did not develop until trauma had piled upon trauma, culminating in the great fear engendered when morbid thoughts caused her to cry excessively as she feared for her son's life.

We have discovered in hypnoanalysis that this seems often to be the case: A person is free from allergic reactions for any number of years, and then suddenly one or more allergies show up, always preceded by strong emotional circumstances.

A year or two after the hypnoanalysis of the hayfever victim just described, her doctor reported to me that she had gone through a couple of hayfever seasons without showing any evidence of allergy. She has recovered completely from her reaction to the pollen, though skin tests still prove she is sensitive to pollen. In addition, her morbid fears were completely erased. I am certainly not claiming that the hypnoanalysis itself was responsible for her recovery. It was supplemented by the work of an excellent doctor who had the good sense to continue working with the patient until her difficulties were completely corrected. The credit belongs not only to hypnoanalysis, but to the intelligent cooperation and further work by a good doctor.

Let me give you another illustration of allergic reaction. I was asked to employ hypnoanalysis with a young lady who had been completely free from any signs of allergy until she had reached the age of eleven, when a severe case of hayfever had developed. The hypnoanalysis revealed that when she was eight years old her mother died and it was a terrible shock to the young child. Eventually, she seemed to have recovered from the shock, and was in excellent health. She showed no allergic reactions. Three years later her father remarried and brought the stepmother to live with the child. That fall she developed hayfever. In the hypnoanalysis she told how bitterly she resented the first appearance of the stepmother. She still deeply missed her mother, and felt that no one could replace her real mother. She would sob herself to sleep at night but, not wanting her father or stepmother to know how she felt, she repressed the tears when she was in their presence. The sobbing continued, and when she was alone at night, she would find herself crying even in her sleep. Then the hayfever season came along and with it her first attack of the illness. At the time I saw the girl, it was in the midst of the hayfever season and what I call the "crying syndrome" was apparent.

In my opinion, every case of hayfever represents a crying syndrome. The eyes tear and get red as from weeping; the nose runs; the throat gets dry and raspy. Frequently, there is gasping for breath. All of these signs appear when a person cries excessively. Hypnoanalysis reveals again and again that victims of hayfever and many other respiratory illnesses have undergone traumatic experiences that caused prolonged crying. Consciously, these people have stemmed back the tears, but at a level below conscious awareness the tears persist. The crying apparently affects a change in sensitivity to allergens, and the allergic reactions develop in the crying syndrome of hayfever.

I believe that, just as it is possible for a person to repress unpleasant thoughts, it is possible to repress the emotions which stem from those thoughts. Tears are one of nature's relief mechanisms. If thoughts bring tears and the tears are repressed—that is, the mechanism is not permitted to operate —many respiratory illnesses can and often do result. If you had seen this crying syndrome in literally hundreds of emotional illnesses, I believe you would agree with me that the crying syndrome is worthy of further medical research and study. Find the cause of the syndrome in every patient, and you will probably be able to help many people who suffer from respiratory conditions.

There are exceptions, however. A doctor once brought his son to class, an eleven-year-old boy who was a victim of asthma and hayfever. He had been taken to Denver, where notable work is being done with asthmatic patients. Unsuccessful there, the father took the boy to a distant state where a specialist was reputed to be doing remarkable work with asthmatics. Again, all treatment failed. The boy still had his asthmatic condition. Then the father became a student of hypnosis and one night he suggested that we might uncover the cause of the asthma by means of hypnoanalysis.

I agreed to try, but stipulated that neither parent must be present in the room while we were working with the boy. As I explained to him, we have found it advisable not to have loved ones present when hypnoanalysis is done. Patients who are emotionally involved won't speak freely when family members are present for fear of saying something embarrassing to themselves or disturbing to the people they love.

The boy very much wanted help and he responded to hypnosis beautifully. Under hypnoanalysis, he told how when he was a baby all he had to do was to cry and his mother would come running. With the arrival of a baby sister, attention was divided; now mother didn't respond to his crying as fast as she used to. One day he cried so long and hard that his breathing made a "funny sound." The sound didn't disturb him at all, he said, but when his mother heard it, she came running to him, frightened.

"Rales" she called it, and when she told her husband, the doctor, he too became alarmed. Now the child could get attention any time he wanted it simply by crying and making those funny sounds when he breathed. He could make his father and mother pay more attention to him than they did to his baby sister.

The hypnoanalysis did not produce any immediate improvement that I could see. Before the conclusion of the session, the boy volunteered the information that he was certain his parents favored his sister. He wanted their love so badly even asthma seemed a small price to pay for it. When the parents were made aware of the situation, they were shocked. They told me they would do everything in their power to correct the brother and sister problem. I am sure that, gradually, as the sibling rivalry is eased, the boy will "outgrow" his asthma.

In many cases, a patient suddenly begins to have strong reactions to all sorts of allergens, though he has never been troubled by them before. Skin tests may show that he is sensitive to everything from chocolate to ragweed to wool. Judging by these skin tests, I am led to believe that the allergies have always been present, and that only the allergic *reaction* has been affected. The patient who suddenly has an attack of hayfever has probably been allergic to pollen all his life but, the severe reaction was precipitated by an emotional problem. I believe this to be true of any number of allergies.

Since the allergies have always been present and probably always will be, all that can be done in the light of present knowledge is to correct their *effect*. To my knowledge, no way has been found to cure an allergy; when we remove the reaction, we haven't caused the allergen-sensitivity to disappear.

Some years ago, I had in my class an allergist who was an excellent student. He saw me use hypnoanalysis with a number of patients suffering from allergic reactions. He said to me, "You know, Dave, it's very odd the way I became an allergist. I was in medical school, engaged to be married, when along came an allergy that almost killed me.

"It was graduation day and my girl and I were celebrating the fact that we were engaged. A bunch of young grads, along with my girl and I, went out together for a celebration. We decided to have a shore dinner. We were a perfectly happy group, my girl friend and myself and these other boys and girls, all medical students—all finishing college, and enjoying a wonderful shore dinner.

"There were clams, oysters, lobster, you know what a shore dinner is composed of. All of a sudden I got so sick. Everybody else was perfectly well, but I got so sick I almost died. When I found out that I was allergic to clams and that it was the clams that had made me so sick, I decided to find out something about allergies. And so I became an allergist."

I said to him, "Doctor, I would like to find out exactly what happened that night that you had the clams."

He declared, "It's just like I told you, Dave. Everybody was having a wonderful time. Everybody had clams. Everybody was feeling wonderful, but I got sick. It's because I'm allergic to clams."

I told him, "Not necessarily. You had had clams in your life before and they hadn't made you sick. Let's do hypnoanalysis to find out what caused you to react this way."

I regressed him to graduation night. I had him relive the episode little by little. Just before the shore dinner was served, he and his girl had had a terrible fight. She gave him back his ring and told him she was never going to marry him. He felt miserable. Then the shore dinner was served, and he found he couldn't stomach the clams. That is when the reaction to the allergy occurred.

The fact of the matter is that probably this man had always been allergic to clams, but it was not a vile poison for him until the emotional upset came along coincidentally with the eating of the clams.

Many years ago I saw an interesting allergic reaction. I met an actress who had a recurring and disappearing strawberry mark on her forehead. It was just as red as a real strawberry and looked exactly like a strawberry. But the mark only appeared on her forehead during the strawberry season. "Every time I see a strawberry," she told me, "I get this reaction. I don't know why it happens." Her case is reminiscent of the stigmata (more prevalent in Europe than here) brought on by religious ecstacy. Such marks are evidently stimulated by emotional responses.

A somewhat similar case was brought to my attention by a dermatologist who brought to class a patient afflicted with severe hives. The hives were not present at the time, and the dermatologist told me that the patient had only been troubled by such skin reactions during the past couple of years. The hives would disappear for a while and then come back. The doctor believed there was an emotional basis underlying the disorder. In hypnoanalysis this story was revealed:

The patient had held a minor position as a factory

hand. He was an outstanding worker, and after a number of years of holding the same job, the boss suddenly promoted him to foreman. At first, he was very proud and his friends were very happy for him. Now, however, he had to give orders to co-workers who were old friends, and since the boss expected him to turn out a specific number of units a day, he had to exert pressure on them. He was unhappy about being in a position of authority which he really didn't want—and every time the boss needled him to pressure his co-workers, the hives developed.

To find out whether the reaction was strictly emotional, the dermatologist pretended to be the boss during part of the hypnoanalysis. After listening to the doctor give orders for two or three minutes, the patient developed enormous hives on his arms, legs and body. These hives were larger than silver dollars. When we told the patient the boss had left, almost immediately the hives disappeared.

We have worked with several victims of hives, and the symptoms always seem to originate on an emotional basis. While hives may or may not be considered an allergy, they do show an emotional reaction similar to allergic reactions.'

I was visiting at the home of friends one evening and many guests were present. When a dish of candy was passed around, the man seated next to me looked at the chocolates longingly and said, "Sometimes I get such a fierce longing for chocolates that I eat them no matter what, and then I get so sick that I think I'm collapsing. My nose runs, my eyes water and my stomach is upset. But I can't resist eating the stuff."

Following a theory I had, I asked him to resist the candy this time just long enough for me to give him a few hypnotic suggestions. He was most agreeable; I put him into a deep state of hypnosis, and gave him the suggestion that he could eat chocolate without suffering any ill effects, provided he never had them at a time when he was emotionally upset. Then he ate the chocolates, without any ill effect.

The results were astounding, for he has been able to eat chocolate ever since without having any reaction whatever. He is very careful not to eat them at a time when he is emotionally upset. He is, of course, still allergic to chocolate but he is avoiding the precipitating factor which caused him to react to the allergy. Some allergists claim that all allergies have an emotional basis; others insist that *some* do. Hypnoanalytic research, however, leads me to the conclusion that *no* allergy itself is emotionally produced, but *all* reactions to allergies have an emotional basis. There is quite a difference.

For clarification, let's get back to the crying syndrome. I can remember a nurse who came to class with an extensive rash on her hands. Her eyes were watering and itchy. The crying syndrome was apparent. It seems that she had never shown a reaction to allergies of any type, but in April of that year she suddenly developed a rash on her hands and, concurrently, the watering and itching eyes. She tried wearing rubber gloves but they didn't help at all; the rash continued to get worse. Finally she went to see a dermatologist, who made various tests and discovered that the nurse was allergic to antibiotics. He gave her treatment for contact dermatitis, but even this treatment gave her no relief from the rash or the crying syndrome. The doctor then brought her to class.

I questioned her at length, trying to determine if she had ever had any allergic reactions at all prior to the previous April. She had not. Then I asked her how she was getting along at the hospital where she worked and at home. To these questions she answered, "Everything is fine. I have no problems. I'm happy at home and I like my work."

Then I made the remark, "A pretty girl like you must have a lot of boy friends."

She said, "I did have one."

"What happened?"

"We had a quarrel and broke up. I haven't seen him since."

"When did you have this quarrel?"

She said, "Last April," and broke into tears.

The girl didn't realize that the unhappy ending of her romance had anything to do with her allergic reactions. The emotional problem had acted as the trigger mechanism.

I asked the doctor to continue working with the patient privately along these lines, and she soon showed a marked improvement.

The recognition and treatment of an emotional problem do not, however, relieve every sufferer from allergies, asthma, etc. Judge for yourself whether or not emotion was shown to be a causative factor in the development of the following asthma case.

The patient first began to suffer from asthma when she was twenty-four years of age. The condition persisted for seven years, then completely disappeared for a period of another seven years, only to return violently six months before her doctor brought her to class.

I asked the patient many preliminary questions about family life, her work, her marriage, etc., and she responded that everything was just fine. We regressed her and learned that all through her formative years she had experienced no allergic reactions and no asthma. She was married when she was twenty-three years of age. Now read part of the hypnoalysis which followed:

ELMAN: You've been married a few months now. Are you working or are you staying home?

PATIENT: I'm working.

ELMAN: Do you like your job?

PATIENT: Yes, sir.

ELMAN: When I snap my fingers, it will be the first day you've ever had asthma, and you'll know just what's been happening . . . [snaps fingers] What's been happening today?

PATIENT: I'm coughing. I've got a cold.

ELMAN: How are things going at home?

PATIENT: Fine.

ELMAN: How are you getting along with your husband?

PATIENT: Just fine.

ELMAN: This will be the first day you ever got asthma. Something must have happened that caused a common cold to turn into asthma. When I snap my fingers, you'll know what it was that emotionally upset you that day . . . [snaps fingers] What was it?

PATIENT: I don't know.

ELMAN: Now, stay completely relaxed. When I lift your hand and drop it, you'll know exactly what it was, and if you want to tell me you can, and if you don't want to tell me, you don't have to. But you'll know what it is . . . Now, what happened that day? Do you want to tell me? [Patient has become disturbed; begins to weep, apparently experiencing typical crying syndrome.] This is the first day you've ever had asthma. It's five minutes before you have your first attack of asthma. What's been happening?

PATIENT: I just keep coughing and coughing and coughing.

ELMAN: What are you worried about?

PATIENT: I don't like the cough.

ELMAN: Do you have any ideas on your mind that this might be something serious?

PATIENT: No, sir.

ELMAN: Where's your husband? Is he home?

PATIENT: He's with me.

ELMAN: What's he doing about your cough? Anything at all?

PATIENT: No, sir.

ELMAN: How long have you had this cough?

PATIENT: Three weeks.

ELMAN: And still coughing pretty badly. What's been happening these past three weeks?

PATIENT: I was in the hospital.

ELMAN: You were in the hospital? What with?

PATIENT: Pneumonia.

ELMAN: So, you did have pneumonia and you were in the hospital. While you were in the hospital you were pretty sick, is that right?

PATIENT: Yes.

ELMAN: Did you get scared when you were in the hospital?

PATIENT: No.

ELMAN: You knew at all times that you were going to get well?

PATIENT: Yes, sir . . . [Patient sobs, appears to be experiencing violent emotional response.] My boss said that I had tuberculosis. He kept saying that again and again.

ELMAN: Your boss thought you had tuberculosis. Now we're getting to the cause of the fear that was underlying the whole thing, aren't we?

PATIENT: Yes, sir.

ELMAN: And now we're beginning to see where the asthma came from, aren't we? Because way down underneath, he scared you pretty badly when he said that, didn't he?

PATIENT: I didn't think so.

ELMAN: But now that you look back on it, you can see it clearly again. You realize that his words had pretty stunning effects on you, didn't they?

PATIENT: Yes, sir. I quit my job because of it.

ELMAN: Now let's go to your most recent attack, and see if this attack which occurred six months ago has any of the same elements in it . . . What happened about six months ago?

PATIENT: Just like the flu—I had an upper respiratory infection, and then the asthma came back.

*   *   *

Notice the similarity of the events preceding both attacks of asthma, and notice also how the words of her boss gave her morbid fears. At this point in the hypnoanalysis, the patient rejected any further work, and when we attempted to find the reason for the rejection through ideomotor responses, she revealed that she had gained a great deal of insight into her problem as the result of the hypnoanalysis but that she preferred not to go further at this time. Her doctor continued the work with her privately.

Although hypnoanalysis is often fabulously interesting, sometimes it can become dull and discouraging. During one class, I had worked with an asthma sufferer, but without any success. After the class was dismissed, his doctor persuaded me to work with this patient again. This time, to my surprise, he accepted hypnosis readily and quickly went into a deep state of somnambulism. This is another indication that many patients will not reveal their problems before a group of doctors. He had previously, that evening, rejected hypnosis when the class was in session.

He was a man in his forties or fifties, and had been an asthmatic victim since early childhood, he said. I began compounding suggestions by taking him back to the first grade in school, and followed it by taking him to successive grades, hoping that by increasing his awareness, I might be able to discover the cause of his asthma.

He was able to identify every child in the first, second, third and fourth grades. And each time he mentioned the children with whom he studied in those early years, he would mention a boy named Joe. "I like Joe," he said. "We're awfully good friends."

I took him to a week before the first asthmatic attack, and everything was fine. He was a completely happy boy. Three days before the attack, everything was still fine. Two days before the attack, he said, "We're out in the yard playing ball. Joe and I are arguing. Boy, am I mad. I hit him and knocked him down."

"Did that break up your friendship with Joe?"

"Oh no. We're too good friends for that. We made up in a little while and I apologized to him. He said I really didn't hurt him anyway."

Then I took him to the day of the first asthmatic attack and asked him to relate what was happening in the classroom. He started mentioning the names of the boys in class, and then was silent for a moment. Suddenly he exclaimed, "Where is Joe? Joe isn't here?" Then he began to sob violently.

The abreaction was so severe that I decided to terminate it. When I brought him out of hypnosis, he said, "I was talking about Joe, wasn't I? I haven't thought about him for many years."

"Yes," I said, "Tell us about Joe."

He said, "Joe died when we were in the fifth grade. I thought that when I hit him I caused it. I can remember now how many times I cried about it, but I would never let anyone know how I felt. After all, big boys don't go around crying about people who aren't even members of their family."

The crying syndrome was clearly indicated, and was apparently the cause of the first asthma attack.

This case, like many others I have encountered, proves that a guilt complex can exist below the level of conscious awareness. The patient had been carrying that guilt complex ever since childhood. It was the cause of the crying syndrome and the precipitating cause of the asthma.

Chapter 20

DEPRESSIONS

A NUMBER of years ago, a psychiatrist asked me to help him work with a suicidal depressive. Never having worked with such a patient, I was reluctant. However, the doctor explained that he had made little progress and felt that with my aid he could at least learn how this type of person could be handled with hypnotic techniques. This was an assignment I didn't relish, but the doctor was searching for knowledge just as I was, and this was an opportunity to learn what a suicidal depressive was like from the psychiatric viewpoint. The patient, a woman, nearly forty years of age, was not very communicative. At first she only repeated, again and again, "What's the use of living? I want to die."

She accepted hypnosis readily. Now the idea was to find out what caused her to feel the way she did. I couldn't get any answers that seemed to help. She was married, loved her husband devotedly, loved her children. There had been no recent tragedies that might have left her brokenhearted. After the first interview, I was ready to give up. The psychiatrist said, "Work with her some more. I still think you might be able to get at the cause finally." And so I tried again. This time she gave me some information that the psychiatrist had already given me, but she added, "Suicides seem to run in our family. My mother committed suicide and I suppose some day I will—and soon."

I wondered whether her mother's suicide many years ago could have anything to do with the daughter's present depressive state, but I couldn't find any direct connection. Our lack of progress was discouraging. At this point, we called in a doctor who was working for his boards in psychiatry, and who wanted practice in hypnosis though he was already an accomplished practitioner.

I had seen psychiatrists at work, but this was an opportunity to watch a brilliant novice putting into use the studies he had made over many years. He had been in general practice for some time before he began to earn his boards in psychiatry, and had developed a bedside manner I have

228

never seen equalled. In about five minutes he had the patient more at ease than she had been with the psychiatrist and me after hours of work. His words, as I remember them, went something like this: "This lady needs help right now —not later—and she's going to get it right now."

The patient looked up at him and for the first time I saw a look of relief come over her face. She accepted hypnosis even more readily from him than she had accepted it from me or the psychiatrist. It was apparent that she was in deeper somnambulism than she had ever been, and answered his questions more readily. When I had asked her age, she had replied, "Almost forty." But when he asked the same question, she gave her birth date and her exact age. There was quite a difference in the way she answered, and I think it was his bedside manner that caused her to cooperate so fully and quickly.

Then he asked her about her family background. She revealed it without hesitation. When she mentioned her mother's suicide, he said, "Tell me about your mother. What kind of person was she?"

She answered, "Just like me. Always depressed. When I was a little girl there was a flood in our town that killed a lot of people. It depressed her terribly. One day she left the house and when my father came home he asked me, 'Where's mother?' I answered, 'I don't know. Maybe she went down to see the flood.' Daddy got awfully upset. I can remember he almost shouted at me, 'Come quick. We have to find her.' We went rushing down to the flood waters. There was mother, walking further and further out into the flood. She would have drowned if Daddy hadn't plunged in and saved her."

I had never been able to get any detailed information from this patient. Neither had the psychiatrist. But this doctor uncovered the first important clue in a matter of moments. When he questioned her further, she revealed that her father had warned her about her mother's suicidal tendencies.

At this point, the patient began to react violently. The doctor watched her closely. Weeping, she went on, "Every day when I came home from school I'd go looking for mother —always finding her sitting in a chair, looking straight ahead, kind of dazed. One day I came home from school and mother wasn't sitting in the chair as usual. I went all over the house looking for her and calling her, but she didn't answer. Finally I opened a closet door . . . [Here, the patient sobbed almost hysterically.] and there she was—hanging in the closet . . . She was dead."

The doctor and I quieted her down and then the doctor gently asked, "Why didn't you tell this to your psychiatrist? Why didn't you tell it to Mr. Elman?"

"I couldn't—I couldn't—it was too terrible. I didn't want to remember it."

"How old was your mother when all this happened?"

"Thirty-nine."

"How old did you say you are?"

"I'll be thirty-nine next Tuesday."

"Don't you see the connection?"

Still sobbing, the patient answered, "Of course I do. All my life—ever since it happened—I've been thinking that when I reached thirty-nine I'd do just what my mother did —commit suicide. But I don't have to do it, do I?"

After that, treatment was fairly easy. About a year later, I received a telephone call from the patient's husband. He wanted to thank me: she was past forty now, happy and quite well. But without doubt, the entire credit should go to the doctor whose bedside manner and hypnotic skill ended this woman's depression.

In one of my classes there was a handsome young dentist who had a fabulous practice and a beautiful wife. He came to every class session accompanied by his wife. We became quite friendly.

As the session on hypnoanalysis approached, the young dentist came to me and said, "My wife ought to be a good subject for hypnoanalysis. She gets violent headaches occasionally—the migraine type, and when she gets those attacks, I don't know how to help her. Do you suppose you could find out the cause of the migraines?"

Her own physician was there and was very much in favor of having the hypnoanalysis done. Doing hypnoanalysis on this beautiful girl, she revealed nothing. The hypnoanalysis was a complete bust.

Her husband came up to me and said, "Too bad. I know you can't be successful with everyone, but I wish you could have helped her, poor girl. She needs help so badly."

When the class was over and my wife and I were discussing the session, I said, "Too bad about the dentist's wife. She certainly needs help."

My wife said, "I have something odd to tell you. When you finished working with her, she motioned me to come into an adjoining room. When we were alone she said, 'It was useless doing hypnoanalysis on me. I *know* where the headaches come from. I'm terribly worried about my husband. He gets so terribly depressed and does so many erratic things. He won't see a doctor. I love him so dearly. Please talk to your husband about this and try to help us.' "

This was an unusual case . . . We wondered which of the two was right. Maybe they were both right, each causing the troubles of the other.

I was in the midst of a subsequent class lecture when the dentist asked if he could speak with my wife privately. She accompanied him into the adjoining room. When they were alone, he said, "I'm terribly sorry that Mr. Elman got nowhere with my wife on that hypnoanalysis. She needs help so badly. Those headaches of hers keep getting worse all the time. I hate to see her suffer."

My wife took the bull by the horns. She told him what his wife had said—that he was the one who needed help because of the depression, erratic actions, etc.

He smiled charmingly and said, "Mrs. Elman, you should know better than that. After having worked with so many doctors and seen so many patients, you know how these sick people claim there's nothing wrong with them. It's always the other fellow. Of course, my wife says I'm the one who needs treatment. But believe me, she's the one who's sick."

There were three psychiatrists in his class, and after getting this report, I suggested to the dentist and his wife that they both seek psychiatric help. Later, he came to me and said, "We'll see one of your students who is a psychiatrist. Maybe he'll call you in to help with the hypnoanalysis."

That was the way the matter stood when the classes ended and we left town. I assumed they had gone to a psychiatrist. So far as I know, they never saw a psychiatrist.

From what I have told you, wouldn't you imagine it was the wife who was sick? After all, he was such a charming, happy-go-lucky chap, always ready with a smile and a joke. He could always manage to tell an amusing story that would send the other doctors into gales of laughter.

Here comes the somber twist: Two months later, he committed suicide.

A psychiatrist and I became good friends and one day I met him at his office for a lunch date. Before we left, he introduced me to one of his patients, a homosexual with suicidal tendencies.

The psychiatrist had long been working with this young man, but had not utilized any hypnotic techniques as he doubted the psychiatric value of hypnosis.

As soon as the patient was gone, the psychiatrist began describing his problem to me: "I haven't been able to help him. He's been a non-paying patient for almost seven years —and all that time he's been threatening suicide. He keeps saying that some day I'll find him dead on my doorstep."

"Aren't you worried about that?"

"Of course, but people who keep threatening suicide are usually people who are unconsciously asking for help. The ones you have to worry about most are the deeply depressed patients who never mention the subject of suicide."

"But there must be exceptions."

"Of course there are, and he might well be one of them. Every time he commits a homosexual act he gets such a feeling of guilt that he wishes he was dead. Do you think that you could help him with hypnosis? Nothing yet has had any effect on his suicidal threats, and I may be a skeptic but I'm willing to try hypnotic suggestion."

Although I was afraid that suggestion might do no good, at least it could do no harm; and so an appointment was set up. The patient, whom I will call Freddie, was a nice looking chap in his early thirties. There was nothing effeminate about him, though he was wearing slightly garish clothes. Perhaps the outfit would have been appropriate for the stage (he was a singer) but not for street wear.

He said, "I guess the doctor has told you about my problem so we don't have to waste any time. If hypnotism will help me, I'm eager to try it."

Despite this statement, Freddie was one of the most resistant patients I have ever encountered. At that first session, practically all I could do was to talk to him; I could not develop a usable hypnotic state. I managed to discover only that he was a very talented young man, a splendid singer with a great love of music, whose career had progressed no further than a minor role in a Broadway show; he was a chorus boy to be exact.

When he learned that I, too, was a lover of music, he became quite enthusiastic. He didn't want to talk about his problems, but he was more than willing to talk about music. We spent most of the hour talking about our mutual interest. Finally, I signalled to the psychiatrist that there was no use continuing at present, since the patient was completely rejecting hypnosis.

After Freddie was gone, I told the psychiatrist that I didn't think I could get past his rejection, and there wasn't anything more I could do to help.

The doctor insisted that I try again, however, and a second appointment was set up. This time I was quite firm with the patient. I said, "Freddie, if you really want my help, you'll have to follow my instructions. If you won't do that this time, I won't work with you again no matter what the doctor says."

I couldn't induce him to accept hypnosis, but when I offered to teach him autosuggestion, he responded quickly, not realizing that autosuggestion is a form of hypnosis. He became avidly interested in the subject, and when he learned that he could now anesthetize his own hand or leg, he felt that we were making considerable progress. I told him to practice autohypnosis fifty times a day until he had mastered it thoroughly, and that if he mastered autosuggestion, I'd be willing to help him some more. He agreed, and the psychiatrist was pleased.

At the third meeting Freddie said that he was greatly pleased with the results he had obtained from autohypnosis. For the first time in years he was able to get a good night's sleep without waking up time and time again. And bad dreams, which had habitually troubled him, no longer kept coming back.

Then I exposed the fact that autosuggestion, autohypnosis and hypnosis itself were one and the same thing, and that if he could give suggestions to himself so successfully, he ought to be able to take suggestions that were for his good from anyone. This now seemed reasonable to him, and almost immediately I had bypassed his resistance. Thus far the subject of suicide had never come up. Now was the proper time. I steered the conversation around to his suicidal tendencies.

"Yes, some day I'm going to do it—right on the doctor's doorstep."

"Why on the doctor's doorstep? After all, he's been working with you for seven years, never charged you for his efforts, and you know how he's tried to help. Why take it out on the doctor?"

"Because I'm still a homosexual. Why don't the girls in the chorus attract me instead of the boys?"

"You can't blame that on him. You'd be taking your own guilt feelings out on the man who has given you freely of his time, earnestly trying to help you, and yet you resent him. Why?"

"I don't know. I like the doctor very much. I keep coming back to him trying to get help, but I'm getting awfully discouraged and resentful."

I saw Freddie many times after that, always at the doctor's office. I was able to get him over his resentment to the doctor, and to get him over all thoughts of suicide though I didn't know how to correct his homosexuality.

When I got him into deep somnambulism I explained that he must regard homosexuality not as an abnormality, but as an emotional illness; that he must never think of himself as "queer" but as a person who, through no fault of his own, was a victim of illness. I told him that many dedicated men are trying to solve the riddle of homosexuality, and when they succeeded they would be able to help thousands of people like Freddie.

He exclaimed, "You mean I'm just a human guinea pig?"

"Freddie, you are far more than a human guinea pig. You're a symbol—a symbol of your own doctor's dedicated efforts to help people like you. Don't you realize that if he finally succeeds in correcting your homosexuality, you'll be the instrument by which people all over the world can be helped?"

Our conversations during hypnosis often went like that. He would raise the same objections and I would repeat my assurances. After many long sessions, I seemed to have succeeded in calming him and in changing his attitude toward the doctor from resentment to friendliness. I could do nothing more, but at least the psychiatrist now had an amenable patient to work with.

Perhaps this simple technique wouldn't succeed in many cases, but it certainly did in Freddie's case. He began to regard himself as a valiant hero trying to help people who were similarly afflicted.

A number of years later, he was appearing in another Broadway show and he sent passes to my wife and me. We attended the performance and saw Freddie between the acts. I asked him if he ever thought of suicide these days.

He answered, "Good heavens no! I haven't thought of suicide for years—not since you helped me."

In almost every city in which we teach, a doctor will say something like this to me: "Your students claim that with hypnotic techniques they've been able to save lives and restore to normalcy deeply depressed people, patients who have a will to die. They make claims that are hard to believe. Aren't they perhaps talking about cases that are easy to handle? Are they successful with the really difficult cases?"

And I answered them as honestly as I can: "Who is to tell? If a deeply depressed person is restored to normalcy, what better proof is there? Some of the doctors are probably overenthusiastic; some of them are not. Some say they haven't been successful at all. I don't think that every success has been an easy case and it is important to realize that there have been failures as well as successes."

For every failure there have been many successes, but if you suspect that the doctors aren't talking about serious depressions, think of this one:

A number of years ago, a doctor in Jersey City telephoned me about a patient who was in his office. "I've been working with him," the doctor explained, "trying to get him over his despondency, and finally I told him I would call you up to see if you wouldn't come over to help me. Can you do it?"

"Right now?"

"Wait a minute. I'll ask him if he can wait here until you get over."

I could hear him talking to his patient a moment or two, and then the doctor asked me if I could make the appointment for four o'clock on Thursday.

"Well," I said, "if he is very deeply depressed, he shouldn't wait that long. This is Tuesday and it means he is going to be without help for two whole days. We ought to work with him today."

However, the patient insisted he could hold out until Thursday, and that he didn't want to wait for me to drive over now (I lived about half an hour's drive away). This seemed a strange attitude for a patient who was supposedly in urgent need of help. I was puzzled, but I agreed to come on Thursday and I made the appointment with the doctor.

On Wednesday, the doctor phoned again. His first words were, "Cancel that appointment for Thursday. My patient has killed himself."

Fortunately, many deeply depressed people do grasp at help when it is offered to them. And if hypnotic techniques can help some of these people, it is a doctor's duty to employ these techniques.

Hypnosis has prevented suicide in many, many cases. It would be possible to cite additional case histories of depressives helped by hypnosis, but in psychiatry failure is always easier to prove than success. Of a patient who no longer thinks of suicide, it is natural to ask, "Wouldn't he have come back to normal without the use of hypnotic techniques?" Perhaps. "And how can you prove in these so-called successful cases that they were suicidal depressives?" The patient would have to commit suicide to prove the diagnosis was correct. And, of course, suicide only occurs in cases of failure.

However, here is one example of how a deep depression caused illness where, so far as I know, there was no thought of suicide. The doctor explained that the patient had been diagnosed by several physicians as an epileptic. Yet encephalogram readings showed no signs of epilepsy. This patient, a spinster in her forties, was subject to frequent grand mal attacks, and was deeply depressed. She was brought to class. I noted that she looked very weak. She was pale and emaciated, not bad looking, but sick looking. The doctor warned me that she might have a grand mal attack in the midst of the hypnoanalysis, and I was glad he was there to take care of her.

Hypnoanalysis quickly revealed that the seizures were brought on by a guilt complex. I suspected that it was a sexual problem. I therefore terminated the hypnoanalysis and instructed the doctor that this type of case could not be handled in the classroom before a group of people even if they were all doctors and nurses. The doctor agreed, and said that he would continue to work with her in private.

Two weeks later the doctor reported his findings: When he had put her into hypnoanalysis he had quickly confirmed my suspicions. It was a sex problem. She had revealed herself to be a deeply religious virgin with great sexual anxiety. This anxiety caused her to search for sexual relief. The only relief she could find was in masturbation. But after masturbating, she suffered such an intense guilt complex that she developed grand mal attacks diagnosed as epileptic in nature.

A year or two later, the doctor reported, she was in excellent health and was no longer deeply depressed. How he handled this situation was not revealed to me but the *cause* was determined by hypnotic techniques, so that effective treatment could be initiated.

Chapter 21

REVIEW, PRACTICE AND APPLICATION
OF HYPNOANALYSIS

IN STUDYING hypnoanalysis, there is a certain temptation to be avoided by all doctors whose specialties do not lie in the field of psychiatry. The following warning must be remembered at all times: *Leave the work of the psychiatrist to the psychiatrist.*

Your knowledge of hypnoanalysis will be of value to you no matter what your field of medicine is. The dentist will be able to do better work in his field because of a knowledge of hypnoanalysis, the physician will be a better physician, and the psychiatrist will be a better psychiatrist. In the minds of some people the mention of hypnoanalysis brings to mind psychoanalysis, and they consider one the corollary of the other. Actually, there is such a great difference between them that neither could substitute for the other. They have entirely different uses. Psychoanalysis in many cases gives a complete explanation of a complicated behavior pattern. Hypnoanalysis in many cases will reveal the cause of a patient's peculiar reaction to a given set of circumstances. It is the difference between a broad plateau and a pin-point.

Psychoanalysis deals with the material of the unconscious mind which, through special time-consuming techniques, is brought into the patient's consciousness so that he can deal with it. Hypnoanalysis deals with awareness below the level of consciousness which the therapist must help the patient see consciously. It is often a speedier method of therapy. "Unconscious material" is not to be considered a synonym for "awareness below the level of consciousness."

A complete psychoanalysis takes time, years in some cases; hypnoanalysis takes hours. A complete psychoanalysis by means of hypnoanalysis alone would be an extremely difficult procedure. It is doubtful whether hypnoanalysis would lend itself to such a purpose.

238

To illustrate the difference between psychoanalysis and hypnoanalysis, let's take this example: A young boy in school stands up to recite a poem.   He has practiced it a thousand times and knows every word exactly.   Suddenly his mind goes blank; he can't remember the lines.   He sits down in confusion.   Through psychoanalysis, you could find out why the boy forgets; with hypnoanalysis you probably would not get such a complete answer.   You would only find out why he forgot *on that particular occasion*.   The *pattern of forgetting* would be revealed with the use of the first therapy; the *why of the particular occasion* would quickly be revealed with the second.

Let us consider a practical application: A man comes into a dentist's office and says, "I want you to pull all my teeth."   The dentist examines the patient and finds the teeth in excellent condition.   As far as the dentist is able to learn, there is no pathology which requires the removal of the man's teeth.   Here is a most unusual and complicated behavior pattern.   Certainly the case is not one for the dentist.   The psychiatrist is the right man to handle it. And he probably won't use hypnoanalysis or, if he does, it will form only one aspect of therapy.

But suppose another man comes into the dentist's office for dental treatment and it is discovered that he has a most alarming gag reflex.   A gag reflex is considered by most dentists well within the norm of human behavior.   It is not a complicated behavior pattern, but a quirk.   The dentist wouldn't ordinarily send such a man to a psychiatrist.   His patient is merely showing a peculiar reaction to a particular set of circumstances.   Such a case yields to hypnoanalysis in five or ten minutes.   It would yield to psychoanalysis, too, but in a considerably longer period.   Hypnoanalysis makes the patient amenable to dental procedure very quickly, whereas if psychoanalysis is decided upon, the dentist will be unable to work upon the patient immediately, and the patient's mouth condition may deteriorate considerably in the months or years before the psychoanalysis is concluded.

To show that this illustration is more than hypothetical, here is a case history: A doctor brought to class a man with an almost vicious gag reflex.   Ordinary hypnosis and hypnotic suggestions had been tried on him, but he still gagged and vomited. The patient was put into the trance state of hypnosis, and hypnoanalysis was begun. Within five minutes he related how in 1936 he had been the victim of a carbon monoxide incident in which he had almost lost his life. Physicians in attendance at that time inserted a long rubber tube into the patient's mouth, and proceeded to wash out the stomach. It is perhaps an understatement to say the experience was unpleasant. Ever since that time, when any doctor approached with a foreign object to be inserted into his mouth, the patient, at a level below conscious awareness, relived the carbon monoxide incident, and began to gag and vomit. When this was brought to the patient's conscious attention, he was able to cope with the situation instantly; subsequently, extensive dental work has been done on this man and he has never gagged once. In this case, psychoanalysis was not particularly indicated. There was no need for it. This was no complicated behavior pattern needing years for solution; this was an individual reaction to a particular set of circumstances, and, therefore, hypnoanalysis was indicated.

Simple medical problems often call for hypnoanalysis. A man calls on a doctor and gives him a history of migraines dating back to the time when the patient was a boy. He tells how he has gone from one doctor to another. No one has been able to give him relief. He is put under observation in a hospital, given every possible medical test. There is no pathology, but the headaches persist. The new doctor tries hypnoanalysis. Within twenty minutes, he learns that the headaches began when the patient was in the fourth grade at school. He brings on an abreaction of the incidents which occurred just prior to the first headache. He learns that the teacher gave the youngsters an unexpected examination that day for which the boy was not prepared. He flunked the exam miserably. The teacher told him she was going to call at his home after school and have a talk with his mother. The boy was thrown into a panic. He ran all the way home trying to forestall the teacher. Maybe if he was sick when the teacher arrived, he'd have a reasonable explanation for flunking the exam. And so he wished he was sick—wished it so hard and pretended so hard that he actually became sick.

The trick worked. On another occasion he tried it again,

and it worked the second time, too. A habit pattern was created. Now every time an emotional problem comes along, the headache comes along with it. This, incidentally, was an actual case; after the doctor brought the true state of affairs to the attention of the patient's conscious mind, and gave him insight, recovery from the migraines was immediate. The cause had been explained and eliminated. Did another symptom replace the old one? Not at all, for the patient did not want to be sick. He wanted to be well and face his emotional problems squarely. Years have passed since that hypnoanalysis was performed but the patient has not had a recurrence of the migraines, and is in excellent physical and emotional health today.

Let us presume for the moment, however, that the hypnoanalysis had only resulted in a partial success, and that later on the migraines returned, or that the patient showed other symptoms which might be caused by deep emotional conflict. The physician would then know that the patient required more than can be accomplished with hypnoanalysis, and would refer him to a psychiatrist for therapy —perhaps even psychoanalysis.

Mention has been made here of a fairly common neurotic problem in dentistry and a fairly common neurotic problem in medicine. Are these instances isolated? There are few men held in higher repute than Doctor Karl Menninger, whose Topeka Clinic is justly famous. Doctor Menninger made this statement: "Fifty percent or more of the people who go to doctors to be healed of sickness are suffering from neuroses." Many of these people may be helped by hypnoanalysis.

You won't help all your neurotic patients, but if you can merely help *some* of them, the study of hypnoanalysis is worth your time and effort. Let us examine in further detail the recommended techniques in hypnoanalyzing patients. First, *be sure that all organic pathology has been ruled out. This is vitally important.* Next, be extremely careful to arouse no hostility or resistance by committing a blunder in your approach to the trance state. Make no blunt statements of what you intend to do. Don't say, "Sit down, Mr. Jones, we're going to try hypnoanalysis on you." Instead, use the approach which you have already learned, using the term relaxation as the basis of your procedure.

Tell the patient that maybe if he sits or lies down and relaxes a little bit he'll be able to describe his condition much more easily. Show him the advantages of relaxation.

We have talked about the pin-pointing method before. It must be reviewed here, and a definition is in order—pin-point: the starting point of a neurosis. Every neurotic condition had to start somewhere. This starting point has often been referred to as the pin-point. With the pin-point technique, you are trying to locate the particular set of circumstances which acted as the precipitating factor of the neurosis. You may recall Freud's observation that "Amnesias . . . according to our newer studies, lie at the basis of the formation of all neurotic symptoms." Amnesias—inability to remember certain elements of past experiences—necessitate the pin-point procedure. There is no effect without a cause. With the pin-point method, you are attempting to find the initial or beginning cause. *Here are the types of patient problems in which to use pin-pointing:*

1. Where pain persists even after anesthesia has been administered.

2. For migraines or any other specific neurotic symptom causing psychosomatic aches or pains.

3. In the reduction of phobias.

4. For stammering, stuttering, absent-mindedness, etc.

5. For tics, including tic douloureux.

6. In almost all cases where only one specific problem or symptom is involved.

NOTE: The pin-point method is *not* usually indicated in cases where there is a conglomeration of symptoms.

Now for the actual procedure. The first step is to induce the trance state, just as you normally would. Occasionally it is wise to begin with waking hypnosis, inducing the trance state when sufficient rapport has been achieved, but this is something experience will teach you to judge on an individual basis. The next step is to prove to the patient conclusively that in the relaxed state his awareness is greatly increased, that he can remember things which he thought were forgotten. These things were not forgotten—they were merely stored in his memory—and if he is sufficiently relaxed, the early events of his life can be relived with the same vividness and in the same sequence in which they originally occurred.

Perhaps one of the most successful methods of proving to a patient that he can relive these experiences is to bring him back in age to childhood days. Let him attend school again, or an early birthday party, or a Christmas celebration of his childhood. When he begins reliving the event as vividly as though it were taking place now, rapport will increase considerably and you can proceed with the hypnoanalysis.

When you are sure that your patient can relive or recall any specific memory you wish him to have, tell him now that he can remember things about his present condition which will lead him to understand how his illness started. Tell him every illness has a beginning, and all you want to do is to find that beginning in an effort to learn what caused it. Take him back to school again, perhaps to the first grade. Ask him to look around the schoolroom. Ask him if he ever had any symptoms resembling his present ones while attending first grade. Did he ever have the kind of aches or pains which he has as a grown man?

If his answer is yes, tell him that you would like to compare the condition he had then with the condition he has today. Tell him that anything you can produce in this relaxed state can be removed in the relaxed state. All you want to do is to compare symptoms of childhood with the adult symptoms he manifests today. Occasionally a patient will object to reliving previous painful experiences. Reassure him that it is for the purpose of accurate diagnosis and that you will remove the pain instantly. Frequently, this assurance achieves its aim and proper cooperation is secured. In those cases where no amount of reassurance achieves this end pass it by for the moment and return to it later in such a way that the patient does not realize what your suggestions are achieving.

It is important that a comparison be made between the symptoms of childhood and those of adulthood. A headache may be caused by many things, not all emotional. If you are looking for the emotional cause of a headache, a comparison must be made to be sure that an emotional factor *was* the causative factor in the first place and formed a habit pattern which has persisted through the years. For example, a headache in childhood might have been caused by eye strain and subsequently corrected by glasses. Obviously, this would not be what you were looking for, and you would have to continue searching. There is a lot of difference between a pathological condition that causes headaches and an emotional condition that causes headaches.

Perhaps a patient suffers from violent headaches, and is in agony at the beginning of the hypnoanalysis. You have not been able to suggest it away. Now your aim is to compare his present headache with the one he had in childhood. How can you do this if he is distracted by pain while you are talking to him? Tell him that just for a moment you are going to have him imagine that all the aches and pains are flowing out of his body—"as though you are taking wing on a magic carpet." Tell him to imagine how good he would feel if this could actually happen. Explain that it *can* happen, if he will think as you direct him to. Tell him you are going to count to ten, and with every count you make the headache will get lighter and lighter. Count to ten and *count all the way. Do not stop.* Act as though it were the most natural thing in the world for this phenomenon to occur; imply by your confident manner that it always happens, that it never fails. Now, before the patient has a chance to say, "I still have the headache," put in your suggestion: "Notice how much better you feel. That headache is gone completely." The patient in most instances will accept this suggestion since it is a very welcome one, and you have achieved the first partial success.

When the headache is gone or the patient feeling much better, tell him that you would now like to have him imagine he is back in school again, on one of those days when he was sick. Ask him, "Are you in school?" When he says, yes, continue with, "What time of the day is it, early morning or afternoon?" "Morning." . . . "And I suppose you are feeling pretty good?" The patient might answer, "It's morning in school—just before I get sick. I'm starting to feel sick already."

To illustrate technique specifically, here is a hypothetical case, based on a real one and chosen for its own clarity and for the clearcut removal of the symptoms once the cause was understood. Most cases are not as simple and are not as easily solved; because of its simplicity this one lends itself to the teaching of the therapeutic technique. Here is a reconstruction of the conversation between the doctor and his patient:

DOCTOR: What's been happening in school to make you sick?

PATIENT: I don't know.

DOCTOR: What is your teacher doing?

PATIENT: [Might answer anything.]

DOCTOR: What are you doing?

PATIENT: [Tells what he's doing in school.]

DOCTOR: You say you're starting to feel sick in school. What did you have for breakfast this morning?

PATIENT: The usual.

DOCTOR: I'm going to take you back to the time you woke up that morning and then take you right through the day to see just what it was that made you sick. You are fast asleep in bed and it's that morning you felt ill in school. Do you wake up by yourself or is someone waking you?

PATIENT: [Answers.]

DOCTOR: Now you're getting dressed for school. Is anybody helping you?

PATIENT: Yes. Mother.

DOCTOR: And how are you feeling as she helps you?

PATIENT: [Answers.]

DOCTOR: All right, you're dressed now. What is the next thing you do?

PATIENT: [Answers.]

DOCTOR: All right, you're sitting down to breakfast. What room are you in?

PATIENT: [Answers.]

DOCTOR: You're eating in the kitchen. Is anyone eating with you?

PATIENT: [Answers.]

DOCTOR: What are you having for breakfast this morning?

PATIENT: [Answers.]

(NOTE: *From the patient's answers, you can usually judge whether he is actually abreacting or merely recalling. If he appears to be doing the latter, it is necessary for the doctor to stimulate his memory further.*)

DOCTOR: I don't want you to remember. I want you to *be* there. Sitting down at breakfast, that very morning. When I snap my fingers [The doctor can use this or any similar trigger mechanism.] . . . When I snap my fingers, you'll be sitting down for breakfast and it will be that very day and you'll live through everything—just as you did that morning . . . [snaps fingers] Now —you're a little boy and you're sitting there. What are you having for breakfast?

(NOTE: *The patient at this point will usually be able to live through the entire breakfast and the balance of the day's events. Such reliving is known as abreaction, as distinguished from recall. When the patient is halfway through his meal, doctor continues questioning.*)

DOCTOR: Has mother or anybody else said anything this morning so far that in any way disturbs you?

PATIENT: [Answers.]

(NOTE: *It is assumed, of course, that the doctor will be guided by each answer he gets. In this case, the patient's answers showed that nothing upsetting was said by any member of the family up to this point.*)

DOCTOR: Now you're through with breakfast and getting ready to leave for school. What clothes are you putting on?

PATIENT: It's cold outside. I have to put on my coat.

DOCTOR: All right, your coat is on. You're just stepping outside the door. Everything all right?

PATIENT: Yes. Mother is kissing me and telling me to be careful. I'm big enough to walk to school by myself now.

DOCTOR: Are you happy?

PATIENT: Yes—and I'm feeling good, too. Except that I'm kind of scared.

DOCTOR: Scared? Scared about what?

PATIENT: That big dog that lives on the next street. He doesn't like me. He always barks at me. And I got to walk by the house where he is. But mother told me not to worry because he's always inside the screen porch and locked up.

DOCTOR: Then he's probably safe, all right. Now you're crossing the street.

PATIENT: Oh—I'm getting awful scared. The dog isn't chained up this morning. He's on the sidewalk and I got to pass him. I don't want to. I'm going to walk down this side street. Ooh! He's seeing me. He's starting to bark. He's coming after me. I better run. He's going to catch me! He's going to bite me!

(NOTE: *At this point in the actual case, the patient went into near panic. The doctor had to soothe the patient, who began screaming, "Mother! Mother! Help me—help me, oh, please, mister, help me—that dog is after me." The patient finally subsided and continued sobbing.*)

PATIENT: Will you take me to school, mister? Please! And don't tell my mother. Oh, thanks, thanks!

DOCTOR: [Brings abreaction to an end and now substitutes recall.] . . . Did the dog bite you?

PATIENT: No, not really. But I thought he was going to. The man saved me. He was an awfully nice man. He took me to school and nothing happened. He didn't tell my mother or anything.

DOCTOR: [Bringing patient back to abreaction] You're at school now. Are you still scared?

PATIENT: No. I'm all right now. Just a little nervous.

DOCTOR: What's making you nervous?

PATIENT: I got to go home for lunch and I might see that dog—and I got to come back to school. And I got to go home again this afternoon. That's three more trips today—and I—I—I'm getting awfully sick. I got an awful pain in my head. My head hurts. I got a headache. Gee, it's the first time in my life my head ever hurt this way.

(NOTE: *In this case, the doctor was able to learn that the migraine which started in school that day was the forerunner of all subsequent headaches. He was able to compare the first headache with the later ones, and to learn that the dog episode precipitated a habit pattern. At the slightest scare of any kind, the patient—at a level below conscious awareness—relived the frightening incident, and the migraine headache recurred. It is interesting to note how the doctor handled the situation while the patient was still in the trance state.*)

DOCTOR: Well, Joe, you can see how good your mind is when you can recall a thing like that and actually live through it. Can you see now what brought on that first headache?

PATIENT: You mean it was the dog chasing me that did it?

DOCTOR: Yes, but it wasn't quite that simple. Remember when you were in school, worried about having to go home for lunch, and coming back from lunch, and then going home in the afternoon again?

PATIENT: Yes. Gee, I was scared about it.

DOCTOR: Well, you were a little boy trying to escape from a bad situation, having to pass that dog maybe three times more in one day. And there wasn't any escape you could find—and so nature came up with a defense mechanism. If you were sick you wouldn't have to pass that dog again. It wouldn't be necessary. And so you didn't have too much to do with it. Nature did it for you. Nature showed you that by being sick you could escape the dog. And that's how the first headache happened.

PATIENT: Yeah, I guess that's so, all right. But what about all my other headaches? I didn't always have to pass by the house where the dog was, and I still had my headaches. What about those?

DOCTOR: Well, nature sets up peculiar defenses. When you found out you could escape unpleasantness by being sick, a habit pattern was created. From then on, when anything unpleasant came along the headache came with it. Let's see if that's right. When I snap my fingers you'll remember the second headache you ever had— where you were, how it occurred—and everything about it. Now listen for the snap of my fingers . . . [snaps fingers] Now, where are you this second time?

PATIENT: Playing baseball with the kids. Harry's up at bat and it's my turn.

DOCTOR: Then why aren't you up?

PATIENT: He says it's his turn and he's wrong. It's my turn.

DOCTOR: Why don't you tell him that?

PATIENT: If I do, we'll get into a fight again and he's bigger than me. But it's my turn. It's not right for him to take my turn. I'm beginning to feel sick. I'm getting a headache.

DOCTOR: I'll snap my fingers and the headache will disappear . . . [snaps fingers] How about it, Joe, see how a habit pattern works? You're scared this second time, there's no way out that you can figure, and so nature gives you a headache and you avoid the entire unpleasant situation.

PATIENT: It does look that way, doesn't it? But what can I do about it?

DOCTOR: Well, you're a man now, and you don't have anything to be scared about these days, do you?

PATIENT: No, I don't think so.

DOCTOR: Well, all you have to do is decide that when an emotional crisis comes along, you're going to face it squarely. Face up to it, and you'll probably find that you won't have to escape into headaches from now on. Think you can do it?

PATIENT: I can try.

DOCTOR: That won't be enough. You'll have to succeed.
            Now, I'm going to test you and see whether you
            can take an emotional crisis in stride. Here's
            what I'm going to do. I'm going to create an
            emotional situation and see if you can handle it.
            Are you willing?

PATIENT: If you think it will do any good.

DOCTOR: Let's find out. Because if you can face this
            scare, you can face any of them. You're a little
            boy in the first grade of school. How old are
            you, Joe?

PATIENT: Six.

DOCTOR: Do you know any kid named Harry?

PATIENT: Yeah, and I don't like him. He's bigger than me.

DOCTOR: Well, he's talking to you. He's got a chip on
            his shoulder ·and he's daring you to knock it off.
            He says he'll beat you up if you knock it off.
            You can do one of two things—have a headache
            or take a beating. What would you rather do?

PATIENT: I'd rather take a beating. I'm going to knock
            that chip off his shoulder.

DOCTOR: There it is. Knock it off.

PATIENT: [Moves as if knocking chip off shoulder.]

DOCTOR: And you see, nothing happens! You don't get a
            headache, and he doesn't beat you up. That's
            the way most troubles are. Strictly imaginary.
            If you face them, they don't come off. Nothing
            happens. If you remember this lesson, you'll
            probably be able to face any trouble that comes
            along. See what I mean?

PATIENT: Suppose I *do* get my block knocked off?

DOCTOR: Wait a minute, Joe. I'm not asking you to get
            in the path of trouble. If you put your hand
            against a buzz saw you're liable to lose it. The
            idea is that most troubles are minor ones. You
            can face them without worrying about them at

all. Now today when you first came into my office you had an awful headache, didn't you?

PATIENT: Yes—awful.

DOCTOR: Let's find out what caused it. Anything on your mind about home or business that's worrying you?

PATIENT: You might call it that. There are a couple of buyers coming in from St. Louis tomorrow, and one of them expects me to take him out and show him the town. I got a sick baby at home and I don't want to go out with him.

DOCTOR: And so you got a headache thinking about him.

PATIENT: Yeah. There doesn't seem to be any way out.

DOCTOR: But there is. Has it occurred to you that you can tell the buyer about your sick child and ask to be excused this time?

PATIENT: He's an important buyer. We might lose his business.

DOCTOR: Well, how much business do you think you're going to get from him if you're too sick to go out with him, anyhow? Isn't it better to face him and tell the truth, and be a man without a headache than be sick and miserable the way you were when you came into this office?

PATIENT: Yes. I guess you're right. The way things were going I'd have been too sick to go to the office tomorrow, anyhow.

DOCTOR: How do you feel now?

PATIENT: Wonderful. I'm beginning to understand why I get these headaches and from now on I think I can keep them from happening.

DOCTOR: That's what I wanted to hear you say. So long as you face your emotional problems squarely, you'll be a man without a headache. Now, when I snap my fingers, you're going to open your eyes feeling better than you've felt for weeks— months, years. When you get a wonderful feeling from head to toes like you're getting now, that means you're ready to come out of this

dreamlike state. Listen for the snap . . . [snaps
fingers] How do you feel?

PATIENT: Wonderful. Like I've been asleep and just woke
up, but I wasn't asleep because I could hear
every word.

DOCTOR: Well, if you're wide awake and alert as you say,
you ought to be able to tell me all about your
headaches and what caused them. Can you?

(NOTE: *At this point, the doctor reviewed with
the patient all the material which had been
revealed through the hypnoanalysis. By bring-
it to the attention of the patient's conscious
awareness, he doubly fortified the patient
against a recurrence of the migraines. Although this hypnoanalysis occurred many years
ago, the patient has never had a recurrence of
his headache problem.*)

*   *   *

As was stated at the beginning, all cases are not as
simple as this, nor do they always lend themselves so readily
to this type of therapeutic approach. Let us analyze what
happened: By using the pin-point method of hypnoanalysis,
the doctor enabled the patient to guide himself back to the
initial cause of his condition. Having returned to childhood
and having seen for himself what started the habit pattern,
the patient was in a position to choose between two alterna-
tives—he could face his emotional problems and not be ill,
or he could seek escape from them into illness. The average
neurotic when faced with these two choices will choose the
wiser one, a return to normal health. It is a logical conclusion that in a neurotic condition manifesting one specific
symptom only, this symptom is the result of a habit pattern
created by an emotional problem which the neurotic has not
been able to face. Consciously, therefore, he has forgotten
the emotional situation that initially triggered the system.
To repeat Freud's observation, "Amnesias . . . according to
our newer studies lie at the basis of the formation of all
neurotic symptoms."

Doctor after doctor sees cases in which he can find no
signs of pathology and yet illness persists. There are excep-

tions, however, and there is always the question of what *is* pathological and what is *not*. In a previous chapter, I described an asthmatic patient who was brought to class and in a dramatic abreaction revealed that the cause of his illness was his belief that in his grade school years he had caused the death of a friend whom he knocked down.

This case was described to me as asthmatic, and the crying syndrome was apparent. Yet, in tracking down the case for verification of all the facts, I received a letter which revealed that this man was also suffering from many other ailments, including a peptic ulcer. At the time of the hypnoanalysis I did not know that this condition existed. However, you will notice from the following letter that all his symptoms (whether or not they may have been partially pathological) diminished as a result of hypnoanalysis and of the fine work the doctor did in following up the case. Here is what the doctor said in his letter:

"Case of Henry L., about 35-40 years old with intractible peptic (stomach) ulcer of many years. Although this was his presenting complaint, he also had a history of various 'psychoneurotic' complaints of one kind or another. He had seen many doctors and had been a patient at Illinois Research Hospital, which is connected with the University of Illinois Medical School. Under hypnosis you took him back to kindergarten and on through the grades, asking for anything different. At sixth grade when you asked about change he said in a strained voice, 'Joe isn't there. Where is he?' On pursuing that line, it seems that during the summer he had a fight with Joe and gave him a bloody nose. Not long after Joe got sick and died, cause not completely known, but probably an infection, probably meningitis. With your usual technique of bringing this to his conscious attention and with suggestion under hypnosis and in the waking state . . . he improved markedly, particularly in regard to the ulcer syndrome. The rest of his neurotic symptoms also improved, although some mild symptoms remained."

In all the other cases I have mentioned, so far as I know, there was no pathology present, yet these people were undoubtedly ill and they needed help. In my opinion, when a person says he's sick, he's sick. It doesn't matter whether his illness arises from pathological causes or from the stresses and strains under which we live. There are only two things

in the world which can cause a person to be ill, so far as I am
able to learn.   One is evidenced by pathology and is usually
revealable by medical tests.   But when the tests come back
negative, despite pains, aches, fears, repressions, anxieties,
etc., the suffering patient is still entitled to help, and hypnoanalysis is a device which enables the doctor to trace the
cause of the condition in this second type of case.

The reason it's important to trace the cause is that if you
don't know what it is, all you can do is treat the symptoms.
The doctor is in a much better position when he knows what
the cause of the illness is.   Then he can often correct the
condition.

This does not mean that I claim hypnotic techniques
to be a panacea.   I don't think that hypnosis is the last word
in medicine, but I do think it is an important tool.   Sometimes its full importance is obscured under teaching conditions, and only comes to light in clinical—private—use.   This
is our problem in presenting hypnoanalysis before a group
of people.   Many times the patient is unwilling to air his
troubles in public.   For instance, one doctor's wife certainly
had no idea of what caused her headaches or I'm sure she
wouldn't have volunteered to undergo hypnoanalysis during
a class session.   And if her husband had known what caused
the headaches, he wouldn't have let her come up before the
class.   Since he did *not* know, he said, "By all means, work
with her.   She has terrible migraines.   If you can help her,
it will be wonderful."

I got out some of the pertinent material through hypnoanalysis very easily, but her ideomotor response indicated
there was more.   Then, when I saw that I wasn't going to
be able to get the full story, I used hypnosis attached to
sleep, and was talking to her unconscious mind.   Even now,
however, she remained reticent in public.   Finally, I asked
her if she would whisper more information to me and she
said that she would.   She revealed that she was deeply
troubled.   Her exact words were, "I'm so unhappy at home,
I have been contemplating suicide, and I certainly don't want
to talk about it now."   This case obviously had to be handled
by her personal physician privately.   I talked to her husband
about it before they left the class.   Apparently he was unaware of this situation, and was deeply shocked.   He said
he would do something about it immediately.

To further illustrate the technique and uses of hypno-analysis (and especially of abreaction) I would like to tell you about an interesting psychiatric problem, the victim of which was brought to class. The doctor explained that the patient suffered from violent temper tantrums and that he was also a victim of amnesia. He had been shot down in a plane over France prior to the Normandy Invasion during World War II, and couldn't remember anything that had happened after he bailed out of the plane. He knew that some of the crew members were killed or captured, and the others got back across the Channel safely, helped by the French Underground. But he didn't have the slightest idea what happened to him between the time he was shot down and the time he found himself back in England. The psychiatrist felt that there was probably some connection between this amnesic episode and the temper tantrums. Would hypnosis reveal the true situation?

It is interesting to note how good his memory was up to the time he bailed out of the plane, so let's start with part of the interview that preceded the hypnoanalysis:

ELMAN: Give us an idea of what happened so far as you remember?

PATIENT: You mean what occurred that particular day?

ELMAN: Yes. You were in the Air Force at that time?

PATIENT: Yes. We reported to briefing at approximately three-thirty in the morning. And up to that point I had been flying as a crew member—navigator, previously gunner—for about four years. Not once in those four years did I ever turn my personal belongings in to Intelligence, which we were always told to do, but I never did—like most of us. But this particular morning when the curtain was raised and the target was pointed out— the colonel pointed to the target and said, "The target for today is Stuttgart." I got a cold chill. I just knew this was it. After briefing I took all my personal belongings to Intelligence. In fact, I went so far as to repay a pound note to a friend of mine from whom I had borrowed it.

ELMAN: And that's going pretty far.

PATIENT: That's going pretty far. This is the God's honest truth. I handed it to him and he said, "Wait until we get back from the mission." And I said, "No, I'd better give it to you now." He said, "Why?" and I said, "Because we're not coming back." He said, "You're crazy." I said, "Well, take it for me and hold it for me and then it doesn't make any difference." Well, we were what was termed a lead crew for the group. In the American Air Force we bombed in numbers —daylight bombing—so at this time they were using what they called Pathfinder ships. They were the original ships with radar. The Pathfinder ships were the ones that found the target and released the first bombs, and of course, the other ships released their bombs in unison and that was it. In case of a malfunction in the Pathfinder ship, or if the Pathfinder was shot down or got into trouble, the lead ship was to take over. It just so happened this was a long mission. We were the first plane to take off of our group. This was, of course, important later, because we used up more gas than any other plane . . . We had always had a primary target, a secondary target and a third choice target. As we approached the primary target, and we could see our target, the Pathfinder ship called over the radio that their radar mechanism was out. So number two, which was also a Pathfinder ship, took over and they too, reported immediately that they could not get the target on sight . . . We, being the first plane with a bomb sight, it just happened that our bombardier did not have the electricity turned on which would heat up the bomb sight and a cold bomb sight can't be operated properly. *However it was my responsibility to see that he did have it heated up* . . . Therefore, we flew right over the target and no bombs were dropped. We went to the second target and it was covered by clouds, so we couldn't see it. So we went to our third target and dropped bombs.

ELMAN: By this time it had been heated up, right?

PATIENT: Right. On the way back, because we had been fly-
            ing so long, we were practically out of oxygen,
            and we were running low on fuel, too. Because
            we were running out of oxygen we had to lose al-
            titude and at that time the flak got heavy and the
            fighters got thick. On the way back, with us be-
            ing a lead ship now, when I was asked where we
            were and how far we were from shore—from the
            coast—I was completely lost, probably through
            all the excitement. I was asked to give a new
            course and time of arrival and I was off about
            twenty minutes. Part of this was due, of course,
            to the fact that we lost one engine, and then we
            lost a second engine. So, I gave the order to
            head south instead of trying to make it back to
            England. I felt we could never make it back to
            England. We didn't have enough gas. We
            would have had to ditch in the channel and in
            B-24's that was absolutely a death warrant.
            Rather than ditch in the channel, we decided to
            head south. We had one minute's gas left when
            we bailed out . . . *And I don't remember what
            happened after that.*

ELMAN: And when did you notice these severe temper
            tantrums?

PATIENT: When we got back to the States. I spent, I think
            it was five months in Washington for what they
            call their rest cure. And it was during that time
            and mostly after that I would get these temper
            tantrums . . . I've gotten so worked up that on
            one occasion at home, rather than hit my wife,
            I put my fist through a wall—through a plas-
            ter wall.

ELMAN: Our job now is to find out what caused the
            temper tantrums and see if we can eradicate
            them by bringing the cause to your conscious-
            ness, because the cause is lurking down there in
            the unconscious, unquestionably . . . All I want
            you to do now is to follow certain instructions,

and if you follow these instructions, we'll be able to go through it pretty well.

PATIENT: May I ask a question?

ELMAN: Sure.

PATIENT: Usually with this type of analysis, is the patient in many cases helped?

ELMAN: In many cases he is helped, yes. He is never harmed, and he is helped in many, many cases. With our rapid techniques, I can take the time to hear your story and know that in one minute from now we can have you in the state in which it is possible to recall these things, provided there aren't any obstacles in our way— obstacles such as your not following orders, not doing as we ask. You'll find that this will probably help the temper tantrums. It can't hurt them. It won't bring them on, but it will let you see, perhaps, what causes them, and if you are able to understand the cause and cope with it, you'll be able to control yourself.

(NOTE: *At this point, patient was put into somnambulistic state. In the following transcript, note the violence of his abreaction during hypnoanalysis, and especially how the abreaction was terminated.*)

ELMAN: Now, this is the peaceful feeling that you used to know—this nice feeling of relaxation is what you used to have a great deal of. And even today, before you fall asleep at night, those few seconds before you actually fall asleep, this is the feeling that you have—where the mind is relaxed and the body is relaxed and then comes the sleep . . . When a person is relaxed like this, the mind is more aware than it is at any other time. It is in this state, when you're relaxed physically and mentally, that you can relive any episode in your lifetime that's significant to your behavior pattern. For example, at this time I can take you back and let you see exactly what you went through in that mission over Stuttgart, take you back to the time when you were a child and let you see yourself as a kid, and let you see the scenes you saw then. Just to show you how well your mind really works, and how well relaxed you are, I'm going to let you see yourself as a little boy. I'm going to count to three, snap my fingers, and at that point, you'll see yourself back in the first grade of school, and you'll see it as clearly as if you were back in it this very minute. That is, just as if you were in it right now. Now, just stay as relaxed as you are and don't try to remember, because nobody can remember like that. Just say to yourself, "Wouldn't it be nice to be able to see myself back in school when I was in the first grade." You liked school didn't you?

PATIENT: Yes.

ELMAN: I want to show you how you really do remember things, and that any loss of memory that you've had is a defense mechanism of nature. I want to get back of that defense mechanism and let you see yourself as a little kid. Let you see how good your memory really is. I'm going to count to three and take you back to the first year in school. You'll see the teacher, you'll see the desks, you'll see the tables, you'll see the blackboard, you'll see the pictures on the wall, you'll see the windows, and if you walked up to a window you could actually see the same sights you saw when you were a little boy in the first grade. So, just stay as relaxed as you are and we'll get you back to the first grade. Here you are, one . . . two . . . three. There you are in the first grade . . . [snaps fingers] Take a look at the teacher . . . Do you like this teacher?

PATIENT: Yes.

ELMAN: And tell me, what part of the room are you sitting in?

PATIENT: About the middle.

ELMAN: Middle row and middle seat?

PATIENT: Third from front.

ELMAN: Now, mentally, I want you to stand up and turn around and look at the back of the room, cater-corner, to the kid furthest away from you, and tell me who it is. Boy or girl?

PATIENT: Boy.

ELMAN: Now he's going to stand up, as you stand up mentally, and you're going to see who he is. And when I snap my fingers you'll know his name . . . [snaps fingers]   What's his name?

PATIENT: George.

ELMAN: That's good. Then we know the memory is perfect, don't we? Now, I'm going to come up to you as you're sitting at that desk or table or whatever that room had. What were you sitting at?

PATIENT: We had desks.

ELMAN: I'm going to come up to your desk and I'm going to stand alongside you and I'm going to say, "Do you know what a temper tantrum is? Do you ever have tantrums?"

PATIENT: No.

ELMAN: All right, then. Let's go to the fifth grade and you'll see the fifth grade even more clearly than you did the first grade. You'll see the teacher, you'll see the chairs, the tables, you'll see everything. But I want you to notice how the kids have grown up since you were in the first grade. Now, watch . . . one . . . two . . . three . . . [snaps fingers] and there you are in the fifth grade. Do you like school?

PATIENT: Yes.

ELMAN: And are you pretty happy in the fifth grade?

PATIENT: Yes.

ELMAN: Do you like your teacher?

PATIENT: Yes.

ELMAN: How about the kids. Do you get along with them all right?

PATIENT: Most of them.

ELMAN: Do you fight with some of them?

PATIENT: Yes.

ELMAN: Are they hard, nasty fights?

PATIENT: Yes.

ELMAN: What is mostly the cause of the fights?

PATIENT: Neighborhood fights.

ELMAN: But you would call these the ordinary fights of childhood?

PATIENT: Yes.

ELMAN: That fifth grade is pretty vivid, isn't it?

PATIENT: Yes.

ELMAN: Did you go to junior high or eighth grade?

PATIENT: Junior high for one year.

ELMAN: That would be the eighth grade?

PATIENT: Seventh grade, and then we moved.

ELMAN: Let's see you in the eighth grade, after you moved. You see how good your memory is, that you know you moved and you've seen these kids in school; you've seen the teachers; you've seen everything. Now let's go to the eighth grade and let you see that your memory was just as good in the eighth grade—even better. One . . . two . . . three . . . [snaps fingers] Here you are in the eighth grade in the new neighborhood. How do you like this school?

PATIENT: Fine.

ELMAN: Do you like the kids?

PATIENT: Yes.

ELMAN: Have you gotten over the neighborhood fights?

PATIENT: Yes.

ELMAN: So, here we are in the eighth grade and things are going pretty well. How are things at home? Mother all right?

PATIENT: Yes.

ELMAN: Dad all right?

PATIENT: Yes.

ELMAN: I want to ask you something. You're in the
            eighth grade. You're getting to be pretty grown
            up now, getting to be a young man. You know
            what a temper tantrum is in a kid, don't you?

PATIENT: I've seen them.

ELMAN: Ever had them yourself?

PATIENT: No.

ELMAN: So we know then that there was nothing in the
            first years of your life that would cause you to
            have temper tantrums. It must have been some-
            thing later on. So, let's have you graduating
            from high school. I'm going to count to three
            and snap my fingers, and you'll be graduating
            from high school. One . . . two . . . three . . .
            [snaps fingers] Graduation day and you'll see
            graduation exercises. Notice how good it is to
            see graduation exercises again. How do you
            like the graduation exercises? Glad to be here
            today?

PATIENT: Kind of sad.

ELMAN: What's the matter? Sad to leave high school?
            Dad and mother in the audience?

PATIENT: Yes.

ELMAN: Are they kind of proud of you? Are you the
            oldest boy?

PATIENT: No.

ELMAN: The other kids have made high school too, have
            they? And are they in the audience?

PATIENT: My brother is.

ELMAN: This shows that your memory is normal, and can
            go back to your childhood or any part of your life
            and see those things which are important to your
            behavior pattern, and certainly school days were
            important to you . . . Now, it's after high school.
            Have you started college yet?

PATIENT: Yes.

ELMAN: What year is it?

PATIENT: 1936.

ELMAN: What are you studying?

PATIENT: Dairy husbandry.

ELMAN: Now, let's get you to 1940.   Have you graduated yet?

PATIENT: Yes.

ELMAN: You've graduated from college.   You have your full competence now and if you don't want to go any further, you're qualified to go out and make a living in dairy husbandry, is that correct?

PATIENT: Not yet.

ELMAN: Why?

PATIENT: I've changed my course.

ELMAN: What did you change to?

PATIENT: Horticulture.

ELMAN: Do you like that better?

PATIENT: Yes.

ELMAN: You're graduating and majoring in that, is that correct?

PATIENT: Yes.

ELMAN: So you're equipped with an education.   Is that correct?

PATIENT: Yes.

ELMAN: Let's take you to the time when you got your diploma.   One . . . two . . . three . . . [snaps fingers] and there you are, right there seeing the exercises so vividly.   Tell me, are you glad to be graduating?

PATIENT: Yes.

ELMAN: What are your plans?

PATIENT: I have a job.

ELMAN: And you plan on going into that job, is that it?

PATIENT: Yes.

ELMAN: It's in the line you want—the thing you've been
            studying? . . . You're very pleased with it . . .
            Things have gone well at school . . . You're get-
            ting a diploma. All right, while you're getting
            your diploma, I want to ask you a question. Do
            you ever have any temper tantrums?

PATIENT: I think a few—I had a few.

ELMAN: Well then, it wasn't the result of the war at all.
            But there was something that happened that
            caused a boy who had never had a temper tan-
            trum up to the time he finished high school, to
            have them in college. Let's take you back to
            that first year at college . . . You're just finish-
            ing your first year of college. You're studying
            dairy husbandry at this point. Are you happy
            with your studies?

PATIENT: I don't feel that school is giving me enough.

ELMAN: You want more education than you're getting
            is that correct? Tell me, as you finish this first
            year of college, have you had any temper tan-
            trums? Stay relaxed—it's important to stay re-
            laxed . . . You see, we're getting to the cause
            now and since we're getting to the cause let's not
            let any tensions come in. You'll be so much more
            aware when there are no tensions. Have there
            been any temper tantrums in the first year of
            college?

PATIENT: No.

ELMAN: Now you're starting your second year of college.
            Are you still going in for dairy husbandry?

PATIENT: Yes.

ELMAN: But you're not quite satisfied. Is that it? Little
            discontents are creeping in. Let's get you to
            the finish of your second college year. One . . .
            two . . . three . . . [snaps fingers] and it's just the
            end of the second college year.

PATIENT: I quit.

ELMAN: You quit school and you went to another school, is that it?

PATIENT: No.

ELMAN: What happened?

PATIENT: They gave me a scholarship.

ELMAN: In another field?

PATIENT: Just to come back.

ELMAN: There must have been a reason why you quit. What was it?

PATIENT: I thought it was too juvenile. I thought I was man enough to go out on my own.

ELMAN: And they wanted you back to school so they gave you a scholarship to come back and study what you wanted to and that's when the change in studies occurred. Is that it?

PATIENT: Yes.

ELMAN: Up to this point were there any temper tantrums?

PATIENT: Yes.

ELMAN: Apparently something came along that caused that first temper tantrum. It is important that we find out and go to the exact first temper tantrum. And find out when it occurred and what was on your mind at the time. I want to get back to an hour before the temper tantrum, and wherever you were, you will be there again. It will be the first temper tantrum you ever had and it's coming up in about an hour or so. I want you to go back to an hour before the temper tantrum so that we can find out what your thoughts are at that time. Here we go. One . . . two . . . three. . . [snaps fingers] It's an hour before the first temper tantrum. Where are you?

PATIENT: In the dorm.

ELMAN: What's been happening?

PATIENT: The junior classmen in the dorm cut me out.

ELMAN: Cut you out for what?

PATIENT: Activities.

ELMAN: Why did they cut you out?

PATIENT: I was voted out of my letter.

ELMAN: Voted out of your letter for athletic activity, you mean? Why were you voted out of your letter?

PATIENT: Personal, I think.

ELMAN: Had you earned the letter?

PATIENT: Yes.

ELMAN: You had earned it and then they didn't give you the letter. Was this a pretty big disappointment to you?

PATIENT: Yes.

ELMAN: You worked hard to get the letter?

PATIENT: Yes.

ELMAN: We're coming to within about half an hour of that temper tantrum. Where are you and what's been happening?

PATIENT: The athletic board met and one student was the deciding vote and voted that I should not get my letter.

ELMAN: Were you present there?

PATIENT: No.

ELMAN: But you heard about it.

PATIENT: Yes.

ELMAN: And where were you at the time this was happening?

PATIENT: In my room.

ELMAN: In your room waiting for the decision, is that right? And the decision seemed pretty important to you. What had you done or what had you not done that caused these people to vote against you? What happened? Had you said anything? Had you done anything? Had you noticed any personality defect that kept you from making friends?

PATIENT: Some of the students didn't like me because I was given responsible jobs. They had to take orders from me. I assigned students to work.

ELMAN: And you made them do it even though they didn't like to do it.

PATIENT: They had to do it.

ELMAN: And you felt they had to do it.

PATIENT: Every student had to work.

ELMAN: Would you say this was responsible for not getting the letter?

PATIENT: Not all.

ELMAN: What was the rest? Because unquestionably that letter meant a great deal to you; otherwise the temper tantrums never would have occurred.

PATIENT: I used to date my friends' girls.

ELMAN: And they didn't like that.

PATIENT: No.

ELMAN: You wouldn't have liked it either. In your mind, you probably thought it was a big thing to date your friends' girls. But the friends didn't like it any more than you would. Now that you look back at it you can see that if one of those boys whose girl you dated had to make the deciding vote, he certainly wouldn't vote in your favor, would he? Wouldn't you say that you knew as you were sitting there in the room that the vote had to go against you? Didn't you feel as you were in the room that if those friends had to do the voting you wouldn't get the letter? And wasn't there quite a feeling of guilt involved; quite a feeling that if you didn't get the letter, you already knew why?

PATIENT: Yes.

ELMAN: In other words, this was a guilt complex, wasn't it? And the temper tantrum was merely a manifestation of a guilt complex. You really knew why you didn't get the letter. They hadn't been the ones who took the honor away. You had been the one who took the honor away from yourself, and therefore you felt guilty about it. Isn't that right? Am I telling you this or are you telling me this? Are we discussing absolute truth now?

PATIENT: Yes.

ELMAN: Can you understand why a person feeling guilty gets mad at himself? You get so mad you could put your fist through the wall. Isn't that so? You're mad because you say to yourself, "If I hadn't done so and so, this wouldn't have had to happen." But you're not thinking it out loud. You're repressing that sort of thought, but the thought is there, nevertheless, at an unconscious level, isnt it? Now, if this is true, and if we are discussing the absolute truth, you'll find that every temper tantrum you ever had was the result of a guilt complex, where you were really mad at yourself, and took it out on the other fellow. Are you beginning to see what I'm talking about?

PATIENT: Yes.

ELMAN: Let's go to the last temper tantrum you had and see if we're right in assuming that this was really a case just like that of the letter. When I snap my fingers you'll know exactly when it was . . . [snaps fingers] When was it?

PATIENT: About a month ago.

ELMAN: What happened? . . . It's just an hour before . . . What's been happening?

PATIENT: My daughter. A boy has been calling at the house almost every night. And my wife and I discussed it. I didn't feel that this boy should be coming to the house so often. My wife and I got into an argument.

ELMAN: Now, why didn't you feel the boy should be coming there quite often? How old is your daughter?

PATIENT: Fifteen and a half.

> (*Note: I must interrupt the transcript here to point out certain facts. The same kind of situation that had precipitated the first temper tantrum was occurring again. The first incident was precipitated because he was taking the other fellows' girls away from them. The latest flare-up took place because now somebody was taking his girl—his daughter—away from him, in his unconscious thinking. This indicates that further work was required by the doctor in charge of the case, in order to give the patient insight, for at this point, although the patient realized how the latest temper tantrum occurred, he was not associating it with the first one. This should also indicate to the reader how it is often impossible to perform a complete hypnoanalysis in one session. Let me review this case from the beginning: The first temper tantrum was precipitated by his failure in his responsibility to fellow students, as well as frustration at not getting his letter. Remember that in telling about the airplane incident, he said it was his responsibility to have the bomb sight heated up. He had not done this. Again he failed in his responsibility, and the accident that followed left him with a severe feeling of guilt. The third incident, involving his daughter, was triggered by parental jealousy and by his feeling of being responsible for the girl's behavior; when his wife didn't agree with him about dealing with the situation, again he was frustrated, and again he felt guilty about a failure to handle his responsibility. I must point out that we have covered only three temper tantrums. However, the doctor reported that there had been many more. Therefore, we know that a habit pattern had been established. Now let us continue with the transcript; the patient is still in somnambulism as I address him.*)

ELMAN: Now, let's go a little bit further. You'd like to learn exactly what happened to you after that plane crash. Let's see what happened as we have you in the air and the first engine goes out ... You'll find that you'll remember exactly what happened . . . There we are . . . You're there now as I snap my fingers . . . [snaps fingers] Now, tell us what happens and you'll see that the memory comes right back.

PATIENT: I see the railroad yards and we dropped our bombs. We're hitting 320 degrees. I asked for a course and I start working backwards. I can't pin-point.

ELMAN: There's a reason why you can't pin-point. I'll snap my fingers and you'll know the reason . . . [snaps fingers] What is it? Are you nervous?

PATIENT: I got lost on the last turn.

ELMAN: What's happening?

PATIENT: I asked for an ETA to the coast. Time is running out . . . We can't see the coast . . . We just lost number two . . . I'm working back again . . . I can't find where we are . . . still can't see the coast . . . We just lost number three . . . I take a reading . . . We don't have enough fuel . . . I asked should we continue or head south . . . We head south . . . I think I know where we are . . . We only have four minutes of gas . . . We have to get ready for emergency . . . Fighters below are coming . . . I can't get out . . . I climb . . . I got out . . . I'm afraid . . . I open my chute . . . It's long down . . . I'm not going to make it to that farm . . . I try for a road . . . I missed . . . Now I'm stuck up in a tree . . . Germans all over . . . I'm just . . . I'm stuck . . . I can't get out of my chute . . . I get out—I'm out . . . Some Frenchmen are coming . . . They throw me a wire . . . I start down . . . I fall . . . I'm knocked out . . . They tell me to come with them . . . I hide my jacket and my gun . . . I go with them. [*Patient shows violent reaction, begins hyperventilating.*]

ELMAN: You don't have to be so excited about it. You can tell the whole story.

PATIENT: We saw Sergeant Branch in a tree . . . They get him out . . . They chopped down the tree . . . We hide all night . . .

ELMAN: You're much calmer now as you tell the story. The fear's all gone.

PATIENT: [Sounds breathless] There are soldiers all over . . . They're looking for us. I can't speak . . . We got to get out of here . . . We're walking through the woods . . . We're going up the road . . . [breathing heavily again] We see a man on a bicycle . . . We jump in the ditch . . . He comes . . . He stops . . . We go on the other side and hide . . . He comes back, he gives us coffee . . . He told us to go to town, and wait . . . We wait . . . He comes back . . . Talked of the sergeant— Sergeant Warren was killed . . . Brings us his dogtag number . . . His chute never opened . . . We go around town . . . Awful hungry . . . They bring us bread, and cheese . . . We see German soldiers . . .

ELMAN: Now, Im going to count to three and all the nervousness will leave. One . . . two . . . three . . . [snaps fingers] Now the nervousness leaves. You'll calm down, and you'll recall it all, and you won't be affected by it, but you'll recall everything because you see how good your mind is. You realize that, don't you?

PATIENT: Sure.

ELMAN: These are the things that you blotted out of your mind because they were unpleasant.

PATIENT: It hurts.

ELMAN: I'll snap my fingers and you'll feel wonderful . . . [snaps fingers] Now, you feel so good. I'm going to bring you out of this because I think you've had enough of it and you know that you can remember everything. You can remember anything you want to. This was just nature's defense mechanism for making you forget an unpleasant episode. And, of course, it was unpleasant. But it happened a long, long time ago. You're all over it, and you know you came out of it clearly. We don't have to have you go through the whole abreaction now. You know already you've been helped, don't you?

PATIENT: Yes... I'm shaking.

ELMAN: You won't when I have you open your eyes,
            and you'll feel so good for having gotten this
            out of your system, up into consciousness again.
            And now you'll feel like a new man. This is
            what we call a mental catharsis. You'll feel so
            good. All right, you can open your eyes . . . No-
            tice how good you feel. Well, how do you feel?

PATIENT: Tense. Look at my hands—all wet.

ELMAN: You were hyperventilating. That's why I
            stopped it. But isn't it a nice thing to know
            you can remember? And now you know exactly
            what happened.

PATIENT: Yes.

ELMAN: You relived just part of the episode and you
            saw how excited you got, didn't you?

PATIENT: I could feel it.

ELMAN: Of course you could. That's what we know as
            an abreaction. And sometimes it can be pretty
            violent. The reason I didn't let the abreaction
            continue was that you were hyperventilating
            badly.

PATIENT: Am I supposed to be nervous now?

ELMAN: No. You've relived something that was horrible,
            so naturally you would show some signs of strain
            after going through it.

PATIENT: But I didn't remember.

ELMAN: Sure, because you'd blacked it out for so many
            years. Now you know how you got back across
            the channel and everything, don't you?

PATIENT: Yes.

ELMAN: But you thought you had completely forgotten
            it. You hadn't forgotten any of it. Nature had
            just drawn a veil over it as a protection to you.
            In the reliving of it, of course, you hyperven-
            tilated, and you had quite a severe abreaction.
            This isn't as violent an abreaction as we've seen.

> We have had to take people who have gone through military action where their buddies are being shot down all around them; these men were terrified. You were scared. You've seen action. You know what it's like. You've seen fear and you've seen bravery mixed up in one and the same thing.

PATIENT: Bravery comes out of fear.

ELMAN: And the man who says he isn't scared is just not honest. If a man has ordinary imagination, then he's scared . . .

*   *   *

In this case, you can see how frustrating circumstances and a conviction of guilt precipitated the temper tantrums. Although the frustration occurred in the airplane incident prior to the actual bailing out, the habit pattern would cause his temper tantrums to become more violent as he was recuperating during the rest cure. The doctor, of course, had to do further work with this patient before his condition could be entirely corrected.*

Did you recognize how the abreaction was speedily terminated? It is a very simple device, yet it always works. I have never known it to fail. It is done by a change of tenses as the operator speaks to the patient. If you wish to change abreaction to recall, all you have to do is change your tenses. Instead of saying, "What happens now?" simply say, "What happened then?" By this simple means you have substituted recall for abreaction. Many times, when a patient becomes highly excited, I change abreaction to recall, but continue the patient in the hypnotic state for further questioning, perhaps later inducing abreaction again.

---

*I did not have my own tape recorder on during the above hypnoanalysis and must add this footnote in appreciation to the doctor, who kindly sent me his tape recording for inclusion here.

Chapter 22

HYPNOSIS ATTACHED TO SLEEP—
HYPNOSLEEP

A MEEK little man walked hesitantly up to my desk, looked around cautiously for a moment, and then said, "Mr. Elman, could I speak to you privately?"

I walked to the side of the room with him. Once there, he peered cautiously around to make sure no one was listening, and then asked, "Is it true that you teach your doctors how to hypnotize people when they are fast asleep?"

"Yes."

"I have to learn how to do that. It's absolutely necessary. I don't need the rest of your course, but that's one thing I have to learn. It would make life so much easier for me."

"Wait a minute. Let's get this straight. Hypnotizing people when they are asleep requires an extensive knowledge of the subject. You just can't learn part of it and expect to be successful. You have to learn the entire subject."

"Oh, I know hypnosis very well—been using it for years —but no one has taught me how to hypnotize people while they are asleep—and I have to know how."

"Why is it so important?"

Again he looked around cautiously before he answered. "Mr. Elman, Ive been married for over thirty-five years and I hope there are many good years ahead for my wife and me, but all through our marriage I've been faced with an awful problem. It's my wife, really—she's the problem."

"Is she ill?"

"No, not at all. She's in perfect health, and we love each other dearly. But I have a problem that must be corrected. She's always picking on me."

I thought he was ribbing me, but he went on quite seriously. "Do you know what it's like to be married to a domineering woman? I'm what you call a henpecked husband."

"I'm sorry to hear that, but how could hypnosis help you?"

"I've had a plan for a good many years. I've tried very hard, but I can't make it work. I want to hypnotize her and give her the suggestion to quit picking on me. If she knew how much it distresses me, I'm sure she'd stop the henpecking."

"Why don't you tell her that?"

"I have, but it hasn't done any good. She doesn't take me seriously."

"Then what's your plan?"

"Simply this. She won't let me hypnotize her. Now if I can do it while she is fast asleep, she won't even know she's hypnotized. Then I can give her the necessary suggestion, and I'm sure she'll quit picking on me."

I said to him, "Doctor, you have an entirely erroneous impression of hypnosis. No matter what phase of hypnosis you use, the patient has complete power of selectivity and if the patient doesn't want to accept the suggestion, he won't. We demonstrate that very clearly in class. Occasionally, when we get the state to which you refer, we intentionally give the patient some kind of suggestion which we believe will be unwelcome to him in order to watch his reaction. Always, the patient either wakes up from his sleep or continues to sleep, but rejects the suggestion. I still think that the best way to handle your situation is by discussing it frankly with your wife. If she won't listen to you while she is awake, she certainly won't while she is asleep. Hypnosis can't be used for such purposes. If this is your only reason for enrolling in the course, please don't enroll."

"All right, Mr. Elman, I'm sure you know more about that than I do. I guess I did have a wrong impression. However, I am going to enroll in the course because I feel it would be to my advantage to learn your techniques for use with my patients."

During the entire course he did not mention the problem he had with his wife. He studied diligently and brought in some excellent reports about the fine work he was doing with his patients. My opinion of his ability increased considerably.

A year later, however, he attended one of my classes in the same city. He asked if he could make an announcement to the new students, and of course I gave him my approval.

Imagine my surprise when he stood up and made the following statements. (Unfortunately, no tape recording was made,
but I'll try to give an approximation of his words.):

"When I enrolled as a student of Mr. Elman, I did it for
only one purpose. I wanted to learn how to hypnotize my wife
in her sleep and give her suggestions to make her stop picking on me and nagging me. Mr. Elman said I couldn't do it—
that I wouldn't be successful. I've been more than successful.
I hypnotized her while she was sound asleep. She'd never
let me hypnotize her while she was awake but I did it when
she was asleep, and she didn't even know it. I talked to her
unconscious mind—told her how much her picking and nagging was disturbing me, and suggested that she never do it
again. She hasn't henpecked me for over a year, and I'm
very proud to say that as a result I've been much happier.
And maybe she has been much happier."

Apparently while she was asleep, he was able to get
across to her the fact that she was making him unhappy,
and she must have wanted him to be happy or she would
never have taken the suggestion.

One of the most interesting techniques of suggestion
(and one of the least familiar to most doctors and laymen
alike) is a phenomenon that I used to call hypnosis attached
to sleep. Recent studies with medical instruments attached
to sleeping patients have prompted me to change the name
to hypnosleep, which is more in keeping with the phenomenon's close relationship to both mental states.

My first personal experience with this phase of hypnosis
involved my son. In 1940, my wife and I had to take a trip
to Canada, and we left our year-and-a-half-old baby in perfect health in the care of a competent nurse. When we
returned, our baby was suffering from asthma. As he grew
older, the asthma and his allergic reactions became worse.
He obtained some symptomatic relief with medication and
care, but each attack became progressively worse. Despite
medical supervision, and although we carefully followed the
doctor's instructions, by the time he was nine or ten years
old, we were distracted parents. When he had an allergic
attack, he'd have to stay in bed for days at a time before
symptomatic relief was afforded.

If he had a fight with a boy at school, by the time he
got home a rash had appeared in the creases of his elbows

and knees. This rash would rapidly spread from shoulders to wrists and from buttocks to ankles. The entire area was raw because he scratched so much. The doctors insisted we weren't following instructions, but we *were* following instructions, precisely. We took care of our youngster the best we knew how. Nothing helped.

In 1949 he experienced an allergic reaction that badly upset us. He was in bed for several days, gasping for breath, and the extensive rash was another presenting symptom. At this time, a group of New Jersey physicians and dentists were urging me to teach them the subject of hypnosis, and consequently the topic was discussed quite frequently in our home. One day, my wife asked me if I couldn't use hypnosis to help our boy. Not being a doctor, and having had no experience with medical problems or patients at that time, I was understandably reluctant.

"Would it hurt to hypnotize him and tell him he won't itch?" she asked. "Is that against your ethics?"

I didn't think any doctor could object to that, so I hypnotized my son and told him the areas that troubled him wouldn't itch any more. The results were miraculous. The itch disappeared completely. In a day or two the raw areas were covered with scabs, and healing had begun. My wife then suggested that I hypnotize him again and tell him he'd get well in a hurry.

I couldn't see any objection to that, so I hypnotized him again, and told him he'd get well very quickly. The symptomatic relief was remarkable. In a day or two he was completely free of symptoms and could return to school. I knew I hadn't corrected the allergies or the asthma, but I had obtained more relief for my son than any medication had been able to provide. I also knew that if he got into a fight at school, he'd get sick again.

I decided to teach my youngster autosuggestion in an effort to prevent the allergic attacks from recurring. He became an adept student and was greatly helped, but I knew he wasn't cured. If any strong emotional experience came along, an allergic attack and the asthma would be precipitated. If I could only get to the root cause of the allergic reactions, I thought perhaps I could help my son permanently. I tried hypnoanalysis on him. He was quite amenable at first, but before I got to the root, he brought himself out of the hypnosis and declared vehemently, "I don't like this. I don't want any more of it."

"But I'm doing it for your own good. Don't you realize that? I want to help you."

"I don't care. I won't do it. Sorry, Dad."

And that was it—a complete rejection. There was no use working with him. If he rejected hypnosis there was nothing I could do. We have found since then that this is not unusual in hypnoanalysis. Parents or near relatives are often unsuccessful with members of their families because these patients are reluctant to divulge their emotional conflicts for fear of embarrassing themselves or hurting someone in the family, especially since so often members of the family are directly concerned with the problems.

In my son's case, months and months went by, without any further attempt at hypnoanalysis. He became more and more adept with autosuggestion and it afforded him so much relief that he was quite satisfied to let things stand as they were. By this time, I had begun teaching doctors the professional use of hypnosis. The subject, naturally, was uppermost in my mind. While reading a magazine one day, I came across an ad that read, "Learn languages while you sleep." It went on to explain that there were recordings which could be turned on at night, to play while you slept, giving language lessons that would be retained when you awoke—and if you continued doing this for a few months, you could learn a language.

I recognized this technique as the development of an experiment that had been conducted in the South Pacific during the Second World War. I had been conducting a radio program at the time, and a Government information office had asked me to interview a doctor who had been working with servicemen on one of the Pacific islands. He had been putting miniature speakers under the pillows of these men, and when he was sure they were sound asleep, he would turn the speakers on by remote control and teach the men to speak Chinese or Japanese. When the men woke up, they didn't realize that this had happened, but in a few months they had learned the languages and could speak them fluently.

The Bureau of War Information suggested that the doctor and several of the men who had been taught this way be brought to New York for the broadcast. I was delighted, but the program was cancelled at the last minute because the War Department suddenly decided that the experiments ought to be considered classified information.

Now, years later, the technique was being used commercially—and apparently with success. If doctors and language instructors can communicate with sleeping people, I thought, I should be able to do it, too, and if I can communicate with a sleeping person, I can hypnotize one, and if I can hypnotize him, I can probably perform hypnoanalysis without awaking him.

Perhaps, with this technique, I could find out what caused my son's allergic reactions and remove the cause. It was worth trying. Of course, there were obstacles. Suppose I woke him up? Suppose he rejected hypnoanalysis even if I succeed in hypnotizing him while he was asleep? How could I hypnotize him without waking him up? And how could I get him to answer my questions while he was sound asleep and hypnotized? I knew I had to hypnotize him instantly. It couldn't be done by prolonged methods. What were the fewest words I could use to bypass his critical faculty and at the same time establish selective thinking? As I climbed the stairs to his room that night, intent on trying the experiment of hypnotizing him while he slept the words to use seemed to come right up out of the unconscious part of my mind. And the amazing thing is that they were the right words, though I had no conscious recollection of ever having used or heard them before.

I entered the bedroom. It was nearly dark but I could see that he was covered from neck to toe. His head protruded from the blanket and the little finger of his right hand was curled around the edge of the covering. I approached his bed. He didn't move. His respiration was slow and easy. There wasn't a sign of asthma that I could notice. Very gently I spoke to him. "You can hear me but you can't wake up . . . You can hear me but you can't wake up . . . You can't wake up . . . I'll know you're hearing me when the little finger that I'm touching begins to move."

Nothing happened even when I touched the finger. I tried it again. I waited. It seemed a very long time. The finger still didn't move. I repeated, again, "You can hear

me but you can't wake up. I'll know you're hearing me
when this little finger begins to move . . . Move it but you
can't wake up."

His little finger began to move, slowly, very slowly. I
knew I was in communication with him and had hypnotized
him while he was fast and sound asleep.

Almost everyone has at some time dreamed that he can't
wake up. You have probably had such a dream, and you
realize that this is a manifestation of bypassing your own
critical faculty. In reality, of course, you can wake up; you
only think you can't. Similarly, I had established selective
thinking in my son's mind. Now the idea was to prolong
the hypnosis and try to perform hypnoanalysis while he was
fast asleep and hypnotized.

I spoke to him very gently: "This is your father talking,
and he's here to help you. He wants to help you so much.
You can talk to me, but you won't wake up. You know how
much autosuggestion has helped you, but there is more help
coming if you will only talk to me and tell me what is on
your mind. Move that finger again, and I'll know you're
hearing me."

The finger moved but he remained asleep. Then the
hypnoanalysis began, still gently, very gently. By this time
I was very excited. I was doing something which, so far
as I knew, had never been done before. I could not afford
to make a mistake. Every once in a while I could get him
to talk to me, to answer my probing questions. As we
approached disturbing material, he moved in his sleep, and
I became alarmed. Fearful of waking him up, I said, "I'm
going to stop talking now and you'll fall fast asleep, and in
the morning when you wake up, you won't even remember
that I talked to you while you were asleep. You'll have no
recollection whatever. But tomorrow night, we'll try this
again and you'll be very receptive."

As quietly as I could, I left the room. I was quite elated
because I felt that now I had found a way to help my son.
The next night I tried again. And again I succeeded. I even
managed to get out some of the disturbing material without
waking him. By this time I was becoming overconfident and
thought the rest of the work would be easy. On the third
night, with supreme confidence now that I could do it, I
hypnotized him in his sleep and proceeded at once to go to

the place in the hypnoanalysis where we had left off the night before. That was the worst thing I could have done. No sooner had I approached a traumatic episode that occurred when he was four years old than he awoke with a start and asked in an excited voice, "What's the matter, Dad? What's the matter?"

I had been caught red-handed. I didn't know what to say or do. I managed to get out a few comforting words: "Oh, you're awake. I've been talking to you quite a while. Were you asleep? You jumped so suddenly you startled me."

"What's on your mind, Dad? What do you want to talk to me about?"

"Nothing important. Go back to sleep. I thought you were hearing me all the time."

"No. I just woke up. What is it Dad? What is it?"

Somehow I convinced him he should go back to sleep, thinking he would probably question me further in the morning. But in the morning he didn't even mention it. Our conversation had been completely forgotten. The odd part of the incident is that on subsequent nights when I tried to hypnotize him in his sleep I merely had to say one word, and he instantly awakened. I have never been able to duplicate the feat since that night with him.

I thought I had made an important discovery and had no conscious knowledge that anyone had ever duplicated what I had done—that is, hypnotize a person in natural sleep. A few years later, however, a doctor showed me a book that described how the feat had been accomplished many years ago by a Scandinavian operator. In fact, several operators in the past have succeeded in doing the same thing. It is quite possible that many years before, in studying hypnosis, I had read that book, had buried the modus operandi in my mind and brought it forth from the unconscious when I needed it.

In one of my early sessions, I happened to mention to the doctors in attendance what I had been able to do with my son. They asked what good had been accomplished. I was able to tell them, "Even with an incomplete hypnoanalysis, the results have been greater than I had dared to hope for. His allergic reactions were less severe and the attacks were further and further apart."

Then the doctors asked me to teach them how to hypnotize a sleeping patient. This might seem simple, but it wasn't. In order to demonstrate how to attach hypnosis to sleep you have to have a sleeping person. How can you have a sleeping person in the classroom? And how could you be certain the person on whom you demonstrated was actually asleep? Before attempting it, I had to study the sleep mechanism of the human mind. It was distressing to find how little had been written about it. Most of the writing was useless since every doctor who had written a book or paper on the subject seemed to have a different theory. None of them explained the sleep mechanism in a way that could be proved reliable. Despite intensive study I am still not satisfied that I have the answer or that anyone else has the complete answer at this time. For the present, all we can do is to accept the observations on which all writers seem to agree, and discard everything on which they disagree. The first thing we did was to say to the doctors, "We are going to try an interesting experiment. Do any of you have patients who fall asleep easily? If you do, will you please bring these patients to class next week. We are going to try to get them to fall asleep here in the classroom." In every meeting room, we had a cot set up to make things easier, but this didn't help, for we found that these people became so interested in the class lectures that they remained discouragingly wide awake. Then we tried to accomplish the feat by giving posthypnotic suggestions. This succeeded in many cases but took an interminably long time to do and some of the patients rejected this suggestion. Sometimes doctors attending the lectures had to wait up to three hours before the posthypnotic suggestion became effective.

Nevertheless, we learned a great deal from these early experiments. When we succeedd in obtaining natural sleep and then attached the hypnosis, we were able to secure a hypnotic anesthesia that was positively amazing. It is in many cases a better anesthesia than can be secured in any other phase of hypnosis. Doctors began reporting that it was much deeper and better anesthesia than it was possible to secure in the Esdaile state of hypnosis. Still we weren't satisfied with classroom procedure, because it took too long to make it practical for the doctor.

One night a doctor asked me what I would do if I wanted to have a person fall asleep instantly as the result of a posthypnotic suggestion. Without thinking, I answered, "Give him a suggestion in the somnambulistic state that he will fall asleep instantly on cue when you rouse him from the state."

My wife asked, if I had known this all along, why had I been trying for the same result by going the long way around. I explained that I wanted to make sure it was natural sleep I was getting and not hypnosis. Attaching hypnosis to hypnosis is just compounding suggestions. I wanted the doctors to see they were working with natural sleep. However, we tried the "falling-asleep-on-cue" idea, and it worked. From then on I used the rapid method of obtaining quickly what we believed was natural sleep. The results were spectacular. Now more and more doctors began using what I called hypnosis attached to sleep.

Undoubtedly, this is a deeper form of hypnosis than has ever been deemed possible, but there remains a great deal of research to be done before we can be sure that it is merely hypnosis and nothing more. For several years, I have instructed my doctors to try to hypnotize the patients they found sound asleep when making their hospital rounds. Doctors who have attached instruments to sleeping patients and then produced the state tell me (and are backed up by charts made with the instruments) that when hypnosis is attached to sleep, the sleep *changes* to hypnosis, and the charts do not show a sleep pattern, but a straight hypnotic pattern. Therefore, instead of calling the state hypnosis attached to sleep, I have labeled it hypnosleep. Now let me tell you how to obtain the state; my assertions and instructions will be based on my own experience, research by myself and my students.

Since the year 1841, the word sleep has been used erroneously in hypnosis under the mistaken impression that *sleep* is part of *hypnosis*. It is easy to understand how this fallacy crept into international acceptance, for the early practitioners of hypnosis only observed the state from the outside looking in. They never examined it from the inside.

In fact, the early practitioners were actually afraid to enter the state themselves. Picture the hypnotic operator of that day. He saw the subject with eyes closed, apparently in deep sleep. And the deeper the operator got the subject into trance, the deeper seemed the sleep. As the patient relaxed more and more, his shoulders drooped, his head sagged, his body became almost inert—and if the patient happened to be sitting, he looked as though he were about to fall off the chair. Certainly, the patient *seemed* to be asleep.

Now consider the fact that the early operator learned that he could say, "You are getting sleepier and sleepier—drowsier and drowsier," and the patient would seem to take the suggestion. He would seem to be getting sleepier and sleepier, and the early operator had no way of knowing that the patient never fell asleep.

However, sleep and hypnosis are really two entirely different states. They are not compatible, when the hypnosis *precedes* the sleep. Those of you who are doctors know from your medical studies that in sleep the bodily functions slow down. Respiration gets slower and deeper, blood pressure and heart action slow down, reflex action slows down. In hypnosis, you will sometimes find the mildest of slowdowns, but most of the time, none at all. In sleep the mental processes slow down considerably, and in deep sleep, there is an apparent loss of consciousness. This does not occur in hypnosis.

If you test reflex action in hypnosis, you will find it quite normal. Respiration does not decrease; heart action remains normal; blood pressure remains normal. It is true that these functions can be made to slow down by suggestion, but you can't get them *all* to slow down simultaneously as occurs in natural sleep. Despite appearances, it is impossible to fuse these two dissimilar states—the normally functioning body in hypnosis and the slow functioning body in sleep.

We have made over ten thousand tests in an attempt to induce sleep in hypnosis. In my own work, I have tried to induce sleep in hypnosis by every known technique, but have yet to see the first success. Our students are told to make similar tests. They are asked to report the first case in which they are able to induce sleep in hypnosis. Perhaps some place in the world there may be an exception to the rule that it cannot be done. It is impossible to believe that several thousand doctors, well versed in hyypnosis, and attempting to find that exception, won't find it, if there is one.

This does not mean that normal sleep cannot be induced *by suggestion;* on the contrary, sleep can be induced by suggestion very easily if the right techniques are used. But you cannot turn hypnosis into sleep nor can you leave a patient in hypnosis and expect him to fall asleep.

Since this information is diametrically opposed to the theories in textbooks that have been written on the subject, as well as countless medical articles, it seems only fair to say that if someone, somewhere finds a way to attach sleep to hypnosis, we want to know it and will be ready to modify this present statement of findings. This is a research project worthy of your participation: Try to attach sleep to hypnosis; keep trying until you are satisfied that it can or cannot be done.

Having voiced the foregoing truths, which I believe to be universal, I must add that the statements which follow cannot be considered universal in their exactitude, since individuals vary from any norm: A healthy person breathes during his waking hours at the rate of sixteen to eighteen times per minute. During his sleep, respiration slows down considerably. (One of the exceptions to this general statement is the expectant mother in the later months of pregnancy; her respiration in deep sleep will be perhaps three or four more per minute than before pregnancy, and this should be borne in mind when working with the expectant mother in the sleep state.)

If a patient who normally breathes at eighteen times per minute while awake is put into deep hypnosis and given a sleep suggestion, sometimes the respirations, through suggestion, can be brought down to about three or four times a minute, sometimes even as low as two; but at all times, he will retain full consciousness. Therefore, to insure the success of sleep suggestions, always give them as *posthypnotic* suggestions. Here are the necessary steps:

1. Count the number of respirations in a minute, while the patient is fully awake.

2. Put the patient into deep somnambulism.

3. Give him sleep suggestions to take effect on cue after you arouse him from the relaxed state.

4. Arouse him from the hypnotic state, and let him fall asleep naturally on cue.

5. After the patient responds to the cue, wait until his

respirations are down to seven or eight times per minute. This must occur without the giving of any suggestions of any kind.

Having seen how to bring on sleep by means of suggestion, let us now study the manner of bringing on the hypnotic state during sleep. Strangely, while it is impossible to attach sleep to hypnosis because of the fact that the body will function at a normal pace in hypnosis, and much more slowly in sleep, it is possible to attach hypnosis to a body and mind functioning at any pace. This is because hypnosis adjusts itself to bodily speed, whereas sleep won't adjust. Once a patient is asleep, soundly asleep, it is reasonably easy to attach hypnosis to his sleeping state.

When this is done, the doctor secures the deepest hypnosis of all. In the light state, the patient is perfectly conscious; this is true of somnambulism, too, for the patient's awareness in somnambulism is infinitely increased; even in the Esdaile state the patient has complete awareness. But when he is hypnotized in his sleep and a complete hypnotic state is obtained, the doctor, on many occasions, finds himself talking to the unconscious mind of the patient. Although the unconscious mind is fully aware, and perhaps more com-- pletely aware than at any other time in the patient's lifetime, when the patient wakes up he usually has no recollection whatever of the doctor talking to him, and occasionally, the amnesia cannot be completely removed. When amnesia is encountered in any other state of hypnosis, it can be completely removed by suggestion.

In this connection, I must note that when demonstrating this and other procedures in class, it is sometimes necessary to prod a patient's memory. Despite *apparent* amnesia, the patient is prodded into recalling certain incidents. Under certain circumstances, this would not be done by the doctor using such therapy on a patient. Prodding a patient to recall sometimes destroys the amnesia. If, for any reason, the doctor wants the amnesia maintained, he will not prod.

We have taught that the amnesia which occurs in somnambulism is a *false* amnesia and can be removed at will. However, when the hypnotic state is attached to sleep, the amnesia is usually deep. It is like a dream, says the patient, which he can't remember. It just seems lost. Even when prodded, the patient does not seem to have total recall.

The suggestions given in this state are not lost, however. Anesthesia can be given which is most powerful; preoperative tension and anxiety can be completely removed; and psychiatrists have stated that in this technique they have the perfect device for probing into the mind of the patient who has the memory of traumatic events deeply buried below conscious awareness.

This is a deep state of hypnosis in which insufficient research has been done. It deserves much study. Tens of thousands of doctors will have to use it and report on it before we can possibly gauge its true value—but as of this writing, it promises to be the most exciting phase of all hypnosis, with unquestionably the greatest possibilities.

To obtain hypnosis in sleep, the following steps are necessary:

1. Count the respirations of the patient. Make sure breathing is down to about seven or eight times a minute; six or seven a minute is even better. If the patient is breathing too fast, you will be wise to wait until he is more soundly asleep.

2. Approach the patient very gently, for the aim is to bypass the critical faculty without arousing him from sleep. The bypass must occur instantly. I have found the following speech to be extremely valuable if spoken very gently, but very confidently: "This is [your name] speaking. You can hear me but you can't wake up. You can hear me but you can't wake up. You can hear me but you can't wake up."

3. The patient is usually in such deep sleep that the above must be repeated several times before it seems to penetrate his unconsciousness. Continue: "I'll know you're hearing me when your thumb, which I'm going to touch, begins to rise. I'll know you're hearing me when your thumb moves. You can hear me but you can't wake up."

4. When the thumb responds, continue to talk gently, compounding suggestions as you proceed.

5. When you have finished giving the desired suggestions, or have concluded the hypnoanalysis, your next

step is to remove the hypnotic state so that the patient can continue an entirely natural sleep state until he wakes up by himself. Do it as follows: "When I stop talking to you, you will revert to the state you were in before I started talking to you. You will sleep deeply, and in the morning, you'll awaken completely refreshed—won't even remember I've been talking to you—but you'll feel so much better about the operation [or "will not be bothered any more by this allergic reaction" or whatever suggestion is appropriate]. You won't worry about it a bit. You just know we wouldn't be performing the operation if we didn't know it was going to be absolutely safe for you, and easy for you to take. And you'll get well so fast. Now go to sleep very soundly, and I'll see you in the morning . . . I'll stop talking now."

The amateur working with this state will, in his first attempts, undoubtedly come across instances in which he will arouse the patient before the hypnosis can be attached. Therefore, it is important to make certain that the patient is in deep sleep before proceeding. The expert in hypnosis finds this state easy to achieve; the amateur finds it extremely difficult. Because of this fact the above lesson is not covered in my classes until well toward the end of the course. You should be an adept hypnotic operator before you can expect to learn this procedure.

In the first chapter of this book, I mentioned an interesting incident that occurred in San Antonio, Texas, a few years ago: I was telling my students that people undergoing surgical anesthesia retain their sense of hearing and that the mind functions even at a level below consciousness. One of the men, Doctor William Torres, expressed disbelief, declaring that he had undergone an operation for appendicitis some years ago and did not remember anything about it once the anesthesia was started. I told him that in the state of hypnosleep a patient could often relive an operation and repeat what he had heard or felt during complete general anesthesia. The doctor didn't believe this was possible until his own voice proved it to him.

He had brought a tape recorder with him, as many of my students do, and he turned it on before we proceeded to investigate his ability to relive his experience in surgery. Doctor Torres is not a native of this country. Like many naturalized citizens he has spoken our language long enough so that he usually thinks in English—although Spanish idioms sometimes crop up in his speech. Now and then he has some slight difficulty in expressing himself in English, but I believe when you read his words, his meaning will be clear at all times. Recently, I asked him to send me a transcript of the tape recording made in class when he experienced hypnosleep. Here is his reply:

"You phoned me regarding the copy of the recording of the hypnoanalysis on my surgical case . . . Here it is. If it is useful for you in your teaching I'll be very satisfied. This is your lesson in San Antonio, Texas, on March 3, 1960. The lesson was in progress when I asked a question and then you answered and put me into trance and made the hypnoanalysis. The transcript follows:"

ELMAN: You can do hypnoanalysis in the sleep state and the patient will repeat the entire conversation that took place in the depths of anesthesia. And if the doctor who did the surgery happens to be there, he'll say, "I forgot that took place. I didn't remember that. I thought the patient couldn't hear." And he'll also say, "I never believed that such a thing was possible."

DOCTOR: When I was operated on for appendicitis I didn't remember anything. They might be moving during the operation, moving instruments and making noises and I don't recall anything. I just recall when I went out after being given the anesthesia.

ELMAN: Would you like to know what happened during that surgery?

DOCTOR: All right.

ELMAN: If I can get a patient into the right state, I can take him through his surgery again. You didn't feel anything during the operation, did you?

DOCTOR: No.

ELMAN: All right. And you say you didn't hear any-thing. You *think* you didn't hear anything. Suppose I tell you that you *did* hear something and suppose I let our doctors hear what you heard.

DOCTOR: That would be a fine thing. I'd like to try.

ELMAN: All right. Take a long, deep breath and close your eyes. In just a moment I'm going to ask you to make the numbers disappear. Just let them go. Are they all gone? Let them go. All right. Now, Doctor, when I have you open your eyes, those numbers will still be gone. You won't be able to find them. Now open your eyes . . . [addressing doctors in audience] This is a good opportunity, incidentally, to check on technique. Notice the check point. Get the somnambulism and prove it before and after eye-closure . . . [to Doctor Torres] Doctor, count down from one hundred, will you please?   [Doctor is silent.] Are they all gone?

DOCTOR: Yes.

ELMAN: All right. Close your eyes again. Now, Doctor, every number will be back again except the number three. That will be gone. It will be as though the number three has never existed for you. You won't remember consciously that I gave you this suggestion, but you will react to it. Want it to happen, and you'll find that number is completely gone. Open your eyes, please . . . Count down from ten, will you please, Doctor?

DOCTOR: Ten . . . nine . . . eight . . . seven . . . six . . .five four . . . two . . . one.

ELMAN: That's fine. Close your eyes again. Now, when I have you open your eyes, any time you see me lift this outine of procedure that I have on my desk, you will instantly fall fast and sound asleep. You won't remember that I gave you this suggestion, but you will react to it. You can forget consciously this whole conversation, but any time I lift that outline tonight, you're going to fall fast and sound asleep. It will happen instantaneously. You won't remember that I gave this suggestion. Forget the whole conversation, but be guided by it. All right, now open your eyes, please. How do you feel?

DOCTOR: All right.

ELMAN: Good. Every doctor here has a copy of this outline . . . Follow the instructions. [Lifts outline and Doctor Torres falls asleep; long pause as doctor goes deeper asleep. Doctor's respirations are counted. Operator addresses him.] I'm going to talk to you. You can hear me but you can't wake up. You can hear me but you can't wake up. I'll ask you questions. You'll be able to talk to me but you won't wake up. I'll know you're hearing me when this thumb which I'm going to touch begins to move. Move your thumb so that I'll know you're hearing me. [After long pause thumb moves.] I'm going to take you back to the day of your operation for appendicitis. I'm going to take you into the operating room right now. You're in the operating room. You're going to be able to tell me everything that happened, even after anesthesia was administered. You'll be able to tell me just how you felt at all times and the words you heard. First, I want you to tell me who was in the operating room with you?

DOCTOR: There were the surgeon, the assistant, the anesthetist, and I see two nurses over there.

ELMAN: I want you to hear them talking. They'll be saying again exactly what they were saying the first time. I want you to pay particular attention to the words that the anesthetist uses as he administers the anesthesia. When I snap my fingers he will be talking. Tell me exactly what he says. This will be fact, not fancy. You have no license to dream. Remember, this is a scientific experiment. Please, above all things, don't use your imagination at all in any direction. We just want fact. You'll find that your unconscious mind knows a great deal more than you think.

So now I want you to hear the words of the anesthetist when I count to three and snap my fingers. One . . . two . . . three . . . [snaps fingers] What's he saying?

DOCTOR: He's saying "And the name of the Father," something like, "In the name of God."

ELMAN: I want you to tell me what kind of anesthesia is being given you. As a medical man, you know.

DOCTOR: Chloroform.

ELMAN: They've got a cone over your face, have they?

DOCTOR: They have a mask.

ELMAN: A mask over your face. And they're dripping it onto the mask, is that what they're doing?

DOCTOR: Yes, that's right.

ELMAN: Now they've started to drip it onto the mask and you're going to find that you can hear every word they say, and you can tell me exactly what they're saying, because you can hear everything that is being said, just as you heard it the first time. You'll hear it below the level of consciousness but be able to repeat it.

DOCTOR: I started talking.

ELMAN: What did you talk about?

DOCTOR: I don't know.

ELMAN: When I snap my fingers you will. It's all there below the level of consciousness . . . [snaps fingers] Now you'll know what you said. Don't try. It will be right there.

DOCTOR: I was talking something in English.

ELMAN: Anything important?

DOCTOR: No. Just scattered words.

ELMAN: Was there any anxiety at all?

DOCTOR: No. None at all.

ELMAN: Was there any excitement stage?

DOCTOR: I don't know.

ELMAN: When I snap my fingers you'll know . . . [snaps
            fingers] Now, Doctor, consciously you cannot
            pay any attention to the words I say. I'm going
            to be talking to your unconscious.

DOCTOR: The surgeon says "confusion of the languages,"
            because I was supposed to talk in Spanish.

ELMAN: Tell me what they're saying now.

DOCTOR: I don't hear anything.

ELMAN: When I snap my fingers, you'll hear. If there
            was any talking, you'll hear it . . . [snaps fingers]
            Who's talking, if anybody?

DOCTOR: I can't hear anything.

ELMAN: When I have you open your eyes, the cue I
            gave you a little while ago will be more effective
            than ever and you'll find this time when I have
            you go to sleep that I will be talking to your
            unconscious mind, and your conscious mind will
            have no memory of what I've talked about. All
            this will happen after I have you open your
            eyes . . . [Note here the compounding of sugges-
            tions.] Now I'll stop talking and you open your
            eyes . . . [Patient opens eyes.] I was talking
            a while ago about this outline and I was say-
            ing that I want everybody to pay very close
            attention to it . . . [Holds up outline; doctor goes
            to sleep.] Now, Doctor, your conscious mind can
            forget everything I'm talking about but your
            unconscious mind can talk to me. It's during
            the course of the operation now; your conscious
            mind is going to sleep but your unconscious
            mind is always aware. I want you to tell me
            what the doctors said, what the nurses said, what
            the anesthetist said, what you said—if anything.
            What everybody said during the course of the
            operation. You can tell me that because now
            I'm talking to your unconscious mind.

DOCTOR: A tremendous noise in my ear.

ELMAN: That's one of the things you get with chloroform
            —a buzzing noise that you get in your ear. All

right, through that buzzing what do you hear them saying?

DOCTOR: Nothing. I just hear buzzing.

ELMAN: I'll remove the buzzing and you'll hear what they say . . . [snaps fingers] The buzzing is gone now. What do you hear?

DOCTOR: Somebody says "we have to make a longer cut."

ELMAN: Did anybody say why? [no answer] Anything else? [no answer] Are they making a longer cut?

DOCTOR: I think so. I don't feel anything.

ELMAN: Now they're doing the surgery; they've made this longer cut; and your unconscious mind hears everything they're saying and you can repeat to me exactly what was said. Now you'll hear everything. Don't try for it. It's there. You'll hear everything. When I have you open your eyes and I lift this outline again you'll go into a much deeper state. Just want that to happen because I know you're as interested in this experiment as any of us. Now I'll stop talking and you'll wake up . . . [Doctor wakes up.] How do you feel?

DOCTOR: All right.

ELMAN: Do you remember anything we talked about just now?

DOCTOR: We were talking about my operation, I guess.

ELMAN: [Lifts outline. Doctor goes to sleep again.] Let yourself go very deep. Let yourself go deeply asleep. Consciously you have no recollection of what took place during the operation. But at a level below consciousness you know everything and I want you to tell me, after they made this longer cut, what happened. Your unconscious mind knows the answer. And your unconscious mind can talk to me now.

DOCTOR: "Sponge," somebody says.

ELMAN: What else? Is the operation proceeding smoothly?

DOCTOR:	Yes. "Here is one," someone said.
ELMAN:	Then what happened?
DOCTOR:	Somebody says, "It's backwards." [Doctor Torres is referring to surgeon's comment regarding abnormal position of appendix, as will be seen.]
ELMAN:	What else?
DOCTOR:	Can't hear any more.
ELMAN:	All right, I'm going to stop talking. You'll wake up. If your unconscious mind wants your conscious mind to know what you heard during the operation, you'll remember. But if your unconscious doesn't want your conscious to know, you won't remember anything. All right, I'll stop talking and you'll wake up. Notice how good you feel, and all cues will be gone; they'll be void and you'll just have the normal state when I have you open your eyes. Now I'll stop talking and you'll wake up . . . [Doctor wakes up.] Doctor, what happened during your operation?
DOCTOR:	Tremendous noise in my ears.
ELMAN:	What did you hear?
DOCTOR:	Somebody said there's a confusion of the languages.
ELMAN:	When you started to talk. And what else?
DOCTOR:	Somebody asked for the sponge. And somebody else said, "Here it is." I think that's all I can remember. What did I say?
ELMAN:	Well, did they make a longer incision?
DOCTOR:	Oh yes, they said "We need a longer incision."
ELMAN:	Do you remember what you said about your appendix?
DOCTOR:	Yes. When they made an x-ray before the operation I think they found it a little deep, a little backwards. The surgeon hadn't seen the x-rays.
ELMAN:	The surgeon hadn't seen the x-rays?
DOCTOR:	No.
ELMAN:	Did you know it was backwards?
DOCTOR:	No. I didn't know. The picture just showed flat.

ELMAN: Did you know before tonight that this happened
            during the operation?

DOCTOR: No. I just remember until they started the
            anesthesia.

ELMAN: In other words, it never dawned on you that
            you could hear during your surgery. Chloro-
            form anesthesia is pretty deep, isn't it?

DOCTOR: Yes, I think it's very deep.

ELMAN: Did you always think that a person lost the
            sense of hearing just because he had chloroform?

DOCTOR: Well, I thought so. And I still think so.

ELMAN: Did the surgeon ever tell you that they had to
            make a longer incision?

DOCTOR: No. He didn't tell me anything, and I didn't
            ask him.

                          *   *   *

It is interesting to note that immediately after the hypnoanalysis Doctor Torres still did not believe that it was
possible to hear under anesthesia. He only became convinced
when he later listened to his own recording. In the letter
he sent me with the above transcript, he mentioned that
since this time he has undergone surgery once again—and
once again he recalls nothing that happened during anesthesia. That is, he *consciously* recalls nothing. But he knows
now that he maintained awareness throughout the operation,
and that he could easily relive it once more in hypnosleep.
I must add that his original doubt was natural in a doctor
for two reasons. First, any physician knows that a patient
usually seems to be unaware during anesthesia; and this impression is not corrected when a doctor is anesthetized himself, since he does not consciously remember his awareness.
Second, a healthy (in other words, objective) skepticism is
necessary to unbiased scientific research, and therefore becomes second nature to most physicians.

The proof of awareness demonstrated by Doctor Torres,
can be—indeed, has been—repeated many times with patients after surgery. It not only shows the potential value
of hypnosleep but the importance of treating a patient tact-
fully even when he is supposedly in a state of deep anesthesia.

Chapter 23

QUESTIONS THAT DOCTORS
FREQUENTLY ASK

THE PROBLEMS encountered in medicine and dentistry (especially those problems involving the mind and the emotions) are as diverse as the personalities of the patients themselves. To the best of my ability, I have used this book to describe techniques that are generally applicable in treatment and specifically applicable when the doctor's words and actions are tailored to the needs of a given patient.

I follow this same procedure in class. Yet there are always physicians and dentists who come up with questions that haven't been answered in lectures and demonstrations during the course. If I attempted here to answer every such question ever asked, the text would probably be as long as all the world's medical dictionaries combined. But the questions most frequently asked are obviously those most puzzling or most important to doctors. I have carefully compiled them and will give my answers here:

DOCTOR: In every hypnosis textbook that I have read there is mention of the sway test for suggestibility. Why haven't you taught it?

ELMAN: Since everyone is suggestible, there is no necessity to test for suggestibility. Moreover, a reliable test would, by its very nature, have to bypass the critical faculty of the patient and place him on the threshold of hypnosis. The sway test doesn't meet this requirement. A person may pass the sway test and yet refuse to accept hypnosis. Therefore, I consider the test absolutely useless.

DOCTOR: If this is so, why do other teachers of hypnosis use the test? Where did they get it and why do they believe it is effective?

ELMAN: They got it from the stage operator. And you must bear in mind that the stage operator is

putting on a show and he does many things
that are really not necessary for hypnosis. He
is not fooled by the sway test; he knows it is
useless but does it for a stage effect, to make
his demonstration more impressive. There have
been a number of papers written exposing the
fallacy of the sway test.

*   *   *

DOCTOR: I have been told by other teachers always to
be sure the patient is in a comfortable position
before starting hypnosis, and so I have told my
patients to uncross their legs and put their hands
in their laps. I have noticed that you don't do
this. Why?

ELMAN: Because it is unnecessary to get the patient into
any particular position. I have hypnotized a
circus performer on a trapeze, hanging by his
knees with his head down. I do advise, however,
that you tell the patient to get into a position
that is comfortable for him. Putting the hands
in the lap doesn't do any harm, but it doesn't do
any good, either. Let the patient choose his own
manner of being comfortable.

*   *   *

DOCTOR: Why does the stage operator usually have his
subjects sit with their feet flat on the floor and
eyes looking at the ceiling? I never notice you
do this in the classroom.

ELMAN: The main reason this is done is that it looks
good from the front. It is unnecessary, but done
to create a dramatic effect, and it has a tradition
of sorts behind it. In the days when fixation
was thought to be the only reliable method of
induction, entertainers would have their subjects
stare up at the lights above the stage proscenium.
While the stage operator waited for fixation to
take effect he would beguile the audience with
demonstrations of other phenomena—such as
the effects of laughing gas—using a second group
of volunteer subjects. When he thought suffi-

cient time had elapsed, he turned back to the first group, by now drowsy from staring at the lights overhead, and proceeded with the hypnosis.

* * *

DOCTOR: Why didn't doctors adopt the techniques of the stage operators?

ELMAN: The answer to that question is found in many old-time textbooks. Let me quote from one of them: "Stage operators appear to get the state in about three minutes in the midst of noisy surroundings. Since we know this is impossible, we know that the stage operator is a fake and pay no attention to him." When doctors read things like that in books written by apparently authoritative men they were inclined to accept the statements as fact. Therefore, they didn't even ask the stage operator to teach them his techniques. Even today, many doctors regard the stage operator as a fake, believing that he uses stooges as his subjects.

* * *

DOCTOR: I had a patient come in the other day and I proceeded to hypnotize her, but she snapped herself out of the hypnosis and said that her eyes felt uncomfortable. Then she told me she was wearing contact lenses. What should I have done?

ELMAN: I think any doctor using hypnosis on a patient wearing contact lenses should tell him to remove the lenses before proceeding with the hypnosis.

* * *

DOCTOR: I have been reading in a book about a scale of depths in hypnosis. Your teachings seem to conflict with this author's. Please explain the scales employed by some hypnotists.

ELMAN: The scales you have read about reflect the views of the authors just as my teachings reflect my own views. I have carefully examined every so-called "scale of depth" that appears in the literature, and I can't agree with any of them. For example, one writer claims there are at least thirty different depths; another says there are twenty; another writer says there are only ten. Although I work with as great depths of hypnosis as anyone has yet induced, I find only five usable depths, and I've covered all of them. One is the light or superficial state. Two is the somnambulistic state which can be compounded to any depth. Three is the coma or Esdaile state, sometimes called the plenary state. Four is hypnosleep. (These four are the so-called trance states.) Five is waking hypnosis—a state which doctors have found extremely valuable as a form of somnambulism achieved without the use of the trance or eye-closure. With these five states anything possible in hypnosis can be done.

*   *   *

DOCTOR: What do I do to quiet a patient who keeps giggling?

ELMAN: Giggling is caused by uncertainty, anxiety, lack of knowledge—in a word, fear. Put the patient at ease by explaining in detail what you are doing and what you hope to accomplish. If the giggling continues, just ignore it and proceed with your work. Pretty soon the patient's attention will be riveted on what you have to say and he will stop giggling.

*   *   *

DOCTOR: Do drugs—sedatives—help to get a better state?

ELMAN: We have found sedatives tremendously effective as long as you don't sedate the patient to the point where communication becomes difficult. Remember, the patient must hear and understand you before he can respond to your suggestions. If the patient has been oversedated I would proceed with hypnosleep, knowing that the patient still retains his or her sense of hearing below the level of consciousness.

*   *   *

DOCTOR: What about the crying, screaming child? I can't get in a word so how can I hypnotize him?

ELMAN: Hypnosis is impossible without communication. If you can't establish communication, there is no help which hypnosis has to offer. Of course, the adept operator realizes that he needs only a few seconds of the child's attention, and if he can get through to the crying child for those few seconds and put his message across, he will have success. Otherwise, there is nothing he can do about it.

                              *   *   *

DOCTOR: How can I answer the patient who says that hypnosis is a lot of "bunk"? This type of person will sometimes refuse to cooperate, or make remarks such as, "No one is going to get control of me."

ELMAN: Hypnosis must be explained very carefully to such a patient. You must make him understand that what you are doing is an accepted method of therapy by the medical and dental professions; that in hypnosis the *patient* is always in control of the situation and can reject any suggestions which are given to him if he objects to them; that at no time does he relinquish control of himself. I have found it very easy to get over this rejection when hypnosis is properly explained, and it takes only a few minutes to do it.

                              *   *   *

DOCTOR: I hypnotized a child last week and got excellent results. The mother brought him in today and said, "Don't ever use hypnosis on my child again." So I gave the child the treatment in the usual manner. He didn't object to the treatment last week when I hypnotized him, but this week he screamed his head off. What should I have done?

ELMAN: All you can do with such a mother is to ask her if she wants her child to have the treatment the easy way or the hard way. First, explain to her what hypnosis is, so that she has no false notions about it. Make it clear to her that, whatever reports she has heard to the contrary, hypnosis is a wonderful and accepted tool in medicine and dentistry today. Then ask her if she wants her child to suffer needlessly. If, after your explanation, she persists in her attitude, you'll just have to treat the child the hard way.

* * *

DOCTOR: Should the parent be present when I'm hypnotizing a child?

ELMAN: I have discussed this question with many physicians and dentists. They tell me that they do their best work with or without hypnosis when the parent is not present. This is because the child leans on the parent as a crutch and makes a nuisance of himself, knowing he will get sympathy from the parent, while making the work of the doctor more difficult and prolonged. Many doctors find some means of keeping the parent in another room while treating their young patients. The same rule applies when hypnosis is used.

* * *

DOCTOR: Should I get the parent's permission before hypnotizing a child?

ELMAN: This is entirely up to you. You don't ask the parent's permission in the writing of a prescription or for a given treatment. You do, however, explain to the parent what treatment will be necessary in your considered judgment. I would not say to the parent that I was going to hypnotize the child to make treatment easy for him but I would say that medicine and dentistry now use medical relaxation to make treatment easy for patients, and that you intend doing the same. From then on, you must be guided by the parent's reaction.

* * *

DOCTOR: I have heard one of your doctors say that he teaches his apprehensive children a little rhyme, and these children say the rhyme and it makes their visit to the doctor much easier; they don't feel anything that the doctor has to do. Have you heard about it?

ELMAN: Yes. Many doctors have had success with this simplified technique. As you know, simple rhymes often help young children to concentrate. They capture a child's imagination, helping him to learn just as some instructive nursery rhymes teach new concepts to small children. Here is the simple rhyme the doctors use:

> Fairy, fairy, prove to me
> Just how easy this can be.
> I'll close my eyes and see you smile
> And watch you dancing all the while.
> While you're dancing in the light
> Everything will be all right.
> Fair, fairy, prove to me
> Just how easy this can be.

I think the best way to use this rhyme is to have the child close his eyes and see a fairy dancing in his mind's eye. Then say to the child, "So long as you see that fairy dancing nothing will bother or disturb you." This technique is excellent for treatment of short duration. It works beautifully for injections. Try it with a child who is apprehensive and I think you will be delighted with the results.

*   *   *

DOCTOR: I had a patient in deep hypnosis and was reducing a compound fracture painlessly. Word got around the hospital of what I was doing and several doctors came in to watch. One of them said, "You can't tell me you're not hurting the patient unless you gave her a sedative before we came in." No sooner were these words out of his mouth than the patient began to wince

with pain. Not knowing what else to do, I had
to use chemical anesthesia. What should I have
done?

ELMAN: Under those circumstances, there was nothing
else you could have done. But this should be
handled in the same way that a hypnotic delivery is handled. You should make sure the
people working with you know how hypnotic
treatments are handled, and if there are persons in the room who don't know the subject
but are merely bystanders, tell them beforehand to please remain silent. After all, it's your
patient and all they have to do is watch. Unless
you are in control of this type of situation, it
will be repeated to the detriment of the patient.
Tell your colleagues either to stay out or be
quiet. You don't want adverse suggestions given
to your patients.

                              *   *   *

DOCTOR: Why are so many people afraid of hypnosis?

ELMAN: They have been exposed to Svengali and Trilby
stories, movies and television shows in which
hypnosis is portrayed as villainous. They are
also exposed to various statements written in
newspapers and magazines by people who know
nothing about the subject. Unfortunately, once
statements are made in print they appear authoritative to the people who read them. These
people are, moreover, exposed to the wrong
attitudes by self-appointed authorities who don't
know the subject. A book was recently written by Doctor Frank Caprio entitled, "Helping
Yourself with Self-Hypnosis." He is a psychiatrist and the writer of many excellent books.
In this one he recommends that people wishing
to be treated by a doctor who uses hypnosis, call
the local medical society for the name of a doctor employing hypnosis in his practice. A lady
called me yesterday to say she had called her local
medical society and had been informed by the
doctor at the society that hypnosis was absolute

nonsense and that anyone who uses hypnosis is a charlatan. He said that if she needed a physician for any specific medical purpose he would be glad to recommend one, but would not recommend anyone who uses hypnosis. He was willing to say this despite the fact that hypnosis is recognized as valid therapy by the American Medical Association and the American Dental Association.

* * *

DOCTOR: I have heard that in several states laws are being formulated to stop the use of hypnosis by anyone but a qualified physician. What do you think about these projected laws?

ELMAN: You can't outlaw the workings of the human mind. You can't keep people from being suggestible, for this is a God-given attribute—nor can you prevent anyone from giving other people suggestions. In other words, you can't enforce a law which is contrary to the laws of nature. Since we are all giving each other suggestions every day of our lives, sometimes without even realizing it, how can this be prevented? This is not always necessarily recognized as hypnosis but quite often that is exactly what it is.

* * *

DOCTOR: I am constantly reading articles about the dangers of hypnosis. These papers are usually written by psychiatrists. You don't seem to feel there are any dangers. Why does your opinion differ so radically from these other opinions?

ELMAN: I have taught thousands of physicians and dentists, and to every one of these students I have said, "If ever you find a danger in hypnosis or have a problem in hypnosis, call upon me. I am interested in your problems as well as your progress." I am proud to say that most of these students have kept in touch with me through the years. Surely, if they contact me with their other problems—and they have—they would contact me with the adverse situations or the dangers. However, I can honestly say I have never had such a report. My students are by no means the only doctors using hypnosis. There are many thousands of doctors in this country using it, and yet you hear no reports of unfortunate instances except from a mere handful who seem to specialize in writing papers on the dangers of hypnosis. These writers have been interviewed and questioned repeatedly, some of them by my own students who have reported to me. The question asked most often of these writers is, "Can you give us some case histories on which we can base our research?" *No one has been successful in getting this information from these writers.* In other words, we must take their word for it. They always talk about the case of a man to whom such and such has happened because he has been hypnotized. Try to find out who that man is and locate him. You can't do it. Always remember that the law of self-preservation is universal and it has never been repealed. It isn't repealed in hypnosis.

*   *   *

DOCTOR: What do I do about the pregnant patient who seems to be so perfectly conditioned for delivery that the doctor is sure she can have her baby under hypnosis, yet she refuses even to relax on her next visit? When the doctor asks what is the matter, such a patient may insist that nothing is wrong—but something must be.

ELMAN: I understand this is a frequent problem with expectant mothers. Let's first cover the reason for such a patient's behavior. We will assume that she was at your office previously and accepted hypnosis. She did so because of her faith in you. You told her this was good for her, and that was all she needed. However, after leaving your office she undoubtedly talked to friends and family about her experience and to her surprise met with several different reactions, some of which disturbed her. Someone probably remarked that *she* would never allow anyone to hypnotize *her*. After all, how did she know what would happen to herself or the baby under hypnosis?

This is enough to upset any prospective mother and yet she would prefer not to embarrass you by repeating the conversation. Therefore, when you asked her what was the matter, she said, "Nothing." I would proceed on the assumption that someone has unsold her on this method of delivery and it is now up to you to resell her by explaining the value of a hypnotic delivery, stressing the fact that as her doctor, you know what is best for her and her baby.

In most instances, this does the trick and you are once again able to hypnotize this patient. Should she not accept your explanation she will just have to have her baby the hard way. I would tell her this, although perhaps not in these words. I would say that she would be receiving every known aid that medicine has to offer to make the delivery of her baby easy and safe, and that hypnosis is a wonderful plus. If she doesn't wish to take advantage of this wonderfull addition, she will have to settle for less. Having said so, leave the decision entirely up to her.

* * *

DOCTOR: One of my patients was conditioned for delivery and she didn't feel anything during labor, but when it came to the actual birth of the baby she snapped herself out of the hypnosis and from then on things were difficult. Is there any way to prevent this from occurring again?

ELMAN: In my experience, there are several reasons why this happens. Fear might have crept in, and since you were unaware of it until too late, there was nothing you could do about it. Another frequent reason is that someone in the delivery room has said something to alarm the patient. You can forestall this by instructing your delivery room assistants in the handling of a hypnotic delivery. But despite all your precautions, you might still come up against such a situation. Here is an unusual one:

An obstetrician came to class and related that one of his patients who was conditioned for delivery was quite comfortable during the entire procedure. She had no discomfort during the contractions and even during the crowning. Then, suddenly, she began screaming at the top of her lungs. This startled the doctor and he said to her, "What's the matter with you? You're not feeling any discomfort; you know everything has been going along just fine, and the baby is here. What are you yelling about?" The patient said, "Mind your own business, doctor. My husband is on the other side of that door and I'm going to get a mink coat out of this delivery or know the reason why." She then resumed screaming. She admitted to the doctor that she had had a painless delivery, but had her reasons for screaming.

* * *

DOCTOR: One of my obstetricial patients had received no conditioning. She was in agony and within an hour of delivery. She'd had all the sedation necessary but she was still yelling and moving around and not too rational. Is there any approach to be used on a patient like that?

ELMAN: If the sedation is to the point where you cannot communicate, you cannot help. But when the doctor can still communicate with the patient, many of our obstetricians tell us they are successful. Past students say to me, "There isn't a patient who comes in for delivery that we can't help to some degree at least; even if the woman is in active labor, even if her contractions are thirty seconds apart, we can still help." You have to work between contractions, but you can do it, and you can do it within thirty seconds.

* * *

DOCTOR: Why do patients sometimes refuse a suggestion given for their own good? I told one that he would wear a dental appliance until the next visit, when I would have to make an adjustment in it. But when he came back I learned he had not even worn the appliance one day.

ELMAN: The way you framed that question makes me suspect that you gave the patient an improper waking suggestion. You were unknowingly hinting that the appliance would be uncomfortable for at least a week. In his mind this was sufficient reason for not wearing it for a week. He preferred to wait for the next visit when you were going to make the adjustment. You could have given the same suggestion in a manner that would have been far more effective and would have helped the patient. You might have said it this way: "This appliance fits perfectly now, and it will not only be comfortable, but you'll actually enjoy wearing it. Your mouth will feel so much better as a result. Come in next week for a checkup." In other words, make your suggestion not only simple, but reasonable; and don't implant doubts in the patient's mind.

* * *

DOCTOR: I'm a fairly new student, but I felt I was ready to try giving a posthypnotic suggestion. So, after I worked with a patient successfully in hypnosis, I gave him an experimental posthypnotic suggestion but he didn't take it. I told him after I roused him he would stand up and shout "hurrah." I'll admit he was a very dignified gentleman but he took hypnosis so well that I don't understand why he didn't take this simple suggestion.

ELMAN: He didn't take it because he didn't want it. Don't ever give a posthypnotic suggestion which is ridiculous or which you feel the particular patient wouldn't be apt to take under ordinary circumstances. The gentleman you gave this suggestion to probably never shouted "hurrah" in his life. Why should he now? Always remember that a patient can accept or reject a suggestion according to his own inclinations, no matter how deeply into hypnosis he goes.

*   *   *

DOCTOR: Why is it that although I have wonderful success with my patients, I can't even get eye-closure with my wife?

ELMAN: There are three likely answers to that question. The first is that your wife knows you are just now studying this subject and doesn't wish to be a guinea pig. When she thinks you know enough about the subject she may let you work with her. The second answer is that she may never let you work with her because, despite all you say, she may believe that the operator has control of the subject and she doesn't want her husband to be in control. And of course, there is also the third possibility that her reason for rejecting hypnosis is the conventional one—fear of the unknown.

*   *   *

DOCTOR: I was using hypnoanalysis with a patient and I took her back to the time before she was born and found out that her headaches developed while she was in her mother's womb. What do you think of that, Mr. Elman?

ELMAN: You were unintentionally giving the patient a dream. You were doing exactly what was done in the Bridey Murphy case. There is no scientific evidence that a fetus has any consciousness whatever or is aware of what is occurring in the womb. Therefore whatever information she gave you regarding that period has no basis in fact.

*   *   *

DOCTOR: I read a paper in a journal saying that a patient who has hysterical paralysis in his arm is using that paralysis as a functional symptom. It serves a purpose and he needs it. The article goes on to say that you can give such a patient a hypnotic suggestion that only one finger will be paralyzed instead of his entire arm. In this way, you are permitting the patient to hold on to his functional symptom but giving him the use of his arm. Having only one finger paralyzed is certainly better than not having the use of the entire arm. What do you think of this?

ELMAN: I contend that such a solution is not a complete correction and will give such a patient only temporary relief. What you are talking about is frequently called transfer of symptoms. I have never known such a transfer to be permanent because this type of suggestoin does not last very long and the patient goes back to his original functional symptom, the one he unconsciously chose for himself. I had a doctor tell me that he had produced such a transfer by suggestion and the suggestion held for ten weeks. Ten weeks may have been a great relief to the patient, but at the end of that time his entire difficulty was back again. I feel that with hypnoanalysis permanent corrections are possible, and I teach my students to work toward that end.

* * *

DOCTOR: Can't we use hypnosis to get patients to pay their bills?

ELMAN: Well, doctor, that might or might not be a welcome suggestion to the patient and, of course, he is in a position to accept or reject your suggestion. I have heard of doctors doing this, and won't presume to judge its ethical aspects, but I don't know how many have tried it without success, nor how many patients have resented such a suggestion.

* * *

DOCTOR: Can hypnosis be used to improve our memories and help us with our studies? I have a college son who does very well except at examination time, when he gets so excited he can't pass the tests.

ELMAN: Such people are easily helped. Superficial hypnotic suggestions will often correct the situation. If that doesn't help the problem, use hypnoanalysis and find out the reason for the panic. And then teach the patient autohypnosis so that he can use it just prior to entering the examination room.

*   *   *

DOCTOR: My wife has what I have always considered a lovable habit. She is always putting things in a "safe place." Usually she can't remember where the "safe place" is. We have always kidded her about it because it just never seemed important. However, two years ago, we were going on a trip when she remembered that we had not put a valuable brooch of hers in the safe deposit box. The bank was closed and she said, "Don't worry about it, dear. I'll put it in a safe place." We went on our vacation and when we returned looked for the brooch. Well, we haven't found it yet. She insists she put it in a "safe place" but we can't find it. Can we find out where the brooch is through hypnosis?

ELMAN: Hypnoanalysis is the only answer I know for that. Take her to the time before she put the brooch away and work up to the actual moment when she put it in the "safe place." You will find that the method is quite effective. It has been tried in several cases and found to be extremely valuable.

There was a similar case involving the loss of some important papers. The doctor insisted that it was his wife who had put the documents away, and his wife insisted he had. Neither of them knew where the documents were. They had gone all through the office and the house in an effort to locate them. We used hypnoanalysis on both the husband and wife and found it was the husband who had put them away and not really in a very safe place. He had put the documents in a box of his son's discarded toys on a top shelf in a closet.

* * *

DOCTOR: What about stage fright and shyness? Can these be overcome by the use of hypnosis?

ELMAN: I have found hypnosis to be extremely valuable in correcting this type of situation. I can remember one instance that occurred many years ago when I was in show business. One of the performers in the stock company I worked for had studied diligently and knew his role very well, but on the night of the first performance he stood at the side of the stage in such panic that he couldn't go on. Using rapid conditioning techniques, I hypnotized him and gave him the suggestion that his memory would be better than ever and that he would remember every line he had studied. The panic disappeared and he gave an excellent performance. I feel the best results are obtained in such cases by using superficial suggestions and then teaching the patient autosuggestion, to be used when necessary.

* * *

DOCTOR: What about enuresis cases? What can be done with them?

ELMAN: We had an interesting experience with enuresis when I first began teaching. We kept statistics on the first seventeen cases reported to us. In eleven of these the suggestions were completely ineffective. In the other six cases, the suggestions were found to be useful. Finally, I began doing hypnoanalysis in enuresis cases and then we began to have more satisfactory results. You'd be surprised at the many different causes of enuresis. Let me list some of them: Sometimes it is a bid for attention which causes the child to wet the bed; sometimes it is fear of the dark; sometimes it's a matter of sibling rivalry. When we have used hypnoanalysis with adult patients suffering from the same problem and traced back the cause, often we have found that the enuresis was precipitated by trauma.

I recall one instance in which an adult patient had been perfectly trained by the time she was three years of age and the child's parents were very proud that their little girl had not wet the bed since she was two. Suddenly she began to wet the bed again, every night. Hypnoanalysis disclosed the fact that one night when she was three, she had to go to the bathroom. She saw a man in her room going through the dresser drawers. He was wearing a mask over his face. She screamed. Her parents came running. There were shots and the man got away. She didn't quite understand what it was all about but there was considerable excitement and many people in the house that night. From that time on, she wet the bed. The patient, at the time of hypnoanlysis, was thirty years of age and a spinster. She had never married because she was ashamed to tell any prospective suitor about her problem. The psychiatrist in charge worked further with her and reported that he was able to correct the problem.

*   *   *

DOCTOR: Recently, I operated on a little girl. One of her toes overlapped another. The surgery was completely successful but after the operation she developed a limp, for which there is no pathological reason. Would hypnosis help in a case like this?

ELMAN: Of course it would. This sounds like a bid for attention, and superficial hypnotic suggestion should correct the situation.

*   *   *

DOCTOR: One of the problems in dentistry is the thumb-sucking child. Can hypnosis be used to stop the habit?

ELMAN: This is a controversial subject between physicians and dentists. Dentists feel very strongly that everything should be done to correct the habit because of the damage it does to the mouth structure. The physician, in many cases, says, "Leave the child alone. She'll outgrow the habit." I prefer not to take sides. However, many physicians and dentists have reported that they have used hypnotic techniques with good success. Some of my students—physicians and dentists alike—prefer to use hypnoanalysis to determine the cause, and in some cases they have been successful.

* * *

DOCTOR: I have heard you state that superficial suggestions are of no permanent value. I must disagree with you. Last year I had a patient who suffered with violent migraine headaches; I suggested one headache away and she hasn't had a headache since. Previously she had been having them every few days. Wouldn't you say this case proves the value of superficial suggestions?

ELMAN: I have never said that superficial suggestions are of *no* value, although they are worthless in certain specific cases. Take your patient with the migraine headaches. Apparently, superficial suggestion has been extremely valuable to her, and I have had many similar reports. But my experience has taught me if she encounters the same circumstances that precipitated the original migraine headaches, her migraines will probably recur. I believe that in such cases hypnoanalysis is a much more satisfactory method of treatment. On the other hand, there are many circumstances in which superficial suggestions are extremely beneficial. This is especially true when the patient needs immediate relief before further therapy can be given.

* * *

DOCTOR: I had a patient on whom I had performed an extraction. She called me by telephone later in the day and told me that she had started to bleed, so I gave her suggestions to stop the bleeding, and it stopped. Do you think this was a wise thing to do?

ELMAN: I have had several reports from dentists who gave such suggestions on the telephone and I am not opposed to the practice if the dentist follows his suggestions with the statement that the patient must come in for an examination as soon as possible; that the bleeding will stop at least until such time as the doctor has been able to check the patient.

*   *   *

DOCTOR: I have attended several hypnoanalysis sessions and have noticed that occasionally when you are working with a patient, even though you seem to be getting along fine, you suddenly terminate the hypnosis and tell the patient's doctor that he will have to continue the work privately. You also add that you will discuss the case privately with him before he leaves the class. Why do you do this? Why don't you tell the entire class what it's all about?

ELMAN: There are several reasons. The most important is that I find myself delving into the patient's personal life. Personal things should not be discussed in public and I don't like to invade the privacy of the patient. Sometimes I suspect there is a sexual problem and certainly this is no topic for discussion before a group of people. When I conduct hypnoanalysis sessions, it is for the sole purpose of teaching the doctors how to use my techniques rather than to effect a correction of the condition at that particular time. When I think I have shown the doctor enough for him to carry on I have no hesitancy in dismissing the patient because I have achieved my aim. It is now up to the doctor to carry on with what I have taught him and treat the patient. Treatment is not within my province.

*   *   *

DOCTOR: I have a patient who menstruates quite heavily. She is a student of ballet and is appearing in a show next week. She's quite upset because her period is due just at that time and she's worried about the heavy flow. Usually, at such times she reduces her activities. How can I help her?

ELMAN: Superficial hypnotic suggestion will help. If the excessive bleeding is not caused by pathology, superficial suggestion will control or stop the flow promptly. Many physicians have reported to me that they can stop the flow and have it start again at a given time.

*   *   *

DOCTOR: I have some patients to whom I have given suggestions for the relief of dysmenorrhea. It works beautifully for that month, but despite the fact that I also give the suggestion that they will never again have this kind of discomfort the following month they are back with the same complaint. Why does the suggestion only work halfway? What am I doing wrong?

ELMAN: Many women greet the approaching signs of menstruation with the thought, "This is my lucky day. I'm not pregnant this month." Consequently, the dysmenorrhea serves a purpose. It is a functional symptom. They are quite willing to get rid of the discomfort once they know they are not pregnant, but the following month they want to be certain *again* that they are not pregnant. Therefore, they reject the suggestion that there will be no signs of the oncoming menstruation. We have found that in many cases— especially among married women and nonvirginal bachelor women—this type of suggestion must be repeated each month. This is not true of the young virgin, and you will find that in many cases the suggestion given to the virgin will last indefinitely if she remains virginal. This type of suggestion can be given over the phone.

*   *   *

DOCTOR: I have a patient who has not menstruated for
            two years. There is no pathology. Can amenor-
            rhea be corrected by hypnosis?

ELMAN: This is one of the easiest situations to correct
            by the use of superficial suggestion. Despite the
            fact that suggestions for the correction of ame-
            norrhea have been given many, many times by
            my doctors, I know of only two instances in
            which these suggestions have not been effective.
            Hypnoanalysis was subsequently used in one of
            these two cases and correction followed. I have
            not been able to secure the history of the oth-
            er case.

                        *   *   *

DOCTOR: I have a newly married patient who says the
            sexual act is very much over-rated. She is truly
            in love with her husband and they get along
            beautifully, but he's complaining. I have exam-
            ined her and can find nothing wrong. Appar-
            ently it is merely an attitude on her part. Can
            this attitude be changed?

ELMAN: It certainly can. If the reason for the attitude
            is known at conscious level, it can often be cor-
            rected by superficial suggestion. However, if the
            patient doesn't know the cause of the attitude,
            you can determine it through hypnoanalysis.
            Once this is revealed to her, the attitude can be
            promptly corrected.

                        *   *   *

DOCTOR: I have a patient who is childless. She has been
            married for over ten years. Since she and her
            husband are both fertile, I can find no reason
            why they can't have children. They have seri-
            ously discussed adopting a baby, as well as
            artificial insemination. This woman feels very
            strongly that she wants her own baby. She
            doesn't care if she gets it by artificial insemina-
            tion but the husband is vehemently against it.
            This marriage may break up if they don't get
            their own baby; the wife is taking the attitude

that she'd better hurry up and do something about it before it's too late. What can the doctor do in a case like this?

ELMAN: We have found that this type of difficulty can very often be corrected through the use of hypnosis. Many doctors have written excellent papers on the subject, and I would suggest that you read these papers and be guided by them. To my knowledge, the writers of these papers are correct in their conclusions.

*   *   *

DOCTOR: I have been using hypnosis in the treatment of dysmenorrhea and amenorrhea with good success. Could hypnosis be used to treat sexual problems in which there is no pathology?

ELMAN: Yes. Doctor Frank Caprio, who is a psychiatrist, has been using hypnosis in the treatment of sexual problems for many years, and has written books on the subject. I personally have been called in to work with patients suffering from dyspareunia, and in each case I have been able to find the cause through hypnoanalysis, resolve the cause and give the patient insight into the problem. The doctors who called me in on these cases have reported success in every instance. I don't believe such conditions can be corrected by superficial suggestion. I believe each case requires hypnoanalysis to find and resolve the cause. Hypnoanalysis revealed that these women often were not frigid; they merely suffered pain at union, and most of the time a specific trauma was directly responsible for the condition. In several cases, the patient had been sexually molested in early childhood. Now, years later, every time she was with her husband, she relived the attack at a level below conscious awareness. The early experience was a painful one and she related pain to the sexual act.

*   *   *

DOCTOR: I read a newspaper article saying that a man
            was arrested for hypnotizing a girl and then
            seducing her. Could he possibly have done this?

ELMAN: I read that article, too, and I also read the follow-
            up article in which it was stated that the case
            had been dismissed. When questioned on the
            witness stand, the young lady admitted that she
            had been having an affair with this man for over
            two years before he hypnotized her. A girl can-
            not be seduced by hypnosis unless she can be
            seduced without hypnosis, in which case hyp-
            nosis is the long way round.

                        *   *   *

DOCTOR: What about nymphomania? Can hypnosis be
            helpful in cases like this?

ELMAN: Yes. Hypnoanalysis is indicated. Nymphomania
            is regarded by many as the opposite of frigidity.
            This is a misconception. They are one and the
            same thing. Only the *reaction* is different. The
            nymphomaniac, being frigid, goes from man to
            man seeking sexual satisfaction. This condition
            is also often caused by trauma.

                        *   *   *

DOCTOR: Quite often, in treating patients, it is necessary
            for the patient to be placed in an awkward posi-
            tion for a long enough period of time to tire him.
            When he gets tired, he is unable to maintain the
            position, making treatment difficult. Is there any
            way in which hypnosis can help this situation?

ELMAN: Yes. I recommend that you get the patient into
            the somnambulistic state before you position
            him, giving him the suggestion that he will be
            able to maintain the necessary position until
            completion of your treatment without difficulty,
            strain or fatigue. Our doctors have reported us-
            ing this technique with success, having had pa-
            tients maintain a given position for several
            hours when necessary.

                        *   *   *

DOCTOR: Patients who have suffered severe burns present a serious problem to the doctor. They are not only in intense pain, but they lose their appetites, which delays healing. Can these patients be helped by hypnosis?

ELMAN: We have had many reports from doctors that hypnosis has been used successfully on such patients, and that recovery has been made much easier and faster as a result. Remember that hypnosis will alleviate pain and that these patients want relief and therefore are receptive to the words of the doctor. After suggestions are given in deep somnambulism for the relief of pain and apprehension, suggestions should be given for improvement of appetite or whatever else is indicated for the patient's welfare. Many excellent papers have been written on this subject. Our findings correspond with these reports.

* * *

DOCTOR: I am in general practice and I have no problems with my patients. How would hypnosis be useful or even applicable in my practice?

ELMAN: Hypnosis can be used on everyone who comes to your office if for no other reason than to put the patient at ease. There is seldom a patient who visits a doctor's office who isn't, to some degree, apprehensive. He is afraid of what the doctor is going to find wrong with him, or of what treatment might be indicated. Even the man who comes in for an insurance examination is worried about what the examination will reveal. This apprehension on the patient's part causes a rise in blood pressure, etc., giving the doctor a false picture of the patient's condition. Hypnosis would relieve such tension, making the findings more accurate and the examination easier for the patient and for the doctor.

* * *

DOCTOR: What is hypnotic anesthesia? I know it is effective because I use it constantly. Can you explain what actually happens that makes it occur?

ELMAN: I believe I can. Just as there is selective awareness in hypnosis there is also selective *un*awareness. I believe amnesia is the manifestation of this selective unawareness and I believe hypnotic anesthesia is also a manifestation of selective unawareness. The patient might receive the pain impulse but is completely unaware of it because he has accepted the suggestion for no pain, thereby making himself unaware of the pain stimuli. This is, of course, purely selective thinking. He has but to think "pain" and it will be there; he has but to think "no pain" and it will not be there.

                        *   *   *

DOCTOR: For relief of postoperative pain you get the patient into the somnambulistic state and he seems to heal better, but the next morning he's hurting again. What can we do about it, and why does it happen?

ELMAN: Apparently, the patient lost the relaxation. Perhaps he didn't sleep well, or something occurred to disturb him. Hypnotize him again and implant additional suggestions for deep relaxation and relief of discomfort.

                        *   *   *

DOCTOR: Many of your doctor-students have reported success in working with apparently intractible pain. I'd like more information about that.

ELMAN: My doctors have reported that they use hypnosis successfully for cancer patients who are in constant and severe pain. They reduce the patient's pain and also reduce the amount of drugs required. In fact, one doctor reports that some of his cancer patients do not even need aspirin. He has just been using hypnotic suggestion for their relief. Nobody would have believed this fifteen years ago, and when I first declared it to be possible many years ago, most doctors laughed. When you are working with "intractable" pain, you have to renew the suggestions at short intervals. You give drugs at short intervals if the patient needs them, and think nothing of it; similarly, you must renew the suggestions every day or two. I'm sure that the doctors who have been so successful with carcinoma victims can't say that none of their patients had the pains come back. These doctors have renewed the hypnotic suggestions at short intervals with excellent success. It's gratifying to be able to keep these patients free of pain for twenty-four hours. As you continue working with hypnosis, you'll find you are able to keep them free of discomfort for as long as a week, two weeks, three weeks. All the time, they can be having other therapy if necessary. And as you get more proficient with hypnosis the suggestions you give will last longer.

* * *

DOCTOR: I understand that in some cases alcoholics have been helped by hypnoanalysis—used to reveal the problems that cause them to drink. However, I wonder if it is possible to work with a person while he is actually drunk?

ELMAN: You can hypnotize a drunk person, but he'll still be drunk. You can rid him of the shakes; you can relieve delirium tremens. You can bring delirium tremens to a conclusion a lot faster. But you can't get him to stop drinking forever, though you can help him a lot. One of our doctor-students worked at a county jail and he told us that he had been able to remove the shakes from a lot of people; he had been able to end delirium tremens for some of them. But you can't cure the alcoholic craving by superficial suggestion. I know of no one who has been successful. As for hypnoanalysis, it will, as you say, reveal the disturbances underlying alcoholism in many cases and may therefore be used as an aid in psychiatric treatment. However, much more clinical research is needed in this area, and even hypnoanalysis will not always correct alcoholism permanently.

*   *   *

DOCTOR: What can we do about the cigarette habit?

ELMAN: Hypnosis is of as little value in permanently correcting the cigarette habit as superficial suggestion is in correcting alcoholism. I have succeeded in giving hypnotic suggestions to people who declared sincerely that they wanted to stop smoking or stop drinking, and I have managed to make the suggestions hold for as long as a month, sometimes for two or three months or even longer. But if you follow up these same cases six months or a year after the hypnotic suggestions have been given, you find that the patients are smoking or drinking as much as ever; the hypnotic suggestions have had no permanent results.

When I was teaching in Brooklyn one of the doctors in class came up to me and said, "Mr. Elman, you implant hypnotic suggestions so deeply that they seem to hold interminably. I want to stop smoking. Believe me, I have tried many times to give it up, but have been unsuccessful. Can you help me?" I told him I could give him a suggestion that would last for a while, but that he would have to use his own will power if he really wanted to stop the habit. He said he was eager to try it, and I gave him the necessary suggestions. In class the following week, he proudly announced that he had not smoked a cigarette since I had given him the suggestions. He made the same report the second week and the third. By this time he was saying to the members of the class and to me, "You see, it isn't true after all that hypnosis has no value in correcting the cigarette habit. I haven't smoked since those suggestions were implanted. I haven't even craved a cigarette. After all, if I haven't smoked for three weeks, it's pretty likely that I'll never smoke again."

The fourth week when he came to class he was smoking a cigarette. This is the usual pattern, yet he believes that because the suggestions worked so well for him for three weeks they can be made to work for anybody indefinitely. He doesn't realize that he had never really given up smoking at all. The craving was still there. This has happened many times and always the patients at first report how well they are doing. Talk to these people a year later and you find that they have resumed the cigarette habit. Those who have taken hypnotic suggestions for giving up cigarettes and have succeeded in so doing permanently could have done so *without* hypnosis. Moreover, since the smoking habit isn't usually based on any very serious emotional disturbance, even hypnoanalysis is of little value. You cannot unearth and correct a traumatic reaction when there *is* no trauma.

Now let me give you an example regarding alcoholism. I have maintained for many years that the alcohol habit cannot be corrected merely by the use of superficial suggestion. In many cases it can be helped, however, by hypnoanalysis, because the victim of alcohol is using liquor as an escape mechanism. If you can give him insight as to what he is escaping from he will often stop the use of alcohol entirely. But merely to hypnotize a person and give the suggestion that he or she will not drink again—no matter what techniques you use—will not have any lasting effect. I recall one incident when I was visiting a friend who knew my views regarding the use of superficial suggestion in the correction of alcoholism. My friend told me about an alcoholic acquaintance and then said to me, "Maybe the man I'm telling you about—and he will be here in a few minutes—is an exception. Won't you please try it on him. He has been a member of Alcoholics Anonymous and despite everything he still continues to drink excessively. Won't you see if you can help him?" Of course, the guest who came in a few minutes later had no idea how I felt about giving such suggestions, but he knew that I was supposed to be quite proficient in the use of hypnosis. He begged me to try to help him. He said that he had not brought his pay checks home in several years. His wife had been forced to go to work to support the family because he spent his checks on liquor. I would be saving a family, he said, if I could help him stop drinking. I told him that if I was going to help him at all, I would have to do it by means of hypnoanalysis. I would have to find out the reason he drank, and maybe if he knew why he had this insatiable thirst for liquor he would understand his problem and that would help him to stop drinking. He said he didn't want hypnoanalysis. All he wanted was to be hypnotized and given the suggestion—implanted strongly—that he would never drink again.

I was finally persuaded to try it. As a result, for the first time in three years he brought his pay check home and had not had a drink. The second week he also brought his pay check home, and by the third week he was so elated about his victory that he told me he would never drink again. If he had been able to stay away from liquor for three weeks, he reasoned that he could certainly stay away from it forever. He said he actually had no craving for alcohol. By this time I, too, was convinced that he was the rare exception and felt certain that I had saved a family. Imagine my distress when shortly thereafter I learned that he was back on the liquor again.

I maintain even now that this man could have been helped by hypnoanalysis, but couldn't be helped by merely trying to accept suggestions in hypnosis that he would have no desire for liquor. The only suggestion this man really took was the one about bringing his pay check home.

This was a suggestion he wanted. He rejected the suggestion he didn't want.

*   *   *

DOCTOR: What about the drug addict?

ELMAN: What we have been able to do for the drug addict is to make the separation pains much easier to bear—almost eliminate them entirely while treatment is going on. Using hypnosis, we can also make the separation from alcohol easier, but we cannot cure the desire for drinking or the craving for drugs by means of suggestion. We can only aid in the treatment by using hypnoanalysis to find the root of the problem.

*   *   *

DOCTOR: One of my patients, a stutterer, was helped tremendously by hypnoanalysis. He didn't stutter at all for six months. Then, suddenly, the stutter came back. Why did this happen?

ELMAN: You didn't make a complete correction. The relapse merely indicates the need for further investigation. Work with the patient again. Go over the same situations and also seek for additional trauma. Then give him further insight into his problems.

*   *   *

DOCTOR: Can a patient lie or conceal facts while in hypnosis? And if so, how would the doctor know, and what could he do about it?

ELMAN: A patient can lie under hypnosis as easily as he can lie, distort or withhold facts without hypnosis. I have found a very good way to detect a lie or an incomplete statement is to tell the patient in somnambulism, that if he deviates in the slightest from the truth, the left side of his face will flush. He will be unable to control or prevent it. Now watch the left side of the patient's face and notice when he deviates from the truth, how the color changes, while the right side remains perfectly normal.

A variation that I have found equally effective and on some occasions even more effective, is to put the patient's finger under the control of his inner mind. If he deviates from the truth or doesn't reveal complete facts, the finger will move. Otherwise the finger can't be made to move, no matter how hard the patient tries to move it. This technique has been found of great help in hypnoanalysis. However, there is nothing in hypnosis that can help you make a patient tell the truth if he doesn't want to. All this technique will do is to let you know that you are *not* getting the truth, and you can then be guided accordingly.

*   *   *

DOCTOR: I have heard that a clinical psychologist in one of your classes made the claim, "In hypnoanalysis, it is not always possible to find the true cause of an emotional problem. In that case, if you give the patient a reasonable explanation for his difficulty—even though it's one that *you made up*—the patient will accept the reasonable explanation and you can help the patient tremendously. In fact you can secure a complete recovery." When he made this statement, you disagreed with him. Will you give an explanation for your attitude?

ELMAN: My experience has taught me that if you do not get the true cause of the patient's emotional disturbances and give him insight into his real problems, you cannot possibly hope to obtain anything more than temporary relief. The doctor must seek the true cause of the patient's difficulties. Otherwise, he is treating an effect; he isn't treating the cause. The conscious mind of the patient might accept a plausible explanation temporarily but his inner mind will reject this plausible explanation unless it is based on absolute truth. No, I cannot accept the theory of the psychologist.

DOCTOR: Can you support your opposition to supplying substitute traumatic causes by citing evidence or clinical examples?

ELMAN: Here is a case illustration that may explain my view. A psychiatrist asked me to help in a case involving the problem of an unconsummated marriage. The young couple were apparently deeply in love, married three years, but with the marriage unconsummated. After an initial interview, the psychiatrist wanted to work with the husband and wife separately, but they were apparently inseparable. If the doctor scheduled an interview with the husband, the wife would show up with him. If he wanted to interview the wife, they would both show up and explain that since it was a mutual problem, they felt the psychiatrist should work with them together. He told them that he must see each patient individually. Finally, they agreed, and now it was possible for him to talk to the man and wife separately. But when he spoke to me, he still hadn't been able to correct the problem. He said, "I suspect there is a guilt complex hidden somewhere but neither one of them will allow me to get at the root cause. I've tried hypnoanalysis without success. Maybe you can get somwhere with them."

I met them at the doctor's office, and while he was working with other patients, I spoke to this couple. They were both apparently anxious to consummate the marriage. In fact, at the first meeting she said she wanted to have children. The husband looked pleased at this, and agreed that he, too, wanted to start a family. I thought the case would be an easy one. However, although they accepted hypnosis and I tried hypnoanalysis, I got no information of value. According to them, everything was perfect, but it was obvious to the psychiatrist and to me that they were concealing something. The problem was how to get these people to talk about their problem. When I reported this to the psychiatrist, he said, "I have an idea that might work. We were talking about your coming here today and each of them expressed an extreme interest in learning the subject of autosuggestion. Would you be willing to teach it to them? They have a feeling it might help."

I agreed, and the husband and wife were delighted. She wanted to make the appointment for the next day. Her husband wanted to make the appointment several days later because he'd be busy the next day. She insisted, however, and the following day she showed up alone at the psychiatrist's office. Please note that when they thought we were not going to delve into their personal problems, they were perfectly willing to make separate appointments. The young lady was eager to learn autosuggestion and took to the subject quickly. A half hour of practice and she was able to anesthetize her hand, and then she gave herself another suggestion and was able to anesthetize her mouth. She gave herself a complete dental anesthesia. I complimented her on her success with autosuggestion and told her she could use it for many purposes. She could even give herself a suggestion to talk more freely about her problems, and if she really wanted to talk more freely the autosuggestion would be readily accepted. She decided to try it. After she gave herself the necessary suggestion, she asked me to work further with her in hypnoanalysis. Information came tumbling out. She talked freely, revealing facts already known but also adding something new. She made the statement, "I'm not the problem—it's my husband. Every time I start making love to him, he becomes violently angry —so angry that I get frightened. Once I got up nerve enough to ask him why he gets so mad and he told me it's none of my damn business and to keep my mouth shut."

The interview ended and I reported to the

doctor what I had learned. He told me to try the same thing with her husband and attempt to learn the reason for his anger. They both came to the office for the husband's appointment. The husband took to autosuggestion almost instantly. I got the young man to give himself an autosuggestion to discuss freely the reason the marriage had not been consummated. He gave himself the autosuggestion and it worked beautifully. Almost immediately, he said, "If my wife will get out of here and wait outside in our car I'll be glad to talk to you."

She departed, and when the door had closed, he said, "Some day I'm going to kill that woman."

I thought he was joking. "What's the matter?" I asked. "Didn't she leave quickly enough?"

"That's not it. But I'm damn glad she got out of here. If that woman doesn't leave me alone, some day I'm going to kill her."

I realized now that he wasn't joking. Under the circumstances, I did the best I could. Through hypnoanalysis, I tried to learn the reason for the violent antipathy.

He said, "Im going to tell you something that even my wife doesn't know."

"What's that?"

"I'm a homosexual. Been that way since I was a kid."

"Are you telling me the truth now, or are you just handing me a lot of nonsense?"

"It's the truth, Mr. Elman. The very thought of having anything to do with a woman repulses me. If my wife starts making advances, I get so mad I want to kill her—and one of these days I'm going to do it."

"Then why did you marry her?"

"I don't know. Maybe to keep people from suspecting my problem. I like her—like her very much—except when she gets amorous. Then I want to kill her."

Tracing the reason for the violent antipathy was fairly easy in hypnoanalysis. When he was a young boy his father had divorced his mother. He felt that his father, whom he loved dearly, had rejected him completely. He wanted his father's love, but after the separation rarely saw him and then only for very short visits. It was a story of absolute rejection. I further learned that his mother and he went to live with an aunt and they shared a small apartment with only one bedroom. This required that he sleep with his mother and aunt, usually between the two women. As he changed from childhood into adolescence, this situation continued and his mother and aunt continued to caress the boy, treating him as a child. One of the startling things he said in hypnoanalysis was, "There were breasts all over the place. They used to hug me while we were in bed. I thought I was going to smother. And I was in constant fear that my mother and aunt would discover that I was becoming excited. Every time they came close, I would get so angry I kept wishing they would get out of bed and leave me alone. I had enough women around me to last me the rest of my life. Is it any wonder I get mad when my wife approaches me? I'm telling you, one of these days when she comes near me I'll get so mad I'll kill her."

This was not a case with which I could give further help, so I closed the hypnoanalysis. The doctor and I discussed the situation at length. He decided that he had sufficient information to continue working with the couple, and that was the last time I saw them. At this point, there was nothing in hypnosis that could alter the situation. The only help these people could be given was extensive psychiatry.

What I want to get across is the fact that this couple would never have accepted a "reasonable explanation" of their difficulties. The husband *knew* what the problem was. Hypnoanalysis certainly has limitations; even psychiatry, in

the light of present knowledge, has limitations,
but it would certainly be a more powerful weap-
on than the techniques within hypnosis.

To illustrate further my position and why
I am averse to supplying substitute causes, no
matter how reasonable, let me give you another
case history: A female patient approaching her
fiftieth year had been suffering from migraine
headaches ever since she was a small child. The
physician in charge informed me that the patient had gone from doctor to doctor seeking
medical aid. In recent months, the headaches
had become so violent that even the strongest
medications didn't relieve her agony. The doctor
wanted to find out if hypnoanalysis would solve
her problem. Investigation revealed an unusual
story. When she was three years old her mother
had once clothed her in a blue dress with blue
shoes and stockings. The father, seeing his
daughter more beautifully dressed than he had
ever seen her before, wanted to take her for a
walk. As they strolled down the street they
passed a baby shop. In the window was a little
blue umbrella. The father and child stopped to
admire it. "That blue umbrella would make your
outfit complete," he said to her. "Would you like
to have it?" The child was delighted. They went
into the store and purchased it. Now the little
girl strutted down the street dressed in blue,
swinging her blue umbrella.

The question was asked in hypnoanalysis,
"Where is your Daddy taking you now?"

She answered, "To Bronx Park Zoo. We're
going to see the animals. I love my Daddy."

And so in hypnoanalysis I took her through
the stroll in Bronx Park. Suddenly she began to
sob. I asked her, "What's the matter?"

Through her sobs she replied, "That little
girl—she wants my blue umbrella. She's stamp-
ing her feet and crying."

"That shouldn't make you cry. What are
you crying about?"

"My Daddy says I have to give it to her. He says she's so sad and I'm so happy. I should share my happiness and give the girl my blue umbrella. I don't want to do it and Daddy's making me do it."

"What happens now?"

"He's taking the umbrella away and giving it to the little girl. He says that will stop her crying."

"Does it?"

"Yes, but that's what's making me cry. I don't want to give it to her. It's my umbrella. He bought it for me."

Now she began to cry more violently. Probing further, I discovered that her father had scolded her, and had followed the scolding with the explanation that he was teaching her a valuable lesson. He told the child that she must learn to share her happiness, and also that any happiness must always be accompanied by a little sadness. She concluded, "He told me that's something I should know and always remember. Oh, my head hurts."

When the patient accepted the explanation that this episode started a trigger mechanism that created her migraines—every time she was happy, a headache appeared—her apparent recovery was like magic.

Her doctor called me and said, "Hypnoanalysis is wonderful. One session and we've corrected a condition that has persisted for forty-seven years." She was free of headaches for six months. Then the doctor called me and asked, "What did we do wrong? The headaches have come back."

We did further work with the patient. This time the hypnoanalysis revealed that her son was getting married and it was necessary for the son to have his birth certificate. This upset the mother, for the date on the birth certificate would show that the son was conceived five months before the mother's marriage. She was afraid her son would think that she had been an indecent woman. He might even think that the man he had always looked upon as his father was not the man responsible for his birth. It was a situation that would give anyone a headache. It was a normal reaction, and the doctor was quickly able to smoothe the situation out. Once more we thought we had done a good job. The headaches disappeared this time for three months. Then I was called in again. "We haven't ferreted out all of the true causes," the doctor said. "Of course, there was the same situation—joy at her son's forthcoming marriage and unhappiness that he might discover the unfortunate circumstances which preceded his birth. But there's something else lurking there that we haven't learned and made clear to her. She needs further insight."

The third hypnoanalysis revealed the balance of the story. The mother, madly in love with her husband, had always been under the impression that he had married her because she was pregnant. Maybe, she thought, he didn't love her at all, but had stood by her all those years because of his innate decency. "He just says he loves me. How can a woman be sure when she's had relations with her husband before marriage? And I want so much to have him love me."

"Have you been happy with him all these years?"

"Of course, I have. But didn't my own father tell me that with every bit of happiness there has to be something sad? And maybe that's what it is—my doubts about my husband's feelings for me."

Now that all the facts were in the open, the patient began to understand her recurring headaches. Although this happened many years ago, she hasn't had a headache since.

Could the doctor have given such a patient a "substitute cause" and expected to get lasting results? This was a case where, even though *some* of the true causes were revealed, further work was needed. I maintain that a doctor should never be satisfied with an apparently reasonable explanation to the patient. The explanation must be the true one.

*   *   *

I have endeavored in this closing chapter to answer the questions I most often hear in the classroom. Since these are generally based on clinical experiences and problems, they seem to me to be the questions for which answers are of the most immediate importance. But there are thousands of questions still to be answered. If this book serves to show even a few doctors the true value—and possibilities—of hypnosis, it will lead to further use of the phenomenon and, hence, to further study. And if it accomplishes this, it will have served its purpose well.

"Hypnotherapy as a Career"
Training in Clinical Hypnosis and Hypnotherapy

- Accelerated Intensives (50 hours in five days) or Weekend Classes (10 hours each Saturday)

- Diplomas awarded as "Master Hypnotist," "Hypnotherapist" and "Clinical Hypnotherapist"

- All diplomas authorized by the California Board of Education

- Approved by the California Board of Behavioral Science Examiners and the California Board of Registered Nursing

- National certification awarded

- One-, two-, three-, and four-week programs available

For details on this exciting and rewarding profession
write for our **free** catalog:

Hypnotism Training Institute of Los Angeles
700 S. Central Ave., Dept. TT
Glendale, CA 91204
or call
(818) 242-1159

LATEST TRAINING VIDEOS
FROM *WESTWOOD PUBLISHING*

1 - HYPNOTISM TRAINING

INSTANTANEOUS INDUCTIONS (STANDING)

PART ONE (two subjects) Total Loss of Equilibrium; Eye Catalepsy/Arm Catalepsy; Deepening by Compounding; Non-Verbal Reinduction; Waking Hypnosis Creating Partial Amnesia; Creating Total Post-Hypnotic Amnesia; Induced Speech Inhibition; Second Instantaneous Induction; Test Eye Catalepsy; Rule of Reversed Mental Effort; Teaching Self-Hypnosis to Subject; Healing Suggestions.

PART TWO -- COLIN - A student from England has never been hypnotized before. Gil Boyne demonstrates Instantaneous Induction (standing), deepening by disorientation, deepening by realization, rule of reverse mental effort, deepening by rocking subject, arm catalepsy, automatic motion, deepening by pyramiding, hand-clasp response, creating somnambulism, creating post-hypnotic proof-of-trance, conditioning for post-hypnotic reinduction by repeated instant inductions, post-hypnotic talk, post-hypnotic reinduction, why *"fully aware"* replaces *"wide awake"*, trance termination, second post hypnotic talk.

PART THREE -- SEATED INDUCTIONS
Includes:
- hand-pressure induction
- trance termination
- two-finger induction
- clearing the mind
- gazing-at-the-moon induction
- arm levitation (eye-catalepsy and heavy left arm)
- reversed hand-clasp induction

107 minutes ● *$75.00*

STAGE HYPNOSIS

PART ONE - From 1960 to 1965, Gil Boyne entertained thousands with his *"Hilarious Hypnosis Stage Show"* in nightclubs throughout the U.S.A. This video tape combines one full hour of highly-skilled stage hypnosis techniques with the hilarious antics of a stage full of subjects.

PART TWO - Ormond McGill, Dean of American Hypnotists, presents a fascinating and mirth provoking one-hour show in his unique style. This is your opportunity to compare and learn from the art of two of the world's great stage hypnotists.

120 minutes ● *$75.00*

HYPNOTISM TRAINING FILM #501
GIL BOYNE TEACHING AND DEMONSTRATING

Hypnotherapist, Gil Boyne demonstrates five methods of Instantaneous Induction and simultaneously explains the processes in non-technical language as he works with ten subjects.

Vivid examples of *Testing and Deepening, Training the Client, Developing Rapid Rapport and Reeducating the Client* are captured live and unrehearsed, using students in attendance. Also includes Arm Levitation, Eye Catalepsy, Arm Catalepsy, Automatic Motion, Key Word Reinduction. Plus ten methods of deepening the trance, post-hypnotic suggestions, and amnesia and other hypnotic phenomena.

105 minutes Special Offer - Our best selling video at a special price: Was $125.00 - now just $39.95. Includes a complete word-for-word transcript of the film absolutely FREE!

GIL BOYNE'S
HYPNOTISM TRAINING FILM #300
Part I Advanced Hypnotic Training

Actual live, unrehearsed demonstrations filmed in a classroom setting using the students in attendance. Gil Boyne teaches and demonstrates Instantaneous Inductions, Testing and Deepening, Training the Client, Developing Rapid Rapport, Reeducation of the Client.

Part II How To Visualize

A frustrating problem for hypnotherapists is the number of clients who report they are unable to visualize or use visual imagery. Here is how you can finally overcome that problem -- forever.

At a training seminar a student informs Gil Boyne that he is unable to visualize. Watch as Boyne hypnotizes the subject and creates a process in which the subject "sees, hears, tastes, feels and smells."

105 minutes ● *$49.95*

TO ORDER CALL (818)242-1159 OR FAX (818)247-9379
Westwood Publishing Company ● *700 S. Central Ave* ● *Glendale, CA 91204*

HOLLY - *YOU SCARE ME* **and**
PAT - *FEAR OF PUBLIC SPEAKING*

Holly, a young woman in her mid-twenties, breaks into tears in the first day of a Clinical Hypnotherapy course. When instructor Gil Boyne questions her she says, "You're scaring me." This seems a paradox since Boyne has not spoken directly to her in the class. He suggests that he hypnotize her to discover the background of her emotional upheaval. In minutes she is regressed to a terrifying scene with a threatening step-father. Abreaction, reeducation, rescripting and closure occur in rapid succession and the projected fear of an animated authority figure is dissipated.

PART TWO - A mature, intelligent female hypnotherapy student reports a fear of public speaking. She states that she "always sounds haughty" when speaking to a group. A comprehensive intake interview fails to reveal any evidence of negative childhood experiences or identifications. Trance is induced and deepened and a highly specialized program of affirmations and visualizations is presented.

46 minutes • $49.95

New THE CASE OF BUNNY
PHYSICAL PAIN FROM EARLY SEXUAL ABUSE

Boyne demonstrates instantaneous inductions with several subjects. While testing one of them by making her upraised arm rigid she exclaims, "It's a miracle." She goes on to say that she has been unable to lift her arm higher than her shoulder for over two years. Boyne hypnotizes her and in an exciting and highly dramatic age-regression he discovers the cause of her arm, neck, and shoulder problems to be a result of early sexual abuse by her alcoholic father. Using several original and unorthodox techniques, Boyne creates a complete release from these disabling symptoms.

58 minutes • $75.00

New THE FEAR OF CRITICISM &
THE CURSE OF PERFECTIONISM

Gil Boyne lecturing teaches the crippling effects of the fear of criticism and the style of perfectionism. He works with two subjects (Miriam, Sam); and discovers "childhood scripts" including the compulsive people-pleaser, "Won't Say No."

53 minutes • $49.95

New GEORGE/BOB

OVERCOMING THE *I CAN'T BE HYPNOTIZED* PROBLEM. George, a university professor from Connecticut, has been many years in the practice of hypnosis but still doesn't know if he has ever been "in a trance" or if his clients have ever been hypnotized. One session with Boyne convinces him of his trance-state to his satisfaction.

FEAR OF FAILURE Bob, a 72 year old Hypnotherapist has been unable to experience trance despite his many efforts to do so. Using age regression, Boyne uncovers mother's early scripts "You'll never amount to anything". Bob enters into a deep trance complete with several tests. Boyne then teaches him self-hypnosis and he comes up from the trance amazed and radiant.

100 minutes • $75.00

THE CASE OF BUD
BORN TO LOSE

A depressed male in his mid-fifties is convinced that he is a loser in life. Suffers from alcoholism, insomnia, low self-esteem, self-isolation and negative thinking. In two one-hour sessions on consecutive days, Bud experiences an amazing personal transformation. Filmed live before a hypnotherapy class of forty-five therapists in Chicago. Shows age-regression, abreaction, Gestalt dialogues and many of Gil Boyne's original uncovering/reprogramming techniques.

120 minutes • $75.00

THE CASE OF LEE
THE SAN DIEGO STUTTERER

In a dramatic two hour hypnotherapy session using age regression and "uncovering techniques" Gil Boyne unveils the "battered child" syndrome and fear of castration as an initial sensitizing event for a life-long pattern of stuttering. Three years later, Lee remains totally free of stuttering. Gestalt dialogues, bodywork techniques and Parts therapy.

95 minutes • $75.00

TO ORDER CALL (818)242-1159 OR FAX (818)247-9379
Westwood Publishing Company • 700 S. Central Ave • Glendale, CA 91204

3 - MARKETING YOUR HYPNOTISM SERVICES

GIL BOYNE'S
HOW TO TEACH SELF-HYPNOSIS
HYPNOTHERAPISTS—
Here's How to Double Your Income!
The Complete Course on Video Cassette

Since 1956, Gil Boyne has taught self-hypnosis to more than 23,000 persons in Southern California. Boyne drew from his vast background of experience to create his most exciting new project — a comprehensive course on "How To Teach Self-Hypnosis" — eight hours of actual teaching on video cassette.

See and hear every element in the successf teaching of self-hypnosis, skillfully demonstrated an actual class setting.

The videos also include a 99-page Marketir Manual and a complete word-for-word transcript the eight-hour video cassette.

8 hours on 4 video tapes PLUS two manuals ● $195.

Also available separately: "How To Teach Se Hypnosis" Transcript/Training Manual, $35.00; a Marketing Manual, $35.00; Both manuals for $50.0(

---

4 - HYPNOSIS FOR HEALING AND PAIN CONTROL

HYPNOSIS FOR MEDICAL
EMERGENCIES
Using spontaneous hypnosis to communicate with the sick and injured to control pain and enhance recovery.

Why is it that conversation at the scene of a medical emergency can have such a critical effect on the patient? This video shows that it is because frightened or seriously injured persons spontaneously enter into a hypnotic state of consciousness that makes them acutely responsive to certain kinds of direct or indirect suggestions.

This program uses dramatizations and graphic illustrations to present guidelines, strategies and techniques for gaining rapport and for giving suggestions and directives that can remarkably help
patients control their own autonomic nervous system responses. These include:

- ●Bleeding
- ●Blood Pressure
- ●Respiratory Functions
- ●Burn Injury Reaction
- ●Pain Response
- ●Immune Response
- ●Inflammation
- ●Heart Rate
- ●Dermatitis

50 minutes ● $75.00

"Don Jacobs video presents proof positive that the use appropriate words in critical situations can not only spe healing but save lives as well.
Gil Boyne, Executive Director
American Council of Hypnotist Examiners
"As this use of hypnosis is extended there will be many li saved."
David Cheek, M.D.
Author, Clinical Hypnotherapist
"Dr. Jacobs' approach to pre-hospital care has the potential having a great impact on treatment outcomes."
Alan V. Brunacini
Chief, Phoenix Fire Dept.
"This tape is on the cutting edge of an exciting and innovat approach to pre-hospital care"
Bennie Cooper, M.A.
Director of Emergency Medical Training, Murr State University

FREE BONUS with "HYPNOSIS FOR MEDICAL EMERGENCIES"
HYPNOSIS FOR HEALING AND PAIN CONTROL
This exciting video shows the use of the pain control method developed by Gil Boyne. Excerpt from three therapy sessions include: 1. The cure of numerous warts in an eight year old girl.
2. The cure of chronic migraine headaches in a 67 year old woman.
3. Controlling limb tremors in a client with Parkinson's disease.

"A Rare Find Unearthed"

FIVE HOURS OF RECORDED HYPNO-ANALYSIS
(Digitally Rerecorded)

By DAVE ELMAN

These extraordinary sessions in hypno-nalysis consist of recordings of actual live ıerapy sessions presented by Dave Elman to hysicians and psychiatrists throughout the Inited States. It is a rare opportunity to learn ˙om the man who taught hypnotherapy to ıore healing arts professionals than any ther instructor before or since.

The package consists of 6 audio cassettes lus a manual in which Davè Elman analyzes ıd explains each session. In addition, the ıanual contains the **Dave Elman Class ˙otes** as a **Special Bonus.** (8 ½" X 11" - ; pp.) **$99.50**

These six sessions of hypnoanalysis include: **The Day of the Kidnapping; An Obesity Problem; When a Husband Is a Headache; Rose Fever and Scleroderma; He Stutters Only When Excited; Hysterical Blindness; Pre-operative Fear in a Child; A Headache and Perfectionism.**

Join the thousands of physicians, nurses and therapists who have experienced the excitement of studying with one of the great pioneers.

"The use of Dave Elman's new concepts and techniques creates a new level of effectiveness."-Gil Boyne, Exec. Dir., ACHE

● ● ● ● ● ● ● ● ● ● ● ● ●

Why does one client stutter? Another ave headaches? Another, cancer phobia? till another, neuro-dermatitis? Why hould an obese client be unable to stay on diet? Why should a client gag and vomit ı the dental chair? Why should a client ˙e subject to attacks of hysterical lindness--or deafness? Why should little ohnny have asthma, and his sister hay ˙ver? Why should a millionaire ıanufacturer and a sewing machine

operator have the same problem of nail biting?

These five hours of recorded Hypno-Analysis effectively demonstrate how Elman's techniques act as a powerful spotlight to illuminate the dimmest recesses of the inner creative mind. You will learn how you can maximize your effectiveness as a hypnotherapist with Dave Elman's personal instruction.

ince these sessions were done in different classes, the sound quality was uneven. Fortunately, we have been able to use ıodern electronic technology to recreate the recordings with the highest possible quality of sound reproduction.

Mail your order to: Westwood Publishing Co. ● 700 S. Central Ave ● Glendale, CA 91204   1

FILL IN AND MAIL ... TODAY

WESTWOOD PUBLISHING COMPANY, INC.
700 S. Central Avenue
Glendale, CA 91204

USE YOUR CREDIT CARD AND ORDER BY PHONE
818-242-1159 or FAX 818-247-9379

Qty	Description		Price	Total

POSTAGE AND HANDLING (USA)

Order Total	Add	Order Total	Add
Up to $25	$2.50	$60.01-$120	$5.75
$25.01-$60	$4.25	Over $120	Free

Calif. residents add 8.25% sales tax.

Subtotal	
Postage & handling*	
Sales tax**	
TOTAL	

❏ Check enclosed for $_____ , payable to Westwood Publishing

❏ Charge my ❏ Mastercard ❏ Visa ❏ American Express

Account No._____ Exp. Date_____

Signature _____

Your Name_____

Address _____

City/State/Zip _____

Daytime Telephone _____

GUARANTEE
You must be satisfied!
You get a 30-day, 100% money-back guarantee
on all books and audio cassettes

Thank you for your order!